Strategies for Selecting and Verifying Hearing Aid Fittings

Michael Valente, Ph.D.

Associate Professor
Director of Adult Audiology
Washington University School of Medicine
St. Louis, Missouri

1994
THIEME MEDICAL PUBLISHERS, INC. New York
GEORG THIEME VERLAG Stuttgart · New York

Thieme Medical Publishers, Inc.
381 Park Avenue South
New York, New York 10016

STRATEGIES FOR SELECTING AND
VERIFYING HEARING AID FITTINGS
Michael Valente

Library of Congress Cataloging-in-Publication Data
Strategies for selecting and verifying hearing aid fittings / edited
  by Michael Valente.
      p.   cm.
   Includes bibliographical references and index.
   ISBN 0-86577-500-1 (Thieme Medical Publishers, New York)
   ISBN 3-13-125801-2 (Georg Thieme Verlag, Stuttgart)
   1. Hearing aids—Fitting.   I. Valente, Michael.
RF300.S76   1994
617.8'9—dc20
                                                                    93-33542
                                                                        CIP

Important note: Medicine is an ever-changing science. Research and clinical experience are continually broadening our knowledge, in particular our knowledge of proper treatment and drug
therapy. Insofar as this book mentions any dosage or applications, readers may rest assured that
the authors, editors, and publishers have made every effort to ensure that such references are
strictly in accordance with the state of knowledge at the time of production of the book. Nevertheless, every user is requested to carefully examine the manufacturers' leaflets accompanying each
drug to check on his own responsibility whether the dosage schedules recommended therein or
the contraindications stated by the manufacturers differ from the statements made in the present
book. Such examination is particularly important with drugs that are either rarely used or have
been newly released on the market.

Some of the product names, patents, and registered designs referred to in this book are in fact
registered trademarks or proprietary names even though specific reference to this fact is not always
made in the text. Therefore, the appearance of a name without designation as proprietary is not to
be construed as a representation by the publisher that it is in the public domain.

Printed in the United States of America.

5   4   3   2   1

TMP ISBN 0-86577-500-1
GTV ISBN 3-13-125801-2

Contents

Preface

This textbook is divided into four parts and is intended for audiology graduate students as well as the practicing dispensing audiologist. The organization of the text is designed to follow the sequence in which decisions are typically made regarding the selection and verification of the amplification needs of hearing impaired patients.

The first section examines numerous issues involved in *selecting* the appropriate gain and output of hearing aids. The first two chapters summarize the numerous procedures available to help audiologists select the appropriate gain using the most widely accepted threshold and suprathreshold procedures. The third chapter deals with the issue of selecting the appropriate output of the hearing aid. These three chapters are intended to help the audiologist select the amplification requirements that will provide good recognition of speech, natural sound quality, and an amplified signal that is comfortably loud.

The second section highlights the issues involved with *verifying* the hearing aid fitting; that is, has the patient received a hearing aid fitting that *reasonably matches* the amplification requirements previously chosen during the selection process? These methods of verification can be used independently (i.e., does the "measured" real-ear gain match the "prescribed" real-ear gain?) or in combination with another method of verification (i.e., using real-ear gain measures in combination with paired comparisons and/or subjective ratings).

The third section describes how the selection and verification procedures can be integrated in the hearing aid fitting for patients having one of six common hearing losses: noise induced, symmetrical, asymmetrical, unilateral, chronic conductive, or profound.

Finally, the fourth section attempts to look into the "crystal ball" and predict how technology and procedures may evolutionize the selection and verification processes in the years ahead.

No project of this magnitude can be completed without the help of many friends. First, I would like to express my deepest gratitude to all the authors for the time and energy they placed into each chapter. Their skills and knowledge are the basis of the success of this text. Second, I thank all colleagues who expended a considerable amount of time and energy in reviewing each chapter and provided numerous suggestions to each of the authors. Their efforts resulted in chapters that are expanded and clearer. Third, I thank Kim Wright, editor at Thieme Medical Publishers, for her enduring help from our initial contact to the completion of this text. Fourth, I thank Margaret Juelich, Judy Peterein, Marti Meister, Belinda Sinks, Kelly Macauley, Mona Sparks, and Lisa Potts. These kind and very talented audiologists allowed me the time necessary to complete this project.

Finally, and most important, I thank my wife Maureen and my daughters Michelle and Anne. Their love and support was essential for the successful completion of this project.

Michael Valente, Ph.D.

Contributors

Ruth A. Bentler, Ph.D.
Department of Speech and Hearing
Science
University of Iowa
Iowa City, IA

Susan M. Binzer, M.A.
Washington University School of
Medicine
St. Louis, MO

Kathryn E. Bright, Ph.D.
University of Northern Colorado
Department of Communication
Disorders
Greeley, CO

Robert de Jonge, Ph.D.
Department of Speech Pathology
and Audiology
Central Missouri State University
Warrensburg, MO

David A. Fabry, Ph.D.
Department of Otorhinolaryngology
Mayo Clinic
Rochester, MN

George A. Gates, M.D.
Washington University School of
Medicine
St. Louis, MO

Dan C. Halling, Ph.D.
Department of Speech and Hearing
Science
Indiana University
Bloomington, IN

Laura K. Holden, M.A.
Washington University School of
Medicine
St. Louis, MO

Larry E. Humes, Ph.D.
Department of Speech and Hearing
Science
Indiana University
Bloomington, IN

Barbara Kruger, Ph.D.
Kruger Associates
Commack, NY

Frederick M. Kruger, Ph.D.
Kruger Associates
Commack, NY

Francis K. Kuk, Ph.D.
Division of Audiology
Department of Otolaryngology
University of Illinois at Chicago
Chicago, IL

Geary A. McCandless, Ph.D.
University of Utah
Salt Lake City, UT

Kelly Macauley, M.S.
Washington University School of
  Medicine
St. Louis, MO

Martha Meister, M.S.
Union Audiology and Hearing
  Aid Services
Van Nuys, CA

H. Gustav Mueller, Ph.D.
University of Northern Colorado
Department of Communication
  Disorders
Greeley, CO

David A. Preves, Ph.D.
Argosy Electronics
Eden Prairie, MN

Lawrence J. Revit, M.A.
Research Audiologist
Frye Electronics
Tigard, OR

Robert E. Sandlin, Ph.D.
Alvarado Medical Center
San Diego, CA

Donald J. Schum, Ph.D.
The University of Iowa
  Hospitals and Clinics
Iowa City, IA

Margaret W. Skinner, Ph.D.
Washington University School of
  Medicine
St. Louis, MO

Robert W. Sweetow, Ph.D.
University of California, San
  Francisco
San Francisco, CA

John E. Tecca, Ph.D.
Hearing Services and Systems
Portage, MI

Maureen Valente, M.A.
Department of Communication
  Disorders
St. Louis University
St. Louis, MO

Michael Valente, Ph.D.
Washington University School of
  Medicine
St. Louis, MO

William Vass, M.S.
Starkey Labs
Eden Prairie, MN

Overview and Rationale of Threshold-Based Hearing Aid Selection Procedures

GEARY A. MCCANDLESS

Introduction

The principle aim of any hearing aid selection and fitting strategy is to ensure that environmental sounds, especially conversational speech, is audible without being excessively loud.[1-3] To achieve a successful fitting, a hearing aid must provide appropriate amplification to maximize speech recognition, provide good sound quality, and provide amplification that is comfortable.[4] To accomplish this, the frequency-gain response of the hearing aid must be shaped to compensate for the loss of loudness as a result of impaired hearing.

Over the years, many procedures have been designed to provide optimum electroacoustic (frequency-gain and output) characteristics for the pathologic ear. One procedure used for many years compared improved pure-tone and spondee thresholds, as well as changes in speech recognition scores derived by fitting several "stock" hearing aids or various hearing aid characteristics while using a master hearing aid.[5] In some cases, hearing aid selection was based solely on user judgments of sound quality or clarity of speech.

A more recent approach has been to calculate desired electroacoustic characteristics based on the results of various psychoacoustic data such as pure-tone thresholds, most comfortable loudness levels (MCL), uncomfortable loudness levels (UCL), and bisecting the dynamic range.[6-13] Prescriptive procedures make the general assumption that, if average conversation speech is amplified to the listeners' comfortable loudness level, the fitting will result in user satisfaction by providing acceptable sound quality, clarity of speech, and comfort.

In this chapter, only threshold-based procedures are discussed, that is, those prescriptive procedures whose formulas exclusively utilize audiometric pure-tone threshold data. Although these methods are based on audiometric thresholds, it is assumed that, even without actually testing these functions, restoration of acuity, equal loudness, or speech spectrum to the ear can be correctly inferred from threshold data.

Basic Requirements of Prescriptive Procedures

To be both practical and effective, the following requirements should be incorporated into any prescriptive procedures:

1. The prescribed frequency-gain characteristics should be based on easily acquired audiologic information, such as pure-tone thresholds.
2. The prescriptive procedure must be based on a defensible rationale such as amplifying all frequency bands to subjective equal loudness, restoring the average speech spectrum to the subject's MCL,[14] or providing operating gain most likely to result in maximum recognition of speech for an individual hearing loss.[15]
3. When the prescribed characteristics are obtained to a reasonable degree, it should provide acceptable sound quality, clarity of speech, and a loudness level that is judged to be comfortable.
4. The prescriptive procedure must be efficient and capable of being administered within the time constraints of a busy office.
5. It should provide characteristics for hearing aid candidates with a wide variety of audiometric configurations, growth of loudness, and degree of hearing loss.
6. The prescriptive procedure should not be so complex as to make it impractical for clinical use.
7. At the time of the fitting, the results must be verified. That is, it is essential to document the extent to which the prescriptive objectives have been achieved. This verification process does not exclude the use of speech or other materials for final subjective verification of sound quality or clarity of speech.

Dispensing Practices in the United States

At present, nearly 80% of all hearing aids purchased in the United States are custom in-the-ear (ITE) hearing aids.[16] Also, about 90% of all current ITE aids are sold to dispensers where the electroacoustic characteristics are selected by the manufacturer, not the dispenser, and use threshold-based prescriptive formulas. Stated differently, the dispenser typically forwards an order form containing the user's pure-tone audiogram to the manufacturer who in turn selects the frequency-gain response based on an internally generated matrix. In these cases, it is the manufacturer who decides which electroacoustic characteristics are considered optimal or, at least, satisfactory. Unless dispenser adjustments are available, hearing aids provided in this manner cannot truly be individualized since the influences of ear canal volume, resonance, loudness recruitment, venting, and other factors cannot be predicted with any acceptable degree of accuracy. The dispensed hearing aid conforms only to the needs of the "average" ear rather than for the needs of an individual.

A smaller number of customized ITE hearing aids have gain and other requirements specified by the dispenser. A variety of prescriptive techniques are used to calculate and specify target gain. As with manufacturer-derived formulas, there is no guarantee that these prescribed characteristics for the ITE are actually delivered to the user's ear due to differences in manufacturing protocols, variations in acoustic coupling, or other unique requirements for a given individual. Small potentiometers on programmable aids can be ordered to make small adjustments. However, rendering a completely different circuit design is often required to achieve the best function and satisfaction.

Questions Relating to Hearing Aid Prescriptive Procedures

The current practice of threshold-based hearing aid evaluation and fitting strategies raises several important questions:

1. What are the basic rationale and assumptions from which each prescriptive formula is derived? Has each prescription formula been validated based on user satisfaction, improved speech recognition, loudness discomfort, sound quality, or other criteria?
2. Are differences present between the various prescriptive formulas that result in significant differences in user satisfaction?
3. Does one prescriptive procedure yield consistently better user satisfaction than others for different audiometric configurations and/or degrees of hearing loss? Are valid measures available by which to compare these prescriptive techniques and evaluate user success?
4. With what precision can a manufacturer deliver specific frequency-gain characteristics to match a prescribed frequency-gain requirement? What flexibility is available to "fine tune" the frequency-gain response and maximum output to achieve compliance to a target prescription.
5. When the prescribed electroacoustic characteristics are provided to a client, do they result in user satisfaction under a variety of listening situations?

Rationale of Prescriptive Procedures

Selective amplification of the frequency-gain characteristics is now a widely accepted principle in selecting and fitting hearing aids. While improved aided speech recognition presented at a level of average conversational levels is a goal of all fitting procedures, speech recognition tests, in themselves, can only demonstrate that a particular set of electroacoustic characteristics are or are not adequate. However, speech recognition testing cannot identify which electroacoustic characteristics contribute to speech recognition ability or which modifications would improve the fitting.

Stated differently, using only unaided speech recognition scores, how can specific electroacoustic characteristics be calculated to yield optimum aided speech recognition? Likewise, after the initial fitting, using only speech recognition tasks as a basis, how can one determine which frequency-gain characteristic needs to be changed in order to improve speech recognition? It must be remembered that improved aided speech recognition is only one factor to consider for a successful hearing aid fitting, and rather large differences in speech recognition scores must be present in order to reflect "true" differences between aids or characteristics of aids.[15]

Prescriptive procedures, using psychoacoustic or audiometric data, have evolved because of the imprecision found in speech recognition-based selection procedures.[17] Demand for valid, efficient, predictive prescriptive protocols have also been required due to the large increases in the number of custom ITE instruments currently dispensed. In the past, the aided benefit from stock hearing aids could be compared in the office or clinic. However, increased popularity of custom hearing aids mandated that individualized electroacoustic characteristics be built into the aid at the time of assembly unless they can be adjusted or externally programmed. The need to preselect the prescribed frequency-gain characteristics was also necessary because ITE and in-the-canal (ITC) hearing aids offered less adjustability due to size constraints. Therefore, it is of particular importance to "order" the frequency-gain characteristics most likely to achieve acceptable clarity, sound quality, and loudness comfort at the initial fitting. The number of aids returned to manufacturers for credit or modifications suggests that these essential criteria are not always met.[18]

Although the use of prescriptive procedures has become popular, no general agreement has been reached as to what measurements should be used to calculate the prescribed gain, (e.g., hearing thresholds, MCLs, or UCLs).[19] However, most dispensers and manufacturers currently use threshold-based procedures for calculation of the prescribed frequency-gain response since the pure-tone audiogram is easily obtained and always available.

Prescriptive Procedures Based on Measures of Most Comfortable Loudness Level

Two broad prescriptive philosophies have emerged that are intended to prescribe the desired frequency-gain response necessary to amplify average conversational speech to the eardrum. One approach specifies that speech signals should be selectively amplified so as to place them within the most comfortable listening range of the hearing aid user. This type of prescriptive formula is based on measuring the MCL or MCL range at various audiometric frequencies. The amount of gain required to amplify the spectrum of average conversational speech to the MCL range determines the prescribed functional or insertion gain.[10,20–22] Others have used UCL measures to calculate the target frequency-gain response.[12] All of these techniques are intended to place the spectrum of average conversational speech within the MCL or preferred listening range of the user.

Prescriptive Procedure Based on Threshold Measures

A second approach is to prescribe sufficient gain to amplify sound, especially speech, to comfortable listening levels using threshold data rather than the more time-consuming MCL measures. With this approach, the MCL, or pre-ferred listening level, is predicted but not actually measured. It is assumed that after fitting desired changes in loudness can be accomplished by use of the volume control. Proponents of this philosophy also believe that a main con-cern with relying on comfortable loudness measures is its relatively poor re-peatability.[23–25] Although some investigations show good reliability of supra-threshold measures such as the MCL, these measures may be difficult for some subjects, cannot be used for fitting very young children or special populations, and are time consuming.

By contrast, threshold-based prescriptive formulas are efficient, easily cal-culated, and applicable to a wide variety of hearing aid candidates, including children and the elderly. Threshold-based formulas assume that the prescribed overall gain increases systematically with increased hearing loss at a predict-able rate.[19] Calculations of the *predicted* MCL, or preferred listening level, made on the basis of threshold data infer that an appropriate amount of overall gain can be accurately specified so as to deliver speech at a comfortable loudness level. One criticism of these procedures is that calculations from threshold data fail to consider individual variations in the amount of desired gain. However, considering that a well-fitted hearing aid has some degree of reserve gain, the volume control can easily adjust the amplified speech spectrum to a listener's comfortable range.[26]

The question arises whether threshold procedures predict the appropriate amount of gain at various frequencies to restore average speech spectrum to the MCL of the pathologic ear. Several comparisons between threshold and MCL-derived procedures have reported that measured outcome and user satisfaction with the two procedures are somewhat equivalent.[26–28] MCL measures are reported to have considerable test–retest variability, and some subjects have considerable difficulty with tests requiring qualitative judgments of comfortable loudness.[23,24] It is for these reasons that threshold-derived formulas were devised. If appropriate loudness can be restored using a pre-scription based on pure-tone thresholds, it is reasoned that assessment and calculation of prescriptive gain requirements can be accomplished more ef-ficiently than those using MCL procedures and yield equivalent or improved results.

Assumptions of Threshold-Based Prescriptive Procedures

No fitting procedure is perfect, especially since conventional hearing aids can only make sounds louder and cannot restore other pathologic deficiencies such as loss of frequency discrimination. The wide diversity of pathologies of the auditory system makes it impossible to predict with precision the needs of each hearing aid candidate, nor can acoustic requirements be generalized to all pathologic ears for all listening situations. Furthermore, not all hearing aids perform alike, even when showing similar frequency-gain responses and out-put characteristics. Subtle, unmeasured differences such as harmonic, transient, or intermodulation distortion, damping characteristics, frequency bandwidth, or smoothness of the gain curve may interact with the patient's functional deficits, resulting in a poor outcome. Prescriptive fitting, when implemented, at best can provide a starting point or close approximation from which minor tuning to the individual's requirements results in an acceptable fitting, from both objective and subjective standpoints. With these considerations in mind, whenever threshold-based prescriptive procedures are to be used, certain assumptions are made.

1. Implementation of threshold-based prescriptive procedures typically require at least three steps:
    a. Calculation of prescribed frequency-gain characteristics, which is based on audiometric data.
    b. Conversion of prescribed target gain values converted into standardized hearing aid coupler measures. That is, the individual real ear prescriptive requirements are converted to $2\,cm^3$ coupler full-on gain requirements and thus to actual hearing aids.
    c. Verifying, with measures of either functional gain (i.e., aided minus unaided sound field thresholds) or insertion gain (i.e., real ear aided gain minus real ear unaided gain) and using probe microphone measures near the tympanic membrane, at the time of fitting that the prescribed gain has been achieved (see Ch. 5).

2. The prescribed electroacoustic characteristics necessary to achieve the prescribed gain are intended to maximize speech recognition and yield acceptable sound quality. It should be stressed that even though a prescriptive target is met, final adjustments of electroacoustic characteristics may be necessary to improve subjective sound quality or clarity of speech.

3. Threshold-based techniques are designed primarily for sensorineural hearing losses, or more specifically, sensory (cochlear) losses. It is assumed that some degree of loudness recruitment is present and that the targeted gain requirements are based on loudness growth functions associated with loudness recruitment. Conductive or mixed hearing losses may require different specifications of frequency-gain characteristics (see Ch. 12).

4. Threshold-based prescriptive fittings assume that the aids are linear or operate primarily on the linear segment of the gain curve. Although nonlinear and multiple channel hearing aids are now available, most hearing aids are single channel instruments with linear input–output functions. In these instruments, gain is linear until the amplifier reaches maximum output, where saturation occurs or output is limited using some method of input or output compression.

5. Threshold-based prescriptive procedures (and some suprathreshold procedures covered in Ch. 2) are appropriate for predicting the "average" gain when the signal at the microphone is at a level of average conversational speech (approximately 70 dB SPL presented in a quiet environment at a distance of 1 m).

6. Many prescriptive procedures do not make corrections for listening conditions other than quiet or for distances greater than about one meter. Stated differently, prescriptive formulae cannot specify frequency-gain

characteristics appropriate for a wide spectrum of listening situations present in the real world.

7. It is assumed that the prescribed frequency-gain characteristics will be closely reproduced with an actual hearing-aid when adjusted to a most comfortable listening level.

Prescribing and Verifying Frequency-Gain Characteristics: Functional and Insertion Gain

Essential to the success in implementing prescriptive fittings is the knowledge of the concepts of *functional* and *insertion* gain. These concepts are discussed in detail in Chapters 4 and 5. It must be stressed that threshold-based formulas assume that, on average, systematic relationships exist between pure-tone thresholds and comfortable, or preferred, listening levels.[29] In most cases, calculating the prescribed insertion or functional gain from audiometric thresholds will provide the amount of gain necessary to amplify average conversational speech when the hearing aid is set to a comfortable listening level.

The term *functional gain* is a psychoacoustic or behavioral measure and usually refers to the difference in decibels between aided and unaided sound field warble tone and/or spondee thresholds (see Fig. 1–1A). It is also assumed that the aided thresholds are measured with the volume control adjusted to a comfortable or preferred listening level. For example, in Figure 1–1A at 1000 Hz, the unaided sound field warble tone threshold is 50 dB, while the threshold with the hearing aid in place with the volume control adjusted to MCL is 25 dB. In this illustration, functional gain at 1000 Hz is 25 dB.

Insertion gain is an electroacoustic rather than a psychoacoustic term and is the difference in decibels between the sound pressure level measured at or

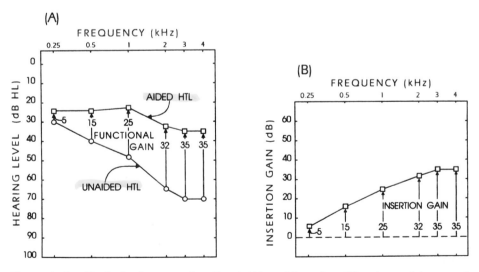

Figure 1–1. Similarity between functional (**A**) and insertion (**B**) gains and how each measure can be plotted.

near the eardrum with and without a hearing aid in place in the ear canal. As with functional gain measures, insertion gain is measured with the volume control adjusted to a comfortable listening level. Figure 1–1B shows the pre-scribed "target" for insertion gain measures for the same hearing loss (i.e., unaided hearing threshold level) illustrated in Figure 1–1A. Note that differing amounts of gain are prescribed each at frequency due to the characteristics of the hearing loss. More gain is provided at frequencies having the greater loss of hearing. Not only will the measured aided thresholds be shifted toward normal threshold levels, but sounds that were barely audible unaided are raised by a similar amount.

Functional or insertion gain measures are used in two important ways in the context of prescriptive hearing aid evaluation and fitting. The first step is *calculation* of the prescribed gain based on threshold data. This was clearly shown as the prescribed aided sound field threshold in Figure 1–1A and as the prescribed insertion gain in Figure 1–1B. The second application is when frequency-gain response is *measured* while wearing the hearing aid. For pur-poses of consistency, it may be desirable to use the terms *target-aided sound field thresholds* or *target insertion gain* when referring to the prefitting calculations and *measured sound field thresholds, measured functional gain,* or *measured insertion gain* when verifying the fitting to ensure that the target criteria have been met.

Figure 1–2B illustrates how this calculation and verification process is used. The prescribed gain is first calculated based on the audiometric thresholds (Fig. 1–2A) and shown as a target curve (Fig. 1–2B; "target insertion gain"). The insertion gain is measured to determine how well the characteristics of the aid conform to the target. Figure 1–2B (relative to the POGO target) shows that the hearing aid is providing inadequate gain above 1500 Hz, which might affect the audibility of the consonant sounds and lend to user dissatisfaction.

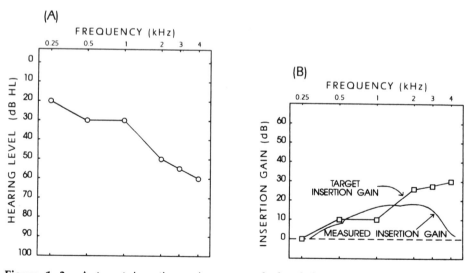

Figure 1–2. A target insertion gain curve calculated from a prescriptive formula (POGO) is shown along with the measured insertion gain. Note the inadequate gain above 1500 Hz.

Measured functional and insertion gain measures may be similar but not identical, since functional gain measures are determined from behavioral (aided vs. unaided) sound field thresholds and insertion gain measures are a physical measure obtained in the ear canal. However, on the average, functional and insertion gains are sufficiently close as to be clinically valid.[30] On occasion, considerable individual differences can be found between these two measures.

Some professionals use the term *real ear* when referring to measured functional or insertion gain. This term is in contrast to *coupler gain*, which is used as a standard reference by manufacturers and is an electroacoustic measure. Coupler gain is the difference between the input level to a hearing aid and the output level measured in a 2 cc coupler. Coupler gain measures are usually performed with either the volume control set to full-on or at a reference test position where the volume control setting is 17 dB down from the high frequency average full-on gain level. Coupler gain is not the same as functional or insertion gain; the latter measures are performed while the volume control of the hearing aid is adjusted to a comfortable level. The 2 cc coupler response, although an acceptable standard, may be a rather poor representation of the aided gain found on an individual ear.[1,31]

Threshold-Based Prescriptive Rules

Since a linear hearing aid provides the same amount of amplification for soft as well as loud sounds, the problem in providing adequate gain in the pathologic ear with recruitment is to arrive at a reasonable compromise. Most hearing aid users have varying amounts of loudness recruitment so the volume control of a linear hearing aid is adjusted to amplify soft sounds to a comfortable listening level but frequently makes louder sounds uncomfortable. When a hearing aid is adjusted to a comfortable level for loud sounds, the softer sounds, including those of speech, are often inaudible.

A logical choice of gain is to prescribe a level that permits hearing sounds that are most important without being excessively loud, that is, near the MCL level. Although an individual's choice of preferred listening level for amplified sound depends on many factors, on the average, preferred listening levels amount to about one-half of the average hearing threshold.[32] For example, an individual with an average loss of 60 dB, or speech threshold near 60 dB, will most often adjust use gain to about 30 dB.

This "half-gain rule" was formalized into one of the earliest threshold-based prescriptive procedures in 1944 by Lybarger,[6,33] whose formula included calculating desired gain at discrete frequencies to compensate for hearing loss. This half-gain rule froms the basis for many current formulas calculated from the hearing threshold level. The formulas that followed the basic principles stated by Lybarger reflect his basic principles wherein various amounts of gain are added or subtracted at specific frequencies based on the severity of loss or audiometric slope. In principle, the half-gain rule states that greater gain is required as hearing loss increases, amounting to approximately one-half the average hearing loss at least for mild to moderate hearing losses.

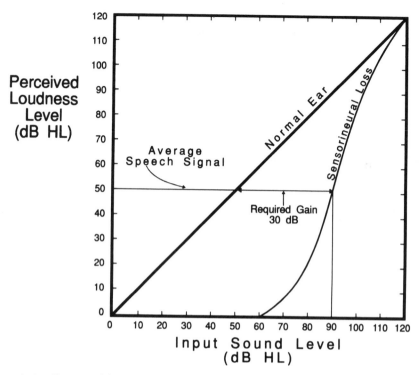

Figure 1–3.   Perceived loudness levels shown for a 60 dB sensorineural hearing loss compared with a normal ear. The gain required to elevate a 50 dB HL speech signal to normal loudness is 30 dB.

The half-gain principle can be illustrated another way, by calculating the amount of gain required to elevate average normal speech spectra to a level comparable to the normal ear. Figure 1–3 illustrates this relationship for a 60 dB hearing loss. It can be seen that the derivation of the half-gain requirement using a linear amplifier corresponds to the gain amounting to about half of the hearing loss up to about 60 dB hearing level. For losses greater than 60 dB HL (hearing level), slightly more than one half-gain may be required. It can also be seen that the level of average conversational speech must be amplified about 30 dB for a 60 dB loss to achieve about the same degree of loudness as found in the normal ear. Figure 1–4, based on Pascoe's data,[29] illustrates how, when applying the half-gain rule, average speech spoken at 55 dB HL (regarding the sound field) is restored to the MCL. Calculation of gain, although made from threshold measures, is clearly seen to restore average conversational speech to the MCL range for hearing losses up to about 60 dB. In this illustration, the average UCL raises about 20 dB for a 100 dB increase in the hearing threshold. The reduced dynamic range, or range of comfortable loudness, is also seen to become smaller with increasing hearing impairment.

The half-gain concept still has clinical utility, especially in arriving at general

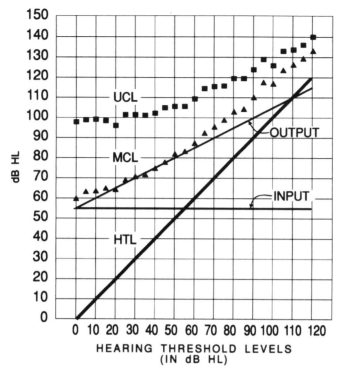

Figure 1–4. Mean MCL and UCL levels for various degrees of hearing loss. Applying the one-half gain rule raises a 55 dB hearing level speech signal to near the average MCL levels for mild to moderate hearing losses. (Based on data from Pascoe.[29])

frequency-gain categories in the preselection of actual hearing aids or in ordering hearing aids from manufacturers, 2 cc coupler specifications, or matrices. It must be remembered that full-on 2 cc coupler data supplied by the manufacturer does not correspond to the target insertion gain, which is measured with the volume control set at a level approximating the MCL.

Comparison of Threshold-Based Hearing Aid Selection Formulas

It is not the intent of this chapter to present the merits of threshold-based versus other types of prescriptive techniques or to argue the relative superiority of one procedure over another. However, it must be realized that, over the years, some 40 or more prescriptive procedures have been published.[1] At least half of these prescriptive procedures are based on audiometric pure-tone thresholds. Since each prescriptive procedure has its own rationale and since the various formulas yield significantly different prescribed gain requirements, not all can be expected to yield equivalent maximum speech recognition, improve sound quality, or maximum satisfactory results. Procedures also differ in their efficiency, ease of computation, and general clinical utility. Some recent reports suggest that not all procedures are equally effective and may result in measurable differences in speech recognition and user satisfaction.[27] It is incumbent on the dispenser or manufacturer to select a prescriptive technique that has a strong theoretical rationale, has good clinical utility and efficiency, results in a fitting acceptable to the user, and provides quantitative evidence of optimum speech recognition.

Of the many prescriptive procedures proposed over the years, only a few are in general use. The popularity of these does not necessarily imply superiority; however, their use seems to be related to ease of calculating the prescribed gain, and they appear to be valid when using linear amplification.

There is considerable difference of opinion as to whether various prescriptive techniques result in significant differences in speech recognition, sound quality, or clarity. One point of view states that minor differences in frequency-gain responses between prescriptive formulas would likely be minimal, especially when adjustment of the volume control is considered.[26,28,34] Others believe that if various prescriptive target formulas are strictly adhered to in the selection of hearing aids, then no two procedures would be equally effective for all individuals.[35] Furthermore, it is argued that, even when allowing for individual volume control adjustments, speech recognition is significantly better with some prescribed target criteria than with others.[36]

To illustrate the similarities and differences between formulas, a comparison of four threshold-based procedures are presented here as applied to two audiometric configurations. The formulas were selected as representing those reported in current use—appearing frequently in the professional literature and commonly found in the instrumentation used to measure insertion gain. The four prescriptive procedures chosen for comparison are (1) Berger[8] (1984), (2) Libby One-Third Gain[9] (1986), (3) NAL Revised (NAL-R)[18], and (4) prescription of gain and output (POGO).[1]

Berger

The Berger procedure is based on the assumptions that amplification should raise sounds toward average conversational speech levels, that amplification of low frequencies should be reduced slightly because of their potential detrimental masking effect on recognition of speech, and that more amplification is required at frequencies having greater hearing loss. Berger et al.[8] further state that speech sounds up to 4000 Hz are relatively important to speech recognition and that overamplification may reduce speech recognition.

The formula was prompted, in part, by what they called the poor reliability of speech recognition tests in the selection of the appropriate hearing aid. They also rejected the use of MCL in prescribing appropriate gain because of its wide inter- and intrasubject variability. Although their gain calculations are based on pure-tone measures, Berger et al. report that the technique produces good speech recognition and patient satisfaction. This technique is one of a few that also includes calculations for prescribing SSPL90.

An appealing aspect of the Berger technique is that it not only provides calculations for target gain and maximum output, but also includes a recom-

Table 1–1. Comparison of Four Threshold-Based Procedures

	250	500	1000	2000	3000	4000	6000
POGO	0.5 (−10)	0.5 (−5)	0.5	0.5	0.5	0.5	0.5
Libby one-third	0.33 (−5)	0.33 (−3)	0.33	0.33	0.33	0.33	0.33
Berger	—	0.30*	0.63	0.67	0.59	0.53	0.50
NAL-R†	0.31 (−17)	0.31 (−8)	0.31 (+1)	0.31 (−1)	0.31 (−2)	0.31 (−2)	0.31 (−2)

* 0.50 for a 50 dB HL.

† Plus 0.05 of hearing level at 500 + 1000 + 2000 Hz (addition for overall gain).

mended testing sequence, rules for when to fit, selection of ear, binaural–monaural selection criteria, and formulas for body, ear level, and binaural aids. The formula, as shown in Table 1–1, is based on pure-tone thresholds and discomfort measures made under headphones. Prescriptions of frequency-gain response are expressed in terms of desired functional gain for 500, 1000, 2000, 3000, 4000, and 6000 Hz (see Table 1–1). The target insertion gain is calculated to which a 10 dB reserve is added at all frequencies.

Libby One-Third Gain

The formula reported by Libby[9] is based on the assumption that gain requirements for mild to moderate hearing losses more closely approximate a one-third rather than a one-half gain rule. Libby also presents a two-thirds gain rule designed for individuals with severe to profound hearing impairment; however, only the one-third formula is discussed here as shown in Table 1–1.

The basic rationale for this study was the suggestion by Libby that mild hearing losses utilize very little gain in real life situations. He concluded that a prescription should reflect the amount of gain actually chosen by the subjects in his study. Contrasted with other formulas based on a half-gain rule, he makes no particular attempt to restore average conversational speech to the average MCL level at discrete frequencies. Calculation for the Libby procedure is one-third the hearing threshold level (HTL) minus 5 dB at 250 Hz, one-third the HTL minus 3 dB at 500, and one-third the HTL at other frequencies between 1000 and 6000 Hz.

NAL-R

The NAL-R procedure is a revision of a procedure first reported by Byrne and Tonnison.[7] Whereas the Bryne and Tonisson technique approximated the half-gain rule, it was felt this original procedure did not meet the aim of amplifying all frequency bands of speech to equal loudness.[18] The revision in 1986 restores a greater amount of desired amplification in the lower frequencies. The general rule was to provide sufficient gain at each test frequency to amplify average conversation speech to the individual MCL when the volume control of the hearing aid was adjusted at a comfortable listening level. Whereas most threshold-based prescriptive procedures calculate gain independently at each frequency, the NAL-R approach uses a half-gain rule combined with a one-third slope rate. The addition of gain constraints is applied to account for cases in which there is considerable steepness of slope. Slope gain modifications are taken into account by multiplying the HTL at each frequency by 0.31, which provides gain corrections for variations in audiometric slopes. In effect, this procedure attempts to control for excessive gain in cases with steeply sloping hearing losses. The NAL-R calculations are considerably more complex than most others, especially when performed by hand. The formula specifies gain calculations from 250 through 6000 Hz using earphone thresholds. The HTL at each frequency is multiplied by $0.31 + [0.05(HTL_{500} + HTL_{1K} + HTL_{2K})]$ minus frequency-specific constants (varies between -17 dB at 250 Hz to $+1$ dB at 1000–1500 Hz) = insertion gain (dB). The basic calculations for this procedure are shown in Table 1–1. However, due to the procedure's greater complexity, it is best to refer to the original article when using it.

POGO

The POGO procedure is based on the assumption that frequency-gain response and SSPL limiting are essential characteristics in a basic prescriptive fitting. Another assumption is that a valid formula can be derived based on pure-tone or other stationary signals that, when appropriately shaped, should result in a frequency response that is pleasant and yields high speech recognition. Furthermore, it is assumed that these measures correlate reasonably well with MCL-derived desired spectra.

The POGO technique first determines the frequency-gain response from the hearing loss measured with an earphone. The target frequency-gain response formula for POGO is given in Table 1–1.

Transformations of prescribed gain for a specific type of hearing aid (i.e., ITE vs. BTE) to coupler gain can be made. A 10 dB reserve gain is also included to assist the dispenser in selecting aids from manufacturer's published $2 \, cm^3$ full-on gain or matrix data. The POGO formula was derived by comparing and assimilating several other successful MCL and threshold-based procedures and integrating real-ear gain data from successful hearing aid users having a variety of hearing losses.

Figure 1–5 is a comparison of the Berger, Libby one-third gain, NAL-R, and POGO insertion gain prescriptions for a mild to moderate sloping audiogram. Figure 1–5B shows the differences in target or recommended insertion gain between formulas. In Figure 1–5C the target curves are normalized at 1000 Hz to illustrate differences in frequency-gain response as might occur when the volume control is adjusted by the use for loudness judgments.

It can be seen that with this degree and slope of loss, the Berger technique prescribes considerably more gain at 1000 and 2000 Hz than the other methods. Gain requirements are considerably less with the Libby one-third gain formula. The NAL-R and POGO target calculations appear somewhat similar in this case.

Figure 1–6B,C shows comparisons of the four formulas applied to a steeply sloping audiogram. The same relationships generally hold between the various formulas; however, the NAL-R and POGO techniques show greater divergence in the high frequencies where the NAL-R specifies less gain.

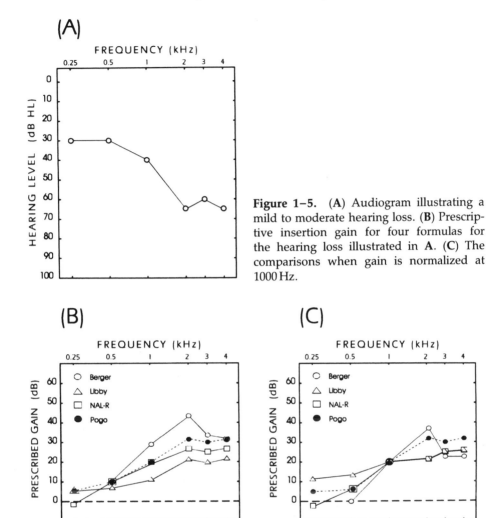

Figure 1–5. (A) Audiogram illustrating a mild to moderate hearing loss. (B) Prescriptive insertion gain for four formulas for the hearing loss illustrated in **A**. (C) The comparisons when gain is normalized at 1000 Hz.

Discussion of methods of output limiting appear in later chapters and thus is not detailed here. However, it is important to note that output specification is essential to the Berger, Libby, and POGO formulas.

Practical Considerations of Threshold-Based Procedures and the Future

This chapter is primarily intended to present the rationale and current uses of threshold-based prescriptive procedures for hearing aid selection and fitting. An obvious question is which, if any, of the several prescriptions is most effective, or at least best suited, for one's particular clinical operation? While many hearing aids will be acceptable based on any of the popular formulas, speech clarity or sound quality may be compromised with some. The findings by Skinner et al.[11] suggest that rather small changes in overall gain, bandwidth,

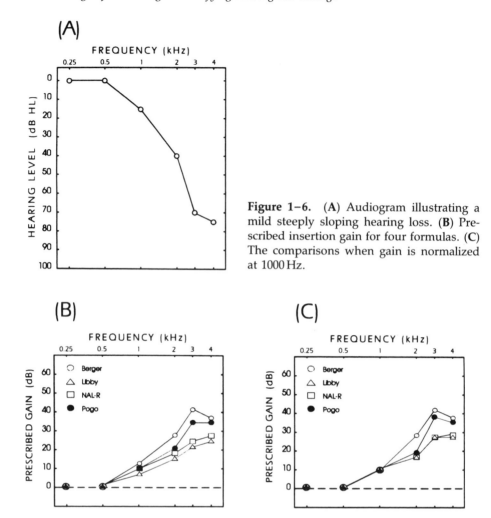

Figure 1–6. (A) Audiogram illustrating a mild steeply sloping hearing loss. (B) Prescribed insertion gain for four formulas. (C) The comparisons when gain is normalized at 1000 Hz.

and frequency response support the notion that no two prescriptive procedures are equally effective. Even when normalized with the volume control, differences in gain between formulae at certain frequencies may be as large as 20 dB. There are but few clinical studies directly comparing the efficacy of different formulas; however, it is difficult to believe that any two prescriptions would be equally effective for all individuals. The fact is, unless specified by the dispenser, selection of frequency-gain response is done by the manufacturer, in which case the dispenser rarely knows the selection procedure used for a given client.

As important as selecting a specific prescription formula for clinical use is the verification process. Providing prescribed gain does not guarantee the user is receiving significant benefit from the hearing aid. Fine adjustments are often required to bring the prescribed characteristics in tune with the subjective impressions of sound quality and comfort.

Although hearing aid selection by threshold prescription for linear hearing aids is the most frequently used procedure today, hearing aid technology has advanced well beyond the current selection and evaluation processes. As newer, nonlinear sound processing strategies become available, new selection procedures will be required that may entail prescriptions and evaluation for several input levels. It should be emphasized that all present prescriptive techniques must be considered temporary and capable of modification or replacement as technical and clinical knowledge expands. We should not expect current practices based on linear hearing aid technology to apply to future hearing aids utilizing nonlinear amplification, multiple bands, noise reduction circuits, or other sound processing strategies. Also needed will be methods to determine gain and output characteristics for multichannel and noise reduction systems. Present selection techniques continue to have particular appeal because of their efficiency and simplicity. Current hearing aid selection procedures based on threshold measures will be used as long as linear amplifiers are utilized. As nonlinear, digital sound processing or other strategies are implemented, new formulas for selection and fitting must be developed.

References

1. McCandless GA, Lyregaard PE: Prescription of gain and output (POGO) for hearing aids. *Hear Instrum* 1983; 3:16–21.
2. Cox RM, Bisset JD: Prediction of aided preferred listening levels for hearing aid gain prescription. *Ear Hear* 1982; 3:66–71.
3. Bryne D: Key issues in hearing aid selection and evaluation. *J Am Acad Audiol* 1992; 3:67–80.
4. Skinner MW: *Hearing Aid Evaluation*. Englewood Cliffs, NJ: Prentice Hall, Inc., 1988.
5. Carhart R: Hearing aid selection by university clinics. *J Speech Hear Dis* 1950; 15:106–113.
6. Lybarger SF: U.S. Patent Application SN 532, 278, 1944.
7. Byrne D, Tonnison W: Selecting the gain of hearing aids for persons with sensorineural hearing impairments. *Scand Audiol* 1976; 5:51–59.
8. Berger KW, Hagberg EN, Rane RL: *Prescription of Hearing Aids: Rationale, Procedures and Results*, ed 5. Kent, OH: Herald, 1989.
9. Libby ER: The 1/3–2/3 insertion gain hearing aid selection guide. *Hear Instrum* 1986; 37:27–28.
10. Pascoe DP: An approach to hearing aid selection. *Hear Instrum* 1978; 29:12–16, 36.
11. Skinner MW, Pascoe DP, Miller JD, Popelka GR: Measurements to determine the optimal placement of speech energy within the listener's auditory area: A basis for selecting amplification characteristics, in Studebaker GA, Bess FH (eds): *Vanderbilt Hearing-Aid Report*. Upper Darby, PA: Monographs in Contemporary Audiology, 1982, pp 161–169.
12. Cox RM: Using ULCL measures to find frequency/gain and SSPL 90. *Hear Instrum* 1983; 34:17–21, 39.
13. Wallenfels HG: *Hearing Aids on Prescription*. Springfield, IL: Charles C Thomas, 1967.
14. Bryne D: The speech spectrum: Some aspects of its significance for hearing aid selection and evaluation. *Br J Audiol* 1977; 11:40–46.
15. Berger KW, Hagberg EN, Rane RL: Determining hearing aid gain. *Hear Instrum* 1979; 30:26–28, 44.
16. Kirkwood DH: 1991 U.S. hearing aid sales summary. *Hear J* 1991; 44:9–11, 14–15.
17. Walden BE, Schwartz PM, Williams DL, et al.: Test of the assumptions underlying comparative hearing aid evaluations. *J Speech Hear Dis* 1983; 48:264–273.
18. Gallagher G: Returns for credit. *Hear J* 1990; 43:13–18.
19. Byrne D, Dillon H: The National Acoustic Laboratories' (NAL) new procedure for selecting the gain and frequency response of a hearing aid. *Ear Hear* 1986, 7:257–265.
20. Bragg VC: Toward a more objective hearing aid fitting procedure. *Hear Instrum* 1977; 28:6–9.
21. Shapiro I: Hearing aid fitting by prescription. *Audiol* 1975; 15:163–173.

22. Skinner MW: Speech intelligibility in noise-induced hearing loss; effects of high frequency compensation. *J Acoust Soc Am* 1980;67:306–317.
23. Berger KW, Soltisz LL: Variability of thresholds and MCLs with speech babble. *Aust J Audiol* 1981; 3:1–3.
24. Christensen B, Byrne D: Variability of MCL measurements: Significance for hearing aid selection. *Aust J Audiol* 1980; 2:10–18.
25. Stephens SD, Bleguad B, Krogh HJ: The value of some suprathreshold auditory measures. *Scand Audiol* 1977; 6:213–221.
26. Humes LE: An evaluation of several rationales for selecting hearing aid gain. *J Speech Hear Dis* 1986; 51:272–281.
27. Byrne D: Hearing aid selection formulae: Same or different? *Hear Instrum* 1987; 38:5–11.
28. Sullivan JA, Levitt H, Hwang JY, Hennessey AM: An experimental comparison of four hearing aid prescription methods. *Ear Hear* 1988; 9:22–32.
29. Pascoe DP: Clinical measurements of the auditory dynamic range and their relation to formulas for hearing aid gain, in *Presbyacousis and Other Age Related Aspects.* 14th Danavox Symposium, 1990, pp 129–147.
30. McCandless GA: In-the-ear canal acoustic measures, in Studebaker GA, Bess FH (eds): *The Vanderbuilt Hearing-Aid Report.* Upper Darby, PA: Monographs in Contemporary Audiology, 1982, pp 170–173.
31. Hawkins DB, Haskell GB: A comparison of functional gains and 2 cm³ coupler gain. *J Speech Hear Dis* 1982; 47:71–76.
32. Berger K, Hagberg N, Rane R: A re-examination of the half gain rule. *Ear Hear* 1980; 1:223–225.
33. Lybarger S: *Simplified Fitting System for Hearing Aids.* Canonsburg, PA: Radioear Corporation, 1963.
34. Humes LE: And the winner is. . . . *Hear Instrum* 1988; 39:24–26.
35. Byrne DB: Recent hearing instrument selection research suggests what? *Hear Instrum* 1988; 39:22–23.
36. Byrne DB, Cotton S: Preferred listening levels for sensorineurally hearing-impaired listeners. *Ear Hear* 1987; 9:7–14.

2

Overview, Rationale, and Comparison of Suprathreshold-Based Gain Prescription Methods

Larry E. Humes, Dan C. Halling

Introduction

The objective of most, if not all, hearing aid fitting procedures is to make speech audible, yet not uncomfortably loud. In other words, the clinician would like to provide sufficient amplification so as to position all amplified speech sounds within the dynamic range of the user at frequencies between 250 and 6000 Hz. Although there are definitions that differ in detail, *dynamic range* can be considered to extend from hearing threshold to some higher sound level at which sound becomes uncomfortably loud.

As noted in the previous chapter, there are several threshold-based methods that share this objective. The primary point of departure between advocates of threshold-based versus suprathreshold-based procedures lies in the relationship between threshold and suprathreshold measures. Consider a hearing aid fitting strategy that has as its objective amplification of speech to the most comfortable loudness (MCL) level. If there is a very strong relationship between threshold and MCL such that knowledge of an individual's threshold will enable accurate estimation of the MCL for that individual, then there is no need to use a suprathreshold procedure, which requires direct measurement of MCL. One would simply measure threshold, estimate MCL, and then amplify speech to MCL. Although this example focuses on a suprathreshold-based method making use of MCL, the same concept would apply to procedures based on other loudness-based measures, such as the upper limit of comfortable loudness (ULCL), which is simply defined by a descending approach to comfortable loudness, or loudness discomfort level (LDL). Advocates of suprathreshold-based methods argue that the relationship between threshold and the desired suprathreshold loudness measure (MCL, ULCL or LDL) is *not* strong enough to permit accurate estimation of these loudness measures for individual hearing aid wearers. For this reason, they must be measured directly.

The limited data available regarding the relationship between threshold and MCL, ULCL, or LDL suggest that the relationship is *not* strong.[1,2] Thus, if the objective of a particular method is to amplify speech to MCL, one must measure the individual MCL directly. Nevertheless, most surveys of current audiologic practices indicate that the most popular prescriptive procedures are threshold based.[3] Why are threshold-based methods, which are less accurate in accomplishing their underlying loudness-based objectives, more popular than suprathreshold-based methods? There are several reasons. First, clinical measurements for suprathreshold-based methods are generally believed to require at least twice as much time as threshold-based procedures. That is, for suprathreshold-based methods it is generally assumed that one must measure both threshold and the particular loudness measure of interest at each frequency rather than just measuring threshold as in threshold-based methods. Although this is true for some suprathreshold-based methods, in particular those that establish amplification targets midway between threshold and some loudness measure,[4,5] it is not true of *all* such methods. For example, if the target is to amplify speech to MCL, then only the MCL needs to be measured for the hearing aid fitting process. However, this still represents additional time because measurement of MCL is not a routine part of the preceding stage of auditory assessment, as is measurement of threshold. It is also important to note that, to date, there have been no studies conducted that demonstrate that hearing aid wearers fit with the more time-consuming suprathreshold-based methods are more satisfied or successful hearing aid wearers than those fit with the shorter threshold-based methods.

The preceding argument, however, assumes that the audiologist is only interested in prescribing the frequency-gain characteristics of the hearing aid in a systematic fashion. Although hearing aid fitting procedures have focused on the prescription of gain, increasing importance is being placed on prescription of the maximum possible sound level or saturation sound pressure level (SSPL). Few would disagree that prescription of the maximum tolerable level for amplified sound should be based on the loudness perceptions of the individual hearing aid wearer. Thus, even proponents of threshold-based methods designed to prescribe frequency-gain characteristics have noted that additional loudness-based measures should be obtained to specify maximum output. Output-limiting controls on conventional single channel hearing aids, however, are typically not frequency specific. Consequently, a single loudness discomfort measure for an amplified broadband stimulus often is sufficient to determine whether the maximum possible output level requires adjustment. This does not, therefore, require a major commitment of additional time. Prescriptive methods based on suprathreshold loudness measures, on the other hand, require that the measurements be performed for narrowband or pure-tone stimuli at several frequencies and consume much more time in the process.

A second reason for the low popularity of suprathreshold-based procedures is related to the information the hearing aid industry requires for manufacturing custom-made devices. Although manufacturers request information in addition to hearing thresholds (e.g., age, previous experience, SRT, WRS, speech MCL and LDL), most manufacturers only *reguire* a patient's hearing thresholds at the audiometric frequencies. A large percentage of those who dispense hearing aids order hearing aids for their patients by supplying only the required information.[6] For example, 80% of the audiologists employed by the Veterans Administration, the single largest employer of audiologists in the United States, order hearing aids in this manner.[7]

A third reason for the relative unpopularity of suprathreshold-based methods is that they can only be used with populations that can make the required loudness judgments. MCL, ULCL, and LDL are loudness judgments that are not easily and reliably made by children or patients with diminished intellectual capacity. Hearing threshold, however, can usually be obtained through behavioral conditioning procedures or estimated from electrophysiologic measurements in these populations, making it possible to use threshold-based methods.

Finally, a fourth reason for the limited use of suprathreshold-based prescriptive methods is related to the reliability of the required loudness measurements. Several studies, in which both hearing thresholds and MCLs were obtained from the same listeners, have found test–retest variability to be two to five times greater for MCL than for threshold.[8–10]

With all of these problems associated with suprathreshold-based methods of hearing aid fitting, why include a chapter on these methods in this book? There are three responses to this question. First, the rationales for various suprathreshold-based and threshold-based methods are identical, and attaining a better understanding of one method will enhance understanding of the other. A second and more important reason, however, is that the hearing aid fitting process used by audiologists is beginning to undergo radical changes. Audiology is moving closer to a process of custom tailoring the frequency-gain and output response of the hearing aid to meet the theoretical objectives of the audiologist *and* the needs of the patient. Two primary factors underlie this change: (1) the emergence of programmable behind-the-ear, in-the-ear, and in-the-canal instruments with extreme electroacoustic flexibility and good fidelity; and (2) the availability of real-ear probe microphone devices to measure directly and efficiently the various real-ear targets on the patient's ear.[11–13] It has been predicted[14] that, in the near future, if a particular hearing aid fitting method has as its objective the amplification of speech to MCL, it will be possible to program the hearing aid to accomplish this objective and to confirm directly its realization in the patient's ear. Threshold-based and suprathreshold-based methods that rely on the use of insertion gain measurements as an intermediary between the specifications required by the hearing aid manufacturer to order the instrument and the realization of the theoretical objectives of the selection procedure on the patient's ear will soon become obsolete.[13,14] Real-ear methods of measuring and confirming amplification of speech to achieve specified suprathreshold targets are beginning to emerge in clinical practice and are likely to become more commonplace in the years ahead.

The third reason for discussing suprathreshold-based methods in this chapter is related to the changing hearing aid technology. Current suprathreshold-based prescriptive procedures are only appropriate for predicting gain for hearing aids having linear amplifiers. Now, with the availability of nonlinear dynamic-range compression hearing aids, these procedures will need to be modified. For these aids, the amount of gain and compression in each frequency region must be adjusted so that soft to loud speech falls within the dynamic range of the individual. Verification will require use of speech spectra at a number of overall levels, with modification of the fit based on the individual's need for sound quality and clarity of speech. Therefore, suprathreshold-based procedures could play an even greater role with nonlinear hearing aids.

Given the foregoing, it is clearly important to understand the theoretical objectives of the suprathreshold-based prescriptive methods. Before proceeding to a discussion of a number of these methods, it would seem appropriate to mention the rather limited application of all prescriptive approaches, whether threshold or suprathreshold based, to "real-world" listening situations. These procedures were developed to predict the average gain required when the input to the hearing aid is average speech at a conversational level (which may be defined differently for each procedure) presented in a quiet, nonreverberant environment at a distance of approximately 1 m. If the actual signal level in the real world of the hearing aid wearer is less than this "typical" level, then the amount of prescribed gain will result in "underamplification." Similarly, if the level is greater than average, then the hearing aid will "overamplify" many real-world sounds. In addition, prescriptive procedures do not make adjustments in their prescriptions for noisy listening conditions, distances less than or greater than 1 m, and so forth. With these caveats about existing prescriptive procedures, the remainder of this chapter reviews and compares several suprathreshold-based prescriptive procedures.

Suprathreshold Prescriptive Procedures

Since Watson and Knudsen[15] first described a suprathreshold-based procedure designed to amplify speech to MCL, a variety of methods have been developed and advocated. Five suprathreshold-based methods have been selected for discussion that have been advocated over the past 15 years and illustrate a wide variety of suprathreshold objectives. Some of the details of each of these methods are summarized in Table 2–1. In the following discussion, the general objectives of these methods are described and then a comparison is made among the resulting prescriptions to determine the degree of similarity among these procedures. For comparison, prescriptions will be generated from two threshold-based procedures that ignore loudness criteria and focus exclusively on the audibility of speech. If, despite being based on considerably different theoretical objectives, these suprathreshold-based and threshold-based methods yield similar prescriptions for frequency-gain characteristics, then the particular set of objectives selected for realization in the patient will be of little consequence.

The suprathreshold-based methods included in this chapter were selected to be representative of a variety of approaches. No intention is made to include

Table 2–1. Summary of Suprathreshold-Based Prescriptive Methods Examined in This Chapter

Method	Objective	Reference
CID	Amplify speech to MCL (gain reduced at 250 Hz by variable amount)*	Skinner et al.[16]
Shapiro	60 dB SPL pure tones amplified (gain reduced by 15 and 10 dB at 250 and 500 Hz, respectively)	Shapiro[17,18]
MSUv3	Amplify speech to a level midway between threshold and ULCL for 250–6000 Hz	Cox[5]
Bragg	Amplify speech halfway between threshold and LDL at 1000 Hz and above, and one-third of this range at 250 and 500 Hz	Bragg[4]
Levitt	Amplify speech to a level 10 dB below LDL between 1000 and 6000 Hz, and 22 and 16 dB below LDL at 250 and 500 Hz, respectively	Levitt et al.[19]

* See footnote below.

every method constructed since the seminal work of Watson and Knudsen.[15] In addition, the indepth procedural details that are required actually to implement any of these methods is not described here. For these details, the original sources (cited in Table 2–1) can be consulted.

MCL-Based Procedures: CID and Shapiro

First, two MCL-based procedures are included in this analysis. One of these procedures has been described in detail by investigators at the Central Institute for the Deaf (CID) and is referred to here as the CID method.[16] Basically, between 500 and 6000 Hz, this method advocates amplifying the long-term root mean square (RMS) average speech spectrum (overall level of 65 dB sound pressure level [SPL]) to MCL.* At 250 Hz, amplification is reduced so that the speech spectrum is amplified to a level midway between threshold and MCL. The other MCL-based method is reported by Shapiro.[17] This method suggests amplifying input signals of 60 dB SPL at frequencies above 500 Hz to MCL. The prescribed gain at 500 and 250 Hz are determined by subtracting 10 and 15 dB, respectively, from the gain prescribed at 1000 Hz. The rationale for using a 60 dB SPL input signal is not clear; it could be a simplified, but inaccurate, representation of the average speech spectrum[17] or an attempt to equate input levels for the prescription with those used to measure coupler gain in a hearing aid test box.[18] Two key assumptions associated with both of these MCL-based methods is that amplifying speech to a level that is most comfortable is a desirable objective and one that overamplifies speech at low frequencies, thereby

---

* The CID prescriptive method has undergone some fine tuning since the Skinner et al.[16] version. In 1988, Skinner[20] recommended amplifying speech to halfway (dB) between threshold and MCL for both 250 and 6000 Hz. More recent changes call for amplifying speech to 90% of this range (threshold and MCL) at 1000–2000 Hz and 80% of this range at 2000 and 4000 Hz. The prescription at 500 Hz has not changed (amplify speech to MCL).

necessitating a reduction in gain (CID method, 250 Hz; Shapiro method, 250 and 500 Hz).

Bisect the Dynamic Range: MSUv3 and Bragg

Two different methods that bisect the listener's dynamic range are also included in this analysis. Cox[5,21,22] has described a method, the most recent version which is referred to as the MSUv3 method, in which the level midway between threshold and the ULCL is defined as the target to which the speech spectrum is amplified. Bragg,[4] on the other hand, establishes the target as halfway between threshold and LDL for 1000–8000 Hz and one-third of the way between threshold and LDL at 250 and 500 Hz. The goal of the Bragg[4] and MSUv3[5,21,22] methods is to position amplified speech at a level midway between the lower and upper limits of the listener's dynamic range expressed in dB (threshold and either ULCL or LDL). Positioning the amplified speech stimulus at a level midway between threshold and some upper limit of the dynamic range, however, may not perceptually bisect the listener's dynamic range. It is well known, for example, that within a 30–40 dB sensation level in a normal or impaired ear, loudness grows much more rapidly than at higher sensation levels.[23,24] Thus, bisecting the dynamic range in dB may not be the same as bisecting the dynamic range in terms of loudness perception.

Levitt Procedure

Another suprathreshold-based method has been described by Levitt et al.[19] This procedure is based on LDL and amplifies speech to a level 10 dB below LDL at 1000 to 6000 Hz and an additional 6 and 12 dB below LDL at 500 and 250 Hz, respectively. The objective of this procedure is simply to *maximize* the audibility of the speech signal at each test frequency while not allowing the amplified signal to be uncomfortably loud (i.e., greater than LDL). In terms of loudness, however, this method may also accomplish the objective of amplifying speech to a level that is one-half the magnitude associated with discomfort. That is, at high intensities in normal and impaired ears, a 10 dB decrease in sound level results in a halving of loudness.[23]

Comparisons Among Procedures

Nine Hypothetical Patients

How similar are the prescriptions generated by the suprathreshold-based methods, both to one another and to other threshold-based methods? To answer this question, audiometric profiles were generated for nine hypothetical patients. The audiometric data from these patients are provided in Table 2–2. Three different degrees of hearing loss (mild, moderate, and moderate to severe) of each of three different configurations (sloping, flat, rising) were combined with the letters S, F and R to represent the type of configuration and with the numbers 1, 2, and 3 to represent degree (1, mild; 2, moderate; 3, moderate to severe). With knowledge of the hearing thresholds, reasonable

Table 2–2.   Thresholds, ULCL, and LDL for Nine Hypothetical Patients*

Case		Frequency (Hz)					
		250	500	1000	2000	4000	6000
S1	T	10	10	10	60	70	70
	U	59	73	77	100	100	94
	L	79	93	95	104	104	98
S2	T	0	15	30	45	60	70
	U	59	87	73	85	100	94
	L	79	102	89	95	104	98
S3	T	20	35	50	65	70	70
	U	73	87	87	100	100	94
	L	88	94	97	104	104	98
F1	T	40	40	45	50	45	45
	U	73	87	87	85	85	79
	L	80	94	97	95	95	89
F2	T	50	55	60	60	60	60
	U	73	91	102	100	100	94
	L	80	100	106	104	104	98
F3	T	65	70	70	70	65	65
	U	77	91	102	100	100	94
	L	86	100	106	104	104	98
R1	T	40	40	30	15	0	0
	U	73	87	73	71	75	69
	L	80	94	89	87	93	87
R2	T	70	55	40	25	10	0
	U	77	91	87	71	75	69
	L	86	100	97	87	93	87
R3	T	70	70	60	50	40	30
	U	77	91	102	85	85	65
	L	86	100	106	95	95	81

* Patients have varying degrees (1, 2, or 3) of sensorineural hearing loss with sloping (S), flat (F), or rising (R) audiometric configurations. All values are in dB HL. T, threshold; U, ULCL; L, LDL.

values for ULCL and LDL were derived using formulas from Kamm et al.[1] MCL was assumed to be 6 dB below ULCL. When the specified target involved the amplification of the average long-term speech spectrum to a specified loudness criterion (true for all methods except that of Shapiro[17,18]), the same speech spectrum[25] (overall level of 70 dB SPL) was used for all methods. Two of the methods require conversion of thresholds obtained under phones to sound field thresholds.[5,16] Any adjustments required to convert from dB SPL in the sound field to dB SPL in the NBS-9A (6 cc) coupler or vice versa were accomplished using corrections published by Bentler and Pavlovic.[26] All prescriptions were generated in terms of real-ear gain, and any values less than 0 dB were converted to 0 dB. All of these assumptions and the audiometric characteristics of the hypothetical patients are consistent with a similar analysis conducted previously on several threshold-based and suprathreshold-based methods.[27]

Two Threshold-Based Procedures

A comparison was made for each of the frequency-gain responses prescribed using these five suprathreshold-based methods, with frequency-gain responses prescribed for threshold-based methods that do not advocate direct measures of suprathreshold loudness levels. That is, even though threshold-based methods such as NAL[28] and POGO[29,30] use threshold to generate a prescribed frequency-gain response, the goal of the prescription is to amplify speech to some suprathreshold loudness level (i.e., 60 phon equal-loudness contour for NAL; MCL for POGO). There are, however, threshold-based methods that have as their goal the optimization of speech recognition based on the Articulation Index (AI)[31] and do not use any loudness-based criteria. Two such methods are the Desired Sensation Level (DSL)[32] and the AIMax[27,33] methods. The objective of both methods is to amplify the average RMS speech spectrum to a level 15–18 dB above threshold at each frequency. According to AI theory, this would allow the full 30 dB range of speech to be audible at each test frequency (if the individual's dynamic range is this wide) and provide maximum speech recognition.

Comparison Among Suprathreshold- and Threshold-Based Procedures

Each of the seven prescriptive methods (CID, Shapiro, MSUv3, Bragg, Levitt, DSL, and AIMax) were used to generate real-ear insertion gain (REIG) values for the nine hypothetical patients listed in Table 2–2. However, all methods utilizing the specified speech spectrum[25] (i.e., all methods except Shapiro) were modified so that the prescribed insertion gain did not amplify the speech spectrum to levels exceeding LDL-12 dB. This criterion was adopted based on the assumptions that the peaks of speech are approximately 12 dB greater than the average RMS level at each frequency[31,34] and that it would not be desirable to have these peaks exceed the listener's LDL. Thus, Levitt's LDL 10 dB target was modified slightly to be LDL-12 dB in these analyses.

Figures 2–1 through 2–3 illustrate the REIG that would be prescribed for *average* RMS speech by each of the seven methods for the sloping (S1–S3), flat (F1–F3), and rising (R1–R3) audiometric configurations, respectively. In each figure, the panels are organized by increasing severity of hearing loss from top to bottom. Before a more detailed analysis of these responses is given, some general features that are obvious from a visual inspection of the figures are noted. First, the Levitt procedure (LDL-12 dB) prescribes the greatest amount of real-ear gain for all patients. Second, the CID method tends to prescribe the next greatest amount of real-ear gain for most patients and unusually high gain at 500 Hz for patients S2, S3, F1, and R1. Third, the Shapiro method prescribes the least amount of real-ear gain in the high frequencies and occasionally in the low frequencies. The remaining four prescriptive methods tend to cluster more closely together. Finally, differences in prescriptions among methods are

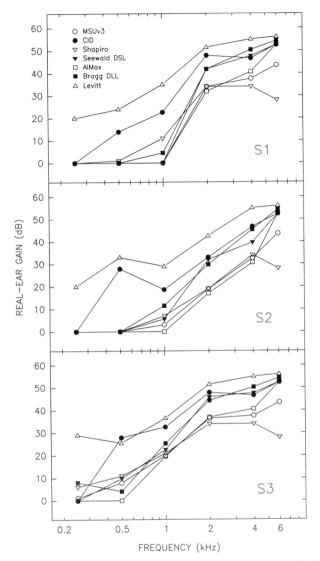

Figure 2–1. Real-ear gain prescribed by each of the seven methods for the three hypothetical patients with sloping sensorineural hearing loss of varying degree (S1, S2, S3).

generally greater for the rising configurations (Fig. 2–3) and for the milder degrees of impairment across all configurations (Figs. 2–1 through 2–3, top panels).

In an effort to analyze similarities and differences among the prescribed frequency-gain responses across methods, three measures were obtained from each prescriptive procedure: (1) low frequency slope (difference in prescribed real-ear gain at 250 and 1000 Hz); (2) high frequency slope (difference in

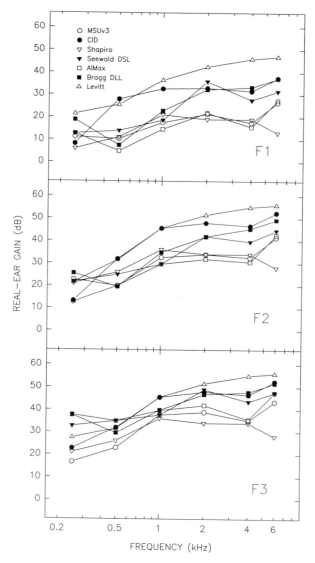

Figure 2–2. Real-ear gain prescribed by each of the seven methods for the three hypothetical patients with flat sensorineural hearing loss of varying degree (F1, F2, F3).

prescribed real-ear gain at 1000 and 6000 Hz); and (3) average overall gain (mean of prescribed real-ear gain at 500, 1000, and 2000 Hz). As in a similar analysis of threshold-based procedures,[35] these values were used to perform a cluster analysis on the various prescriptive methods for each of the nine hypothetical patients. Cluster analysis is a mathematical tool that can be used to group or cluster items according to the degree of similarity of the values observed for specified variables or parameters.

The basic pattern that emerged for six of the nine patients consisted of three

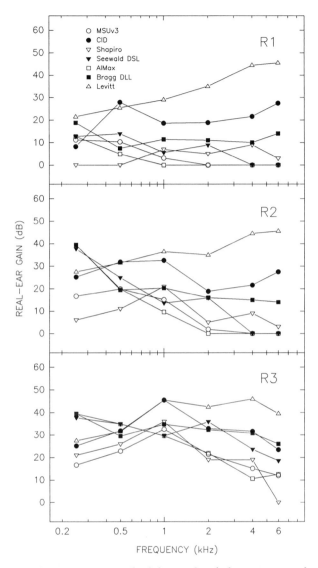

Figure 2–3. Real-ear gain prescribed by each of the seven methods for the three hypothetical patients with rising sensorineural hearing loss of varying degree (R1, R2, R3).

distinct clusters. Cluster 1 contained the DSL, AIMax, Bragg, and MSUv3 methods, Cluster 2 contained the Shapiro method alone, and Cluster 3 contained the Levitt and CID methods. Clusters 1 and 2, moreover, were more alike than Cluster 3. In the remaining three patients (F3, R2, R3) the MSUv3 procedure joined the Shapiro method in Cluster 2. All other aspects of the previously defined clusters remained unchanged. Thus, the cluster analysis tends to confirm that which is apparent from visual inspection of Figures 2–1 through 2–3.

Given a 30 to 40 dB operating range for most volume controls on hearing aids, differences among methods in terms of overall average gain are not as critical as differences in frequency response (*relative* gain across frequency). To highlight these differences in frequency-gain response across methods and audiometric configurations, the prescriptions shown in Figures 2–1 through 2–3 were equalized at 1000 Hz and replotted. A frequency of 1000 Hz was selected since it was used as the pivot point for defining the high and low frequency slopes. The results are shown in Figures 2–4 through 2–6 for the sloping, flat, and rising audiometric configurations. On visual inspection, one of the striking features is the similarity of the high frequency slopes of the frequency-gain responses (gain for frequencies at or above 1000 Hz) across the

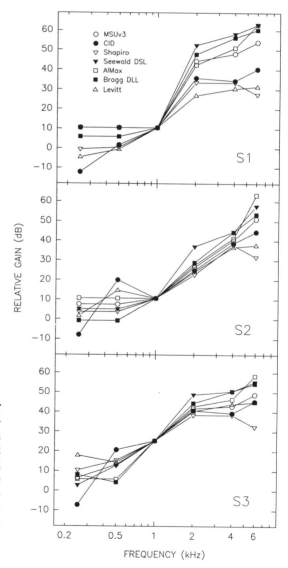

Figure 2–4. Relative gain or frequency-gain responses prescribed by each of the seven methods for the three hypothetical patients with sloping sensorineural hearing loss (S1, S2, S3). The curves in each panel were generated by adjusting the prescribed gain in Figure 2–1 for each method so that all prescriptions were equalized at 1000 Hz.

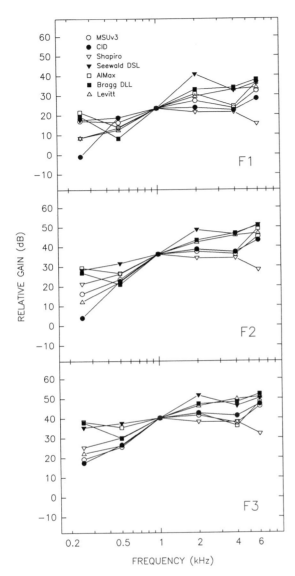

Figure 2–5. Relative gain or frequency-gain responses prescribed by each of the seven methods for the three hypothetical patients with flat sensorineural hearing loss (F1, F2, F3). The curves in each panel were generated by adjusting the prescribed gain in Figure 2–2 for each method so that all prescriptions were equalized at 1000 Hz.

various methods. These slopes were significantly and strongly correlated (r > 0.79) for all methods and configurations. Moreover, with the Levitt procedure eliminated from consideration, these correlations exceeded 0.90.

Such was not the case, however, for the low frequency slopes (gain for frequencies at or below 1000 Hz). Only a few of the correlations of low frequency slope values across prescriptive methods were strong and statistically significant. Discrepancies among prescribed low frequency slopes are probably greatest for the rising audiometric configurations (Fig. 2–6). These large between-method differences in low frequency slope result mainly from the use of constant adjustments in gain at the low frequencies in some methods[17,18,24]

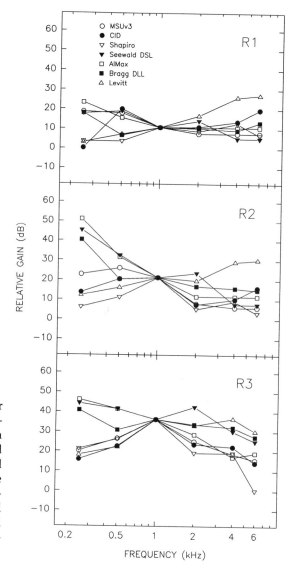

Figure 2–6. Relative gain or frequency-gain responses prescribed by each of the seven methods for the three hypothetical patients with rising sensorineural hearing loss (R1, R2, R3). The curves in each panel were generated by adjusting the prescribed gain in Figure 2–3 for each method so that all prescriptions were equalized at 1000 Hz.

while not in others. Although a constant attenuation of low frequency amplification by X dB may be desirable to reduce possible spread of masking effects in sloping and flat losses, it is not beneficial in cases of rising configurations in which the hearing loss is greatest at the same frequencies.

Table 2–3 summarizes some of the similarities and differences among the seven suprathreshold- and threshold-based methods in terms of low frequency slope, high frequency slope, and average overall gain. Relative (i.e., geometric mean) and absolute (i.e., low and high frequency slope and overall gain) measures of each of these parameters are provided for each prescriptive method. The relative measure is the geometric mean of the method's ranking for that

Table 2–3.   Geometric Mean (GM) Rankings and
Arithmetic Means of Corresponding Parameter Values for Each
Method Computed Across the Nine Hypothetical Patients*

GM Ranking	Method	Parameter Value
LF slope (dB/octave)		
1.1	CID	10.9
2.2	Shapiro	6.6
2.5	Levitt	7.1
3.9	MSUv3	4.0
4.5	Bragg	0.9
4.5	DSL	0.3
5.8	AIMax	−1.2
HF slope (dB/octave)		
1.4	DSL	6.8
1.4	AIMax	6.4
1.8	Bragg	6.8
4.2	Levitt	5.3
4.3	MSUv3	4.1
5.3	CID	3.7
7.0	Shapiro	−1.1
AVG gain (dB)		
1.0	Levitt	37.2
2.0	CID	32.4
3.4	DSL	23.4
3.4	Bragg	22.9
4.7	Shapiro	18.9
5.9	MSUv3	17.7
6.2	AIMax	17.4

* Parameters studied are low frequency slope (LF), high frequency slope
(HF), and average overall gain (AVG).

parameter across all nine configurations evaluated. Thus, if a method prescribed the greatest amount of average overall gain for all nine configurations,
it was ranked number 1 in each case and the geometric mean of these rankings
appearing in Table 2–3 would be 1. This was the case, for example, for the
Levitt method (Table 2–3; note that the CID method was consistently ranked
second in terms of average overall gain). For each of the parameters examined
(low frequency slope, high frequency slope, and average overall gain), the
methods are rank ordered from top to bottom by their average ranking across
configurations. The arithmetic mean of the prescribed values for each parameter are also provided for each method (far column to the right). As would be
expected, these values tend to decrease in an orderly fashion from top to
bottom for each parameter in Table 2–3. Note that the greatest differences
among methods appear in average overall gain and low frequency slope with
little difference observed in high frequency slope. Consistent with the cluster
analyses described previously, the data in Table 2–3 reveal different characteristics associated with various subgroupings of methods. The CID and Levitt
methods, for example, tend to prescribe the steepest low frequency slopes, the

greatest average overall gain and shallow or moderate high frequency slopes. However, it should be noted that the calculated low frequency slope for the CID procedure does not reflect the relatively high real-ear gain at 500 Hz. This high gain at 500 Hz also contributes to this procedure having high average gain. The AIMax, DSL, and Bragg procedures, on the other hand, tend to prescribe the shallowest low frequency slopes, the steepest high frequency slopes and the least amount of average overall gain. This pattern is essentially a mirror image of the CID and Levitt procedures. Finally, the Shapiro and MSUv3 methods tend to fall somewhere in between these two subgroups.

Summary of Comparisons

The preceding analyses clearly indicate that the seven methods reviewed here may be placed into three separate groups, each with distinctly different prescriptions. Six of the seven methods can easily fit into the three groups or clusters. The CID and Levitt methods comprise one group; the AIMax, DSL, and Bragg methods comprise another; and the Shapiro procedure comprises the third. It is unclear whether the MSUv3 method is more closely associated with the Shapiro procedure or the AIMax/DSL/Bragg procedures. Based primarily on the cluster analyses for six of the nine patients (representing five of the six patients with either sloping or flat audiometric configurations) and the fact that the MSUv3 method reverts to a threshold-based (NAL) procedure when ULCLs cannot be measured, the MSUv3 method has been placed in the group with the two threshold-based methods (AIMax and DSL). It is interesting to note that the two dynamic-range bisection methods (MSUv3 and Bragg) are grouped with the two AI-based methods.

Of the group consisting of AIMax, DSL, Bragg, and MSUv3, the latter two require measurement of both threshold and either LDL (Bragg) or ULCL (MSUv3), whereas the other two methods require measurement of only threshold. Parsimony would suggest that the simpler methods should prevail given the equivalence of outcomes with each of these methods. Furthermore, since the AIMax and DSL procedures are both based on the same AI-based concept and the latter method has been better refined for clinical application with both adults and children, the DSL method emerges as the method of choice among this group.

In the group of suprathreshold-based procedures comprised of the CID and the Levitt (LDL-12 dB) methods, the latter has never been advocated as a clinical procedure, but was contrived for research purposes to examine the usefulness of maximizing the audibility of all sounds. Clinically, the goal of amplifying all sounds as loud as possible for a given patient is fraught with difficulties. Thus, the CID method has emerged as the representative of this group of prescriptive methods.

Of the three remaining methods that are representative of the three distinct subgroups of procedures (DSL, CID, Shapiro), probably the most difficult to justify on a theoretical basis is the Shapiro method. As stated by Shapiro,[18] "gain was determined by subtracting 60 dB, which is the customary input SPL for measuring hearing aid gain, from MCL . . ." (p. 211). A constant 60 dB SPL input signal at all frequencies, while representative of standardized testing of hearing aids in couplers, is not informative as to the function of this instrument with meaningful real-world input signals, such as speech. Thus, although the prescriptions generated in this analysis with the Shapiro method are distinct from those generated by the DSL and CID methods, the Shapiro method lacks theoretical justification and will not be considered further as a viable alternative.

This leaves two prescriptive methods to consider: one (the DSL method) based on threshold and designed to calculate the minimum gain needed to maximize speech recognition and one (the CID method) based on threshold and suprathreshold measurements (MCL) that is designed to maximize the listening comfort of the hearing aid wearer by amplifying speech to MCL at all frequencies. Which of these methods is best? Unfortunately, no data are available at the present time with which to address this question. Both methods have firm theoretical foundations and have undergone several revisions to improve their accuracy and clinical usefulness.

There have been no systematic evaluations or comparisons of the success achieved by hearing aid wearers using instruments prescribed by either the MCL-based CID procedure or the threshold-based DSL method. One study, however, did compare the speech recognition and speech quality performance of the MCL-based CID procedure with several other threshold-based methods and found little or no difference in performance across methods.* An additional study by Byrne[37] compared the speech recognition performance of one threshold-based method, four MCL-based methods, and one LDL-based method and observed no significant differences in mean speech recognition performance for the group of listeners associated with the different methods, but did note some significant differences within individual listeners. Similar conclusions have also been reached when the speech recognition performance obtained from hearing aids prescribed by other suprathreshold-based and threshold-based methods was compared,[38] although variations in the actual gain obtained across methods in this study were considerably less than those prescribed by each method, especially at high frequencies. At present, there are no data that clearly support the superiority of one prescriptive method over another in terms of the frequency of successful fittings or the magnitude of success achieved in individual cases.

It may well be that both methods have appropriate places in the hearing aid fitting process. It has been suggested,[39] for example, that it might be desirable initially to adjust a hearing aid for the wearer to maximize listening comfort (i.e., near MCL in the CID method) or sound quality. Then it may be necessary to adjust the frequency-gain response of the instrument gradually to match more closely the response designed to maximize speech recognition (i.e., DSL or AIMax methods). However, for the CID method to be used in this manner, it would be necessary to validate that this method (or a modification of it)

---

* It should be noted that the study by Sullivan et al.[36] used a substantially different version of the CID procedure than is used in the comparisons in this chapter.

does generate a prescription that is most comfortable and one that is initially preferred by patients.

Finally, it should be noted again that the prescriptive methods described in this chapter have been developed for the fitting of hearing aids with linear amplification. With the introduction and widespread utilization of new hearing aid options, such as nonlinear dynamic-range compression, these procedures will need to be modified.

References

1. Kamm C, Dirks D, Mickey R: Effect of sensorineural hearing loss on loudness discomfort level. *J Speech Hear Res* 1978; 21:668–681.
2. Cox RM, Bisset JD: Prediction of aided preferred listening levels for hearing aid gain prescription. *Ear Hear* 1982; 3:66–71.
3. Martin FN, Morris LJ: Current audiologic practices in the United States. *Hear J* 1989; 42(4):25–44.
4. Bragg VC: Toward a more objective hearing aid fitting procedure. *Hear Instrum* 1977; 28(9):6–9.
5. Cox RM: The MSUv3 hearing instrument prescription procedure. *Hear Instrum* 1988; 39(1):6–10.
6. Hawkins DB: Current approaches to hearing aid selection. *J Can Speech Hear Assoc* 1992 (in press).
7. Bratt GW, Sammeth CA: Clinical implications of prescriptive formulas for hearing aid selection. In Studebaker GA, Bess FH, Beck LB (eds): *The Vanderbilt Hearing-Aid Report II*. Parkton, MD: York Press, 1991, pp 23–33.
8. Stephens SDG, Blegvad B, Krogh HJ: The value of some suprathreshold auditory measures. *Scand Audiol* 1977; 6:213–221.
9. Berger KW, Soltisz LL: Variability of thresholds and MCLs with speech babble. *Aust J Audiol* 1981; 3:1–3.
10. Skinner MW, Miller JD: Amplification bandwidth and intelligibility of speech in quiet and noise for listeners with sensorineural hearing loss. *Audiology* 1983; 22:253–279.
11. Cox RM, Alexander GC: Evaluation of an in situ output probe-microphone method of hearing aid fitting verification. *Ear Hear* 1991; 11:31–39.
12. Kiessling J: In situ audiometry (ISA): A new frontier in hearing aid selection. *Hear Instrum* 1987; 38(1):28–29.
13. Humes LE, Houghton R: Beyond insertion gain. *Hear Instrum* 1992; 43(3):32–35.
14. Humes LE: Hearing aid selection and evaluation in the Year 2000. *J Can Speech Hear Assoc* 1992 (in press).
15. Watson NA, Knudsen VO: Selective amplification in hearing aids. *J Acoust Soc Am* 1940; 11:406–419.
16. Skinner MW, Pascoe DP, Miller J, Popelka GR: Measurements to determine the optimal placement of speech energy within the listener's auditory area: a basis for selecting amplification characteristics. In Studebaker GA, Bess FH (eds): *The Vanderbilt Hearing-Aid Report*. Upper Darby, PA: Monographs in Contemporary Audiology, 1982, pp 161–169.
17. Shapiro I: Hearing aid fitting by prescription. *Audiology* 1976; 15:163–173.
18. Shapiro I: Comparison of three hearing aid prescription procedures. *Ear Hear* 1980; 1:211–214.
19. Levitt H, Sullivan JA, Neuman AC, Rubin-Spitz JA: Experiments with a programmable master hearing aid. *J Rehab Res Dev* 1987; 24:29–54.
20. Skinner MW: *Hearing Aid Evaluation*. Englewood Cliffs, NJ: Prentice-Hall, 1988.
21. Cox RM: Using ULCL measures to find frequency/gain and SSPL90. *Hear Instrum* 1983; 34(7):17–21, 39.
22. Cox RM: Hearing aids and aural rehabilitation: A structured approach to hearing aid selection. *Ear Hear* 1985; 6:226–239.
23. Stevens SS: *Psychophysics*. New York: John Wiley and Sons, 1975.
24. Humes LE, Jesteadt W: Models of the effects of threshold on loudness growth and summation. *J Acoust Soc Am* 1991; 90:1933–1943.
25. Cox RM, Moore JN: Composite speech spectrum for hearing aid gain prescriptions. *J Speech Hear Res* 1988; 32:102–107.
26. Bentler RA, Pavlovic CV: Transfer functions and correction factors in hearing aid evaluation and research. *Ear Hear* 1987; 10:58–63.

27. Humes LE: An evaluation of several rationales for selecting hearing aid gain. *J Speech Hear Dis* 1986; 51:272–281.
28. Byrne D, Dillon H: The National Acoustics Laboratories' (NAL) new procedure for selecting the gain and frequency response of a hearing aid. *Ear Hear* 1986; 7:257–265.
29. McCandless GA, Lyregaard PE: Prescription of gain/output (POGO) for hearing aids. *Hear Instrum* 1983; 35(1):16–21.
30. Schwartz DM, Lyregaard PE, Lundh P: Hearing aid selection for severe-to-profound hearing loss. *Hear J* 1988; 41(2):13–17.
31. French N, Steinberg J: Factors governing the intelligibility of speech sounds. *J Acoust Soc Am* 1947; 19:90–119.
32. Seewald RC: The Desired Sensation Level method for fitting children: Version 3.0. *Hear J* 1992; 45(4):36–41.
33. Rankovic CM: *An Application of the Articulation Index to Hearing Aid Fitting*. Ph.D. dissertation, University of Minnesota, 1988.
34. Dunn HK, White SD: Statistical measurements in conversational speech. *J Acoust Soc Am* 1940; 11:278–288.
35. Humes LE: Prescribing gain characteristics of linear hearing aids. In Studebaker GA, Bess FH, Beck LB (eds): *The Vanderbilt Hearing-Aid Report II*. Parkton, MD: York Press, 1991, pp 13–22.
36. Sullivan JA, Levitt H, Hwang J, Hennessey A: An experimental comparison of four hearing aid prescription methods. *Ear Hear* 1988; 9:22–32.
37. Byrne D: Effects of frequency response characteristics on speech discrimination and perceived intelligibility and pleasantness of speech for hearing-impaired listeners. *J Acoust Soc Am* 1986; 80:494–504.
38. Humes LE, Hackett T: Comparison of frequency response and aided speech-recognition performance obtained for hearing aids selected by three different prescriptive methods. *J Am Acad Audiol* 1990; 1:101–108.
39. Humes LE: And the winner is. . . . *Hear Instrum* 1988; 39(7):24–26.

3

Selection and Verification of Maximum Output

H. Gustav Mueller, Kathryn E. Bright

Introduction

Measuring a patient's tolerance for loud sounds and the subsequent selection of a hearing aid's maximum saturation sound pressure level (SSPL90) have long been recognized as two, if not *the* most critical elements, of the hearing aid selection procedure. Failure to select and adjust the hearing aid's maximum output appropriately can result in hearing aid rejection. For example, Franks and Beckmann[1] found that in a group of geriatric patients who rejected their hearing aids, the leading complaint was that the hearing aids "made sounds too loud." This finding, in fact, was reported by an overwhelming 88% of the patients.

While inappropriate selection of maximum output might not always lead to rejection, it nearly always results in a negative experience for the patient. Usually the hearing aid user will adopt one of the following four maladaptive strategies (modified from Hawkins[2]). The patient will:

1. Constantly rotate the volume control wheel (VCW) to adjust for different input levels; patients usually tire of this approach and try the next strategy.

2. Use the hearing aid only in quiet environments where input levels are low. Most individuals, however, would like to use their hearing aids in a variety of listening conditions, so they try another strategy.

3. Always use a low VCW setting so that the hearing aid gain plus the input level does not exceed the loudness discomfort level (LDL) of the patient. Using this approach, average conversational speech (especially the high frequency components) often is not audible, and the user will derive little benefit from the hearing aid. This leads to the final strategy.

4. *The patient will simply stop using the hearing aid.*

38

In general, if the SSPL90 of the hearing aid exceeds the patient's LDL, the fitting is not appropriate. On the other hand, arbitrarily setting the SSPL90 at a reduced level to avoid tolerance problems may result in an unnecessarily reduced dynamic range. In this case, segments of speech signals may not be amplified adequately to be audible, and the hearing aid user will receive a distorted signal due to frequent saturation of the hearing aid, causing inter-modulation and harmonic distortion (see Preves[3] and Fortune and Preves[4] for review). The optimal SSPL90 setting, then, is slightly below the LDL, but as high as possible to prevent limiting the amplified dynamic range.

Measurement of LDLs has historically been an integral part of the hearing aid evaluation procedure. For example, as early as the 1940s, Watson[5] discussed the use of loudness growth functions for individual hearing aid selection. He described the importance of establishing the patient's range of comfortable loudness (RCL) as a fundamental principle of prescribing hearing aids. The classic papers of Carhart[6] and Davis et al.[7] also emphasized the importance of ensuring that the maximum output of the hearing aid did not cause discomfort to the user.

Given the recognized importance of selecting the appropriate maximum output of the hearing aid, one might think that this task would occupy a significant portion of the audiologist's time during the selection and fitting evaluations. We suspect, however, that in some instances, the maximum output of the hearing aid receives little attention. Recently, we reviewed over 600 consecutive orders for custom hearing aids from three manufacturers to observe how the maximum output was prescribed. For 18% of the orders, the dispenser selected the peak 2 cc coupler maximum output using the manufacturer's matrix (presumably this selection was based on LDL measurements). In 3% of the orders, the prescribed output was expressed either in frequency-specific 2 cc coupler values or in frequency-specific LDLs (in dB HL). In the remaining 79% of the orders, either no information concerning maximum output was provided (17%) or only an LDL for speech (dB HL) was made available (62%). There appear to be three possible interpretations of these survey findings: (1) the selection of a hearing aid's maximum output is not critical (we have already discussed that it probably is the number one reason for hearing aid rejection); (2) manufacturers can reliably make the appropriate maximum output selection from the pure-tone thresholds or from a speech LDL (we will discuss later why this is not possible); or (3) the maximum output can be adjusted to match the patient's LDL at the time of the hearing aid fitting (although a reasonable and good idea, this interpretation can be ruled out, as manufacturers report that few dispensers (less than 10%) order a maximum output potentiometer for their in-the-ear (ITE) or in-the-canal (ITC) instruments).

Paradoxically, then, it appears that the hearing aid parameter that many believe is the most important often receives little attention during the hearing aid selection process. We can further assume that if selection of the maximum output is not considered important at the time of the hearing aid order, then adjustment and verification at the time of the fitting probably is also haphazard.

One could argue that maximum output selection becomes less critical when the hearing aid has some form of automatic signal processing, and in some instances this is true. In the survey mentioned above, however, over 80% of the orders were for linear, peak-clipping instruments. This finding is in agreement with that of Hawkins,[8] who found that, in 1991, 82% of the custom hearing aids ordered in the United States had peak-clipping circuitry. Will the increased use of digitally programmable hearing aids make a difference? To some extent yes, as most programmable instruments have some form of compression, which might help to prevent the SSPL90 from exceeding the patient's LDL. On the other hand, many programmable instruments have adjustable compression limiting circuitry, or input compression with adjustable knee-points and/or compression ratios, often requiring independent adjustments in two or three different channels. The success of the fitting often is dependent on the appropriate adjustment of these features, and therefore an even greater understanding of loudness growth functions is required.

Perhaps some dispensers devote little attention to SSPL90 selection because they have heard that LDL measurements are not reliable, that clinical measurements correlate poorly with realworld listening environments, or that the resulting patient benefit is too minimal to justify the time investment. We believe that these claims are unfounded and that measurement of LDLs and hearing aid maximum output selection deserves a greater emphasis in the audiologist's hearing aid selection and fitting protocol. In this chapter, we review some of the variables associated with conducting LDL measurements, present clinical guidelines for conducting these measurements, and discuss how LDL testing can be used for hearing aid maximum output selection and SSPL90 adjustment at the time of the hearing aid fitting.

Variables Associated with LDL Measurements

Instructions

Considering the apparent confusion among hearing professionals regarding loudness discomfort and how it should be defined and measured, it is not surprising that hearing aid candidates are often baffled by the procedure and do not understand what is meant by terms such as *too loud* and *uncomfortable loudness*. Because the determination of LDLs is a behavioral task that requires a subjective response, the instructions given to the listener play an important role. How the instructions are phrased can influence the listener to accept extremely uncomfortable signals or to reject sounds that are only slightly above MCL.

Instructions that have been reported in the literature for determining LDLs have been classified into three categories:[9]

1. Initial discomfort. Examples of this category of instructions suggest that the *first* point at which discomfort is experienced is the level being sought. Individuals may be instructed to respond at "the point where sound first becomes annoying."[10]
2. Definite discomfort. A more pronounced level of discomfort is implied in this category of instructions. Individuals are instructed to respond "when

the sound is so loud that you would choose not to listen to it for any length of time."[9]

3. Extreme discomfort. Instructions in this category suggest pain or other physiologic signs of discomfort such as dizziness or tactile sensation. Examples include telling the individual to respond when the signal "becomes so loud that you are afraid it will hurt your ear."[11] One bold hearing professional even suggested that "as soon as you see the muscles around his eyes start twitching, you have your measurement."[12]

Beattie et al.[13] compiled LDL results for normal-hearing listeners from a number of studies. Their compilation revealed that as the instructions changed, so did the LDLs. For example, the LDLs for speech stimuli obtained using different instruction sets ranged from 90.5 dB SPL (initial discomfort) to 137.9 dB SPL (sharp pain), although differences in psychophysical methods probably also contributed to the variability in results.

Beattie et al.[14] and Hawkins[2] recommended that the instructions for determining LDL include the following features:

1. A clear description of the purpose of the test
2. An explanation of why the test is important
3. Terms and descriptors of loudness in common everyday language.

In addition, it should be remembered that the goal of the LDL procedure is to determine a subjective measurement that will aid in setting the SSPL90 of the hearing aid. If a low LDL is obtained using instructions of the "initial discomfort" type, the SSPL90 may be set too low, thereby restricting the headroom of the hearing aid unnecessarily. On the other hand, if a high LDL is obtained using instructions that imply extreme discomfort, the SSPL90 may be set too high. It is recommended, therefore, that instructional sets attempt to approximate the middle ground of LDLs, that is, the "definite discomfort" category.

LEVELS OF LOUDNESS

Painfully Loud

Extremely Uncomfortable

Uncomfortably Loud

Loud, But O.K.

Comfortable, But Slightly Loud

Comfortable

Comfortable, But Slightly Soft

Soft

Very Soft

Figure 3–1. Descriptive anchors of loudness categories for LDL measurements. (From Hawkins[2] and Hawkins et al.[38])

The following is a sample instruction set suggested by Hawkins[2] that includes a list of terms to be given to the listener in written form (Fig. 3–1). The use of this list is designed to clarify and simplify the process of obtaining LDLs.

> We need to do a test to determine where to set the amplifier on your hearing aid. We want to set it such that sounds do not become uncomfortably loud. You will hear some sounds, and after each one I want you to tell me which of the loudness categories on this sheet [see Fig. 3–1] best describes the sound to you. So after each sound tell me if it was "Comfortable," "Comfortable, But Slightly Loud," "Loud, But OK," or "Uncomfortably Loud" etc. I will be zeroing in on the uncomfortably loud category because that is where we want the hearing aid to stop and not get any louder. So after each sound, tell me which category best describes the sound to you. (p. 28)

In an effort to clarify the task, some instruction sets also include a statement about the length of time the listener should expect to tolerate the stimulus. Finally, some researchers have suggested that there may be a practice or learning effect for LDLs[15,16] and that the listener should be tested and instructed accordingly. The following summary paragraph from an instruction set recommended by Beattie et al.[14] illustrates both of these features:

> Remember, I want to find the highest level [at which] you would be willing to listen to an important speech message for at least 15 min. You can control the loudness by pointing upward for louder, downward for softer, or the speech will remain constant if you move your hand horizontally. Be sure to search thoroughly around your upper listening level before making a final decision. Are there any questions? (p. 205)

Instructions for Children

Attempting to determine LDLs for young children is challenging but can be done given some modifications in procedure and instructions. Kawell et al.[17] reported obtaining reliable aided LDL measures from hearing impaired children between ages 7 and 14 years using an instruction set that includes a pictorial representation of the loudness categories (see Fig. 3–2A). The recommended instructions are as follows:

> We're going to see how loud this hearing aid makes sounds. You will hear some whistles and I want you to tell me how loud the whistle is. [Go over the descriptor list, explaining each choice, starting with "Too Soft."] When the sounds are "Too Loud," this is where you want the hearing aid to stop and you do not want the sounds to get any louder. Now, for every whistle, tell me how loud it sounds. (p. 136)

Recommendations for testing children have also been made by Skinner.[18] Figure 3–2B shows two sets of pictures developed at Central Institute for the Deaf for use with children.[18] The pictures on the right can be quickly and easily drawn to give school-aged children a reference for defining loudness levels.

Types of Signals

LDLs have been obtained for a variety of stimuli, including speech (connected discourse, spondees, sentences, nonsense syllables), pure tones, warble tones,

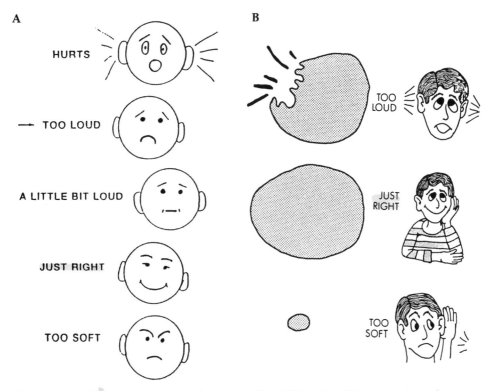

Figure 3–2. Pictures developed for use with children in obtaining loudness judgments. (**A**, from Kawell et al.[17]; **B**, from Skinner.[18])

narrow bands of noise, and filtered speech. Arguments can be made both for and against use of each type of stimulus. Speech stimuli have frequently been used because they represent a real-life situation. Speech signals are also important for determining individual loudness summation, which could influence the maximum output selection. On the other hand, pure-tone stimuli provide frequency-specific information that can be compared with hearing aid SSPL90 curves. While we do not often listen to pure tones in the real world, we do listen to ringing telephones, sirens, whistles, music, and various other tonal signals. It might be useful, therefore, to use different types of input signals to measure different aspects of loudness judgments.

PSYCHOACOUSTIC EFFECTS OF SIGNAL TYPE

In a 1976 study, Dirks and Kamm[19] reported no significant difference between LDLs for spondee words and pure tones for normal-hearing subjects, and Beattie and Boyd[20] found no difference in LDLs for speech and pure tones for a group of hearing impaired subjects. Hawkins[21] evaluated the influence of several types of signals on LDLs of normal-hearing listeners. Although the LDLs for 250 Hz stimuli (pure tones, narrowband noise, and filtered speech) were somewhat higher than for other frequencies, he found no significant

Table 3–1.   Mean LDLs (dB SPL) S.D., and S.E. for 18 Stimuli

Stimuli	*Mean*	*S.D.*	*S.E.*
Pure tones			
0.25	118	7.9	1.8
0.5	111	8.6	2.0
1	107	10.2	2.3
2	108	10.1	2.3
4	106	10.5	2.4
Narrowband noise (center frequency in kHz)			
0.25	117	8.8	2.0
0.5	111	8.5	1.9
1	112	7.7	1.8
2	108	10.3	2.4
4	108	9.6	2.2
Filtered speech (center frequency in kHz)			
0.25	115	9.8	2.2
0.5	112	9.0	2.1
1	110	9.5	2.2
2	109	8.9	2.0
4	108	9.6	2.2
Wideband signals			
White noise	109	10.1	2.3
Sentences	108	7.7	1.8
Spondees	110	10.1	2.3

(From Hawkins.[21])

difference in LDLs for a group of 19 subjects who listened to pure tones, narrowband noise, filtered speech, wide band noise, sentences, and spondees (see Table 3–1). The similarity in LDLs for various stimuli can be explained by considering equal loudness contours. For high level signals, the contours flatten across frequency. In addition, it is well known that for high level signals such as those used to obtain LDLs, the bandwidth of the stimulus has less effect on loudness summation than at moderate intensities.[19,22,23] According to a number of psychoacoustic studies, this pattern is just as likely to occur for individuals with sensorineural hearing loss.[20,23,24] Although Hawkins[21] reported no significant difference between stimulus types for the group data, he did note substantial intrasubject differences. This finding suggests that no one signal be regarded as the signal of choice when obtaining LDLs.

In contrast to the studies cited above, Bentler and Pavlovic[25] found a difference between normal-hearing and hearing impaired subjects' LDLs to pure tones and multitone complexes. They selected combinations of 2, 4, 8, or 16 pure tones spaced across the frequency range 250–4000 Hz. For both subject groups, the LDLs for multitone complexes were lower than those for pure tones, presumably due to loudness summation. The hearing impaired subjects, however, showed more loudness summation than the normal-hearing group.

In further study, Bentler[26] reported that LDLs obtained with ten different environmental stimuli were not equal and were not directly related to the crest factors of the stimuli. She also found that ratings were significantly different for the quality dimensions of annoyance, harshness, loudness, noisiness, and tinniness for the different environmental sounds.

A final and important issue concerning signal type (and test environment) relates to test validity of the LDL procedure, that is, the extent to which the clinically measured LDL accurately predicts real-world judgments of LDL. This topic was studied by Filion and Margolis,[27] who compared clinical loudness judgments of environmental sounds (e.g., nightclub noise, machine noise, air gun noise) to subjects' LDL ratings of these sounds in their social or work setting. They found that intensities that exceeded subjects' clinical LDL values were seldom judged to be uncomfortable in the real-world setting. These findings led the authors to conclude that clinical LDL measurements are not a satisfactory basis for selection of the maximum output of hearing instruments.

EFFECTS OF SIGNAL TYPE ON HEARING AID RESPONSE

In contrast to the psychophysical response, a hearing aid will go into saturation or reach its peak output at different levels for the two types of high intensity stimuli—tonal and complex signals. This factor is discussed later as part of the hearing aid verification protocol.

Procedures

PSYCHOACOUSTIC APPROACHES

The methods used to obtain LDLs may be divided into two main groups: clinician-controlled procedures and listener-controlled procedures. In both cases, an adaptive technique is typically used in which the level of the stimulus is varied depending on the listener's response to the previous stimulus.

CLINICIAN-CONTROLLED PROCEDURES

In the clinical setting, LDLs usually are determined using either the simple Up–Down Procedure or the ascending approach.

Simple Up–Down Procedure. This procedure, suggested by Levitt,[28,29] is a modification of the classic psychoacoustic method of limits. It is a combination of ascending and descending approaches. Stimulus levels are increased or decreased (in 2 or 5 dB increments) depending on the listener's previous response. When this procedure is used for obtaining LDLs, each time the listener indicates that the stimulus is uncomfortable, the intensity is decreased, and each time the listener indicates that the stimulus is comfortable, the intensity is increased. In this manner, alternating ascending and descending runs are accomplished and the LDL is taken as the point at which 50% of the responses indicate an uncomfortable loudness level.

Ascending Approach. This is a variation of the Hughson-Westlake technique for establishing threshold.[30] It is also called a *bracketing technique*. When this procedure is used to determine LDLs, the intensity of the stimulus is increased (usually in 2 or 5 dB increments) until the listener indicates uncomfortable loudness. The intensity is then dropped to a comfortable level and then increased (in 2 or 5 dB increments) until it is again uncomfortable. The LDL is taken as the highest level indicated on two out of three trials.[19]

LISTENER-CONTROLLED PROCEDURES

Method of Adjustment.   Adjustment is a classic psychophysical technique in which the listener adjusts the level of the stimulus until it just becomes uncomfortable (ascending) and then adjusts it until it just becomes comfortable (descending). The stimuli are varied continuously rather than in discrete steps, and the LDL is taken as the average value of a series of such adjustments.

Bekesy Tracking Method.   Bekesy tracking is a variation of the method of adjustment in which a Bekesy audiometer is used to control a continuous, fixed-frequency pure tone or a sweep-frequency tone that ranges from 100 to 10 000 Hz. The listener continuously adjusts the level of the stimulus so that it is alternately just above or just below the LDL.

Several investigators have specifically attempted to measure the effect of psychophysical methods on LDLs for pure-tone stimuli.[15,31–36] In general, Bekesy tracking methods result in LDLs that are approximately 10 dB higher than those obtained with other methods,[35,37] and there is very little difference among the other techniques compared.

Because there is no apparent difference in results among the clinician-controlled procedures, we recommend using the Hughson-Westlake ascending technique, also called *bracketing*. This is a method that is familiar to audiologists, and LDLs to both speech and tonal stimuli can be quickly obtained using this procedure in conjunction with the loudness chart described earlier (Fig. 3–1). In addition, Hawkins et al.[38] have shown that, using this procedure, the stability of LDL measurements over time is good.

TRAINING EFFECT

Several investigators have suggested that a practice or training effect may occur for LDL measurements. Using pure tones, Morgan and Dirks[15] noted a 6–8 dB increase in LDLs over the first four of six test sessions for normal listeners. Walker et al.[39] reported that hearing impaired listeners showed an increase in LDLs of about 8 dB across test sessions a few days apart. Sammeth et al.[40] also reported a tendency for LDLs to increase over time for 15 hearing impaired subjects who were tested on several occasions. An advantage of today's digitally programmable instruments is that even for ITC fittings the maximum output of the hearing aid easily can be altered on repeat visits.

Within a single test session, there is also evidence that the LDL may be raised by exposure to intensities above those that were initially uncomfortable.[35,41,42] Consequently, we recommend that several searches for LDL be made for each patient before a level is accepted.

NONBEHAVIORAL APPROACH

The obvious advantage of using an objective approach for estimating LDLs is that the audiologist does not have to observe and interpret a behavioral response in order to determine the appropriate maximum output for the hearing aid. An objective LDL measure would be especially helpful when evaluating young children. Some researchers have suggested that the acoustic reflex threshold can be used to predict a person's LDL.[43-45] Other investigators, however, have failed to show a consistent relationship between the LDL and the acoustic reflex threshold.[46-49] In general, the conclusions of these latter studies were that the acoustic reflex threshold is too variable to be used as an indicator of the LDL and that it is not a clinically feasible alternative to LDL measurement. Hence, there does not appear to be a reliable objective method for estimation of LDL.

Clinical Selection of Prescribed SSPL90

In this section, we discuss methods that can be used to prescribe the maximum output of the hearing aid. For most patients (80% are fitted with custom instruments), this involves the selection of 2 cc coupler values, or at least the peak 2 cc coupler value for ordering or preprogramming an ITE or ITC instrument.

Before embracing a formalized procedure of LDL measurements as part of the hearing aid selection protocol, it is reasonable to question whether such testing is an efficient use of clinic time. In a recent article on this topic, Hawkins and Schum[50] argued that, although they agree that an appropriate SSPL90 is important for successful hearing aid use and benefit, they do not believe that it is necessary to measure LDLs prior to fitting the hearing aid. Rather, they contended that if an approximate SSPL90 is first selected using a prediction from the pure-tone thresholds (they report using the method of Kamm et al.[23]) and then ordering a hearing aid with an output potentiometer with a large range of adjustment (e.g., 15 dB), an appropriate SSPL90 setting can be obtained at the time of the hearing aid fitting. In the same article,[50] they defended the role of LDL measurements in the hearing aid selection protocol by pointing out that many hearing aids do not have a potentiometer with a large range, and in these cases unaided LDL measurements lead to a reasonable initial "best guess" of an appropriate SSPL90.

In our opinion, the long-term payoff for obtaining unaided LDLs as part of the hearing aid selection protocol is well worth the minimal time investment (e.g., 5–10 minutes). Consider, for example, that in 1992 approximately 25% of all hearing aids fitted in the United States were ITC instruments,[51] and this number continues to increase. For ITC hearing aids, in many instances there is room for only *one* potentiometer. Given the desirability of features such as an active tone control or an adjustable input compression kneepoint, how many dispensers will choose an output control as the one potentiometer? Even when an output control *is* selected, the range of adjustment is less than 10 dB for most ITC models. This places increased importance on "getting the maximum output right" at the time of the hearing aid order.

While the discussion thus far has centered primarily on the penalties encountered when a hearing aid is fitted with an SSPL90 that is too high, selecting an SSPL90 that is too low also has its own set of problems that can lead to hearing aid rejection. There are at least four overall goals, therefore, associated with the appropriate selection of SSPL90 (modified from Hawkins et al.[52]):

1.   Physical discomfort from auditory signals is minimized (or even eliminated) for speech, noise, and environmental sounds in everyday life.

2.   Perceptual discomfort from auditory signals, including one's own voice, is minimized.

3.   The dynamic range available to the listener is sufficiently wide and maximized whenever possible.

4.   The hearing aid output is limited below the level that will cause additional hearing loss.

Selecting SSPL90 From Pure-Tone Thresholds

When SSPL90 are selected from pure-tone thresholds, actual LDL measurements are not conducted prior to the hearing aid fitting. Rather, the LDL is predicted from the pure-tone thresholds, and then correction factors from average group data are used to determine the desired SSPL90. As mentioned in the Introduction, this is the method that custom hearing aid manufacturers often must use, as many audiologists order hearing aids without providing any LDL information.

In general, research has shown that there is a nonlinear function between a patient's hearing loss and the LDL (see Kamm et al.[23] and Pascoe[53] for reviews). Until hearing loss exceeds 40–50 dB HL, average LDLs for individuals with cochlear hearing loss do not differ substantially from those people with normal hearing. This relationship is illustrated in Figure 3–3, which shows scatterplots of individual data and best-fit curves for LDL for pure tones at 500 and 2000 Hz and for spondaic word stimuli. Perhaps the most important clinical information displayed in Figure 3–3 is not the nonlinear function of the hearing loss to LDL relationship, but rather the large individual variability shown for all three stimuli for all degrees of hearing loss. Individual variability of 20 dB or more is common. Considering that the range adjustment of output limiting for many ITE or ITC instruments has a range less than 10 dB, it is clear that even if the audiologist orders an output-limiting potentiometer, appropriate adjustment of the SSPL90 would not be possible for many patients. The research findings of Kamm et al.[23] led them to conclude that *LDL cannot be accurately predicted from the measured hearing threshold and must be measured directly.*

In some cases it is not possible to obtain valid LDLs for a given patient, yet pure-tone thresholds are available. This is most often the case when fitting young children. Two popular hearing aid prescriptive approaches that allow for predicting the patient's LDL and the hearing aid SSPL90 from the pure-tone thresholds are the (MSU) procedure[54] and the Desired Sensation Level (DSL) procedure.[55–57] Discussion of these approaches can be found in Chapter 2.

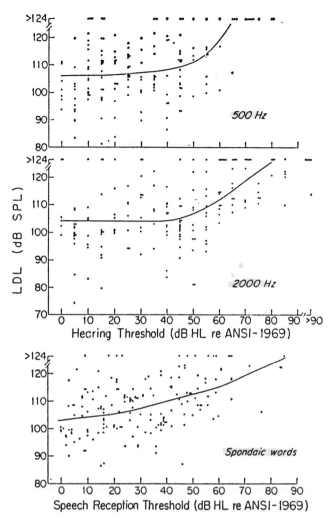

Figure 3–3. Scatterplots of individual data and computer-generated best fit curves for LDL as a function of hearing threshold for 500 and 2000 Hz and for spondaic words. (From Kamm et al.[23])

There are several other approaches to prescribing the desired 2 cc maximum output of a hearing aid besides the MSU or DSL methods. One might question if different maximum output values would be obtained if different methods were used on the same patients? The answer is *yes*. Hawkins et al.[52] compared six popular SSPL90 selection procedures and found that significantly different recommended output values resulted. For each procedure, Hawkins et al.[52] used the test administration they described; hence, the resulting differences could have been a factor of instructions, stimuli, transducer, psychophysical methods, or correction factors. Figure 3–4 shows the mean prescribed SSPL90 values for 500, 1000, and 2000 Hz for the six procedures. Note that the largest difference in mean SSPL90 (approximately 8 dB) is between the prescription of

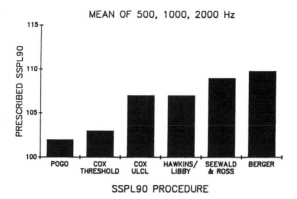

Figure 3–4.   Prescribed SSPL90 values at 2000 Hz from different SSPL90 selection procedures. (From Hawkins et al.[52])

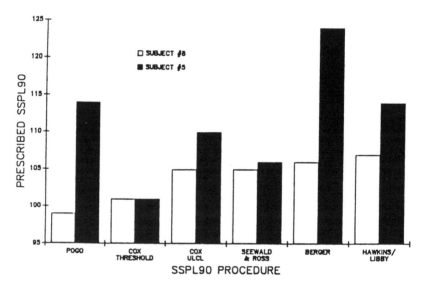

Figure 3–5.   Comparison of prescribed SSPL90 at 2000 Hz for two subjects from different SSPL90 selection procedures. (From Hawkins et al.[52])

gain and output (POGO) and the Berger methods. Hawkins et al.[52] also point out that individual differences can be quite large. Shown in Figure 3–5 are individual SSPL90 selections for two different subjects for the six procedures. While one subject had recommended SSPL90 values within 5 dB for all procedures, the other subject's testing resulted in recommended SSPL90s ranging from 100 to 125 dB. Clearly, these data suggest that the procedure that is used can influence what hearing aid circuitry is ordered. Careful evaluation and postfitting verification is needed to determine which procedure results in predicting the SSPL90 that is best for the patient.

Clinical Protocols for Prescribing Maximum Output

As discussed in the preceding section, whenever possible it is best to measure actual LDLs rather than to predict 2 cc coupler maximum output values from the pure-tone audiogram. The following is a step by step protocol that can be used successfully with the majority of patients to determine appropriate maximum output values.

1. Provide the patient with concise and easy to understand instructions that describe the purpose of the test and the desired response. Key aspects of the instructions should be written down to ensure that the instructions are consistent and complete for each patient.

2. Provide patients with a list of descriptive anchors (see Fig. 3–1) and describe how these terms relate to the sounds that they will hear.

3. Conduct pure-tone testing for the frequencies 500, 1000, 1500, 2000, and 3000 Hz. If a single channel instrument will be fitted, and the frequency at which peak output will occur is known, then it usually is satisfactory simply to conduct LDL measurements only at this frequency.

4. Use the ascending method with bracketing for each frequency (2 dB increments are good, 5 dB increments are sufficient). Record the LDL as the point midway between the "Loud, But OK" and the "Uncomfortably Loud" categories (these categories usually are only separated by 4–6 dB).

5. Convert the audiometric LDLs from dB HL values to 2 cc coupler SPL values.

6. Use the derived 2 cc coupler values to order the custom hearing aid, to select an appropriate matrix, or to select a behind the ear (BTE) hearing aid from a specification sheet. For example, if the prescribed 2 cm^3 SSPL90 is 105 dB, and the hearing aid has an output potentiometer with a 10 dB range, select a 110 dB maximum output for the hearing aid, as this will allow for a 5 dB adjustment in either direction of the predicted value, which should account for any measurement error.

Although there is some intrapatient variability associated with LDL measurements, the above procedure will usually result in a close approximation of the appropriate SSPL90. If conducted carefully, intrasubject variability for the LDL should be 5 dB or less.[19,32,58] As described earlier, there also might be some practice or training effect (which will cause an increase in LDLs), and some researchers have advocated adding an additional 3 dB to account for this variable.[2,59,60]

As noted in step 5 of our LDL protocol, it is necessary to express the patient's LDL in terms of 2 cc coupler SPL so that a direct comparison can be made with the manufacturers' hearing aid specifications. When making these corrections, it is important to consider the transducer and measurement method that is used. Clinicians have the option of using one of three procedures.

Table 3–2.   Conversion Values from dB HL to dB SPL in a 2 cc Coupler

Frequency (Hz)	TDH-39	TDH-49 and 50
250	20.7	21.7
500	9.9	11.9
750	7.3	7.8
1000	5.5	6.0
1500	2.5	3.5
2000	5.2	7.2
3000	5.7	5.2
4000	−0.5	0.5
6000	−0.2	−2.2

(From Hawkins.[61])

PROCEDURE 1: USE OF TDH EARPHONES AND AVERAGE
CORRECTION FACTORS

Although the use of insert earphones is increasing, many audiologists continue to use the TDH series earphones for conducting LDL measurements. These earphones are calibrated in an NSB-9A 6 cc coupler. Hearing aid maximum output, on the other hand, is specified relative to an HA-1 or HA-2 2 cc coupler. Hence, when we are faced with selecting the appropriate SSPL90 based on TDH earphone LDLs in hearing level (step 5 of the maximum output prescription procedure), we not only have to correct for the difference between hearing level and SPL, but also the difference between a 6 cc and a 2 cc coupler.

To assist the audiologist in making these corrections, Hawkins[61] has published data that allow for direct conversion from earphone LDLs to dB SPL in a 2 cc coupler (for additional correction factors, see the research of Bentler and Pavlovic[25]). The Hawkins[61] values for the TDH series earphones are listed in Table 3–2. The numbers in the chart are added to the earphone LDLs to obtain the desired 2 cc SSPL90 values (e.g., if a patient's earphone LDL was 98 dB HL for 1000 Hz, the prescribed hearing aid maximum output in the 2 cc coupler would be 104 dB SPL). While it is not possible to match perfectly the prescribed output at each frequency with the hearing aid's SSPL90 curve, a close approximation, at least to the peak output, usually can be achieved.

PROCEDURE 2: USE OF INSERT EARPHONES AND MEASURED
CORRECTION FACTORS

An earphone type that is better suited for LDL measurements than the TDH series is the ER-3A insert earphone. The ER-3A earphone has the advantages of greater listener comfort, reduced chance of collapsed ear canal, easier use with simultaneous probe-microphone measures, and, most importantly for hearing aid work, calibration in a 2 cc coupler.

With insert earphones there is little reason to use average correction values, as it is possible to determine precise correction values for the audiometer(s)

used for LDL measurements. By placing the insert receiver in the 2 cc coupler, the output of the audiometer can be measured for a given dial setting. For example, a 70 dB HL signal at 1000 Hz might equal 74 dB in the 2 cc coupler. The LDL HL/2 cc conversion in this case would be +4 dB. This procedure is repeated for all frequencies of interest and will account for any calibration deviation of the audiometer. This procedure is not conducted for each patient, only initially to establish correction factors for a given audiometer and earphone set.

PROCEDURE 3: USE OF INDIVIDUALIZED REAL-EAR/2 cc COUPLER
CORRECTION FACTORS

Probe-microphone measurements have a distinct role in the verification of hearing aid performance, but these measures also can be used during the selection of SSPL90. Rather than use either of the correction procedures described above, it is possible to measure an individual real-ear coupler difference (RECD) and use these values to convert to prescribed 2 cc coupler maximum output (see Mueller[62] and Fikret-Pasa and Revit[63] for reviews of RECD procedures). In a comparison of different clinical methods for predicting ear canal SPL at LDL, Zelisko et al.[64] have shown that use of the RECD will provide predicted ear canal values that correlate highly (e.g., 0.988 or higher) with measured ear canal LDL SPL values. Hawkins and Mueller[65] have provided a suggested protocol for conducting RECD measurements:

1. Equalize the sound field and (if necessary) calibrate probe microphone.
2. Place the probe tube in the ear canal 25–30 mm past the tragal notch.
3. Place the hearing aid on the patient and set the VCW to a middle position. Obtain a real-ear aided response (REAR) with a 60 or 70 dB SPL signal (level is important only in that the hearing aid should not be in compression or saturation).
4. Remove the hearing aid without changing the VCW.
5. Measure the 2 cc output of the hearing aid using the same signal type and intensity as used in the REAR measurement.
6. Subtract the 2 cc coupler response from the REAR, producing the RECD.

Once the RECD calculations have been made, the following steps will complete the protocol for determining the prescribed 2 cc maximum output:

1. Obtain LDLs for pure tones at the desired frequencies.
2. Using the probe-microphone equipment with the loudspeaker disabled (either through systems software or by manually unhooking the speaker wires), measure SPL in the ear canal for each LDL.
3. Subtract the RECD from the real-ear SPL values to obtain the prescribed maximum output values for the hearing aid.

This procedure works most effectively with insert earphones. If necessary, the probe tube can be threaded through the foam to help maintain proper position in the ear canal. If your probe-microphone equipment is not located next to your clinical audiometer, a small portable audiometer can be used to deliver the pure-tone stimuli for the LDL measurements.

Selecting Maximum Output For Children

In many ways, it is even more critical that an appropriate SSPL90 is selected for children than for adults. For young, nonresponsive children, it is especially important that a hearing aid output is selected that is low enough to prevent additional hearing loss from overamplification (although it is often difficult to know what this upper-limit SSPL90 value should be).

As previously discussed, an LDL procedure especially for children was developed by Kawell et al.[17] (see Fig. 3–2A and the instructions on page 43). In studying 20 children with hearing impairment, aged 7–14 years, Kawell et al.[17] reported that there was no difference in LDL values between children of this age and an adult population with similar levels of hearing loss. Additionally, the authors report that the reliability was as good as has been obtained for adult LDL measurements (e.g., collapsed across frequency, LDLs were repeatable within 8 dB 95% of the time).

In conjunction with probe-microphone measurements, Stuart et al.[58] reported, using an insert earphone and the child's personal earmold for stimulus delivery. This approach allows for real-ear saturation response (RESR) target to be obtained simultaneously with the LDL measurements. When selecting the

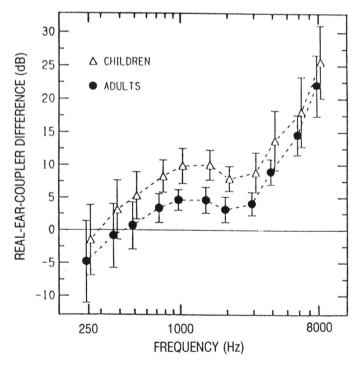

Figure 3–6.   Real-ear/2 cc coupler differences for children and adults. (From Feigin et al.[66])

SSPL90 for children, it is important to remember that, due to the child's smaller ear canal and the reduced residual volume after the hearing aid is placed in the ear, the discrepancy between 2 cc coupler and real-ear output is even greater than for adults. Feigin et al.[66] studied the real-ear/2 cc coupler differences for children and adults, and their findings are displayed in Figure 3–6. The authors report that individual deviation from 2 cc coupler gain was as much as 15 dB or more for some of the children for the 1000–3000 Hz frequency range. This means that a hearing aid selected with an SSPL90 of 128 in a 2 cc coupler could produce an output of 143 dB or higher in a child's small ear canal. Clearly, this points out the necessity of using probe-microphone measurements for measurement of output when hearing aids are fitted to a child's ear (see Hawkins and Northern[67] for a review of specific procedures).

Clinical Verification of SSPL90

Verifying that the hearing aid's SSPL90 is appropriate is an essential component of the hearing aid fitting procedure. The verification is simplified if careful measurements were taken during the selection procedure, and/or the hearing aid has an output control that allows for a large range of adjustment. The following is a clinical LDL/SSPL90 verification protocol that incorporates both behavioral testing and probe-microphone measurements:

1. Provide the patient with concise and easy to understand instructions that describe the purpose of the test and the desired response. Key aspects of the instructions should be written down to ensure that the instructions are consistent and complete for each patient.

2. Provide patients with a list of descriptive anchors (see Fig. 3–1) and describe how these terms relate to the sound that they will hear.

3. Position the patient in front of the loudspeaker (e.g., at a 1 m distance). The sound delivery system must be calibrated to determine the dial setting that corresponds to a 90 dB SPL output for each frequency.

4. Adjust the hearing aid's VCW to 5 dB above patient's use gain or to 5 dB above the prescriptive target gain for new users (this will allow for the possibility that the patient will use greater gain for some listening conditions).

5. Present pure-tone signals at 90 dB SPL for the desired frequencies. If the SSPL90 is set correctly, the patient will point to "Loud, But O.K."

6. If the patient points to categories above the "Loud, But O.K." descriptor, use the output potentiometer to lower the output until the signal is rated in the "Loud, But O.K." category (for some instruments, maximum output can be lowered by adjustment of the compression kneepoint or the compression ratio).

7. If probe-microphone equipment is available, measure the RESR for cross-check. The RESR values should correspond with the target RESR obtained during the SSPL90 selection procedure.

8. As a final verification, expose the patient to intense connected discourse

and to environmental sounds of various types outside of the test booth before the patient leaves the office. These sounds should include both transient and sustained signals. At no time should the patient state that any sound is uncomfortably loud.

There should not be any major surprises during the LDL verification procedure: *If* the unaided LDLs were conducted carefully, *if* the corrections from HL to SPL in a 2 cc coupler were conducted carefully, *if* the correct circuit was selected, and *if* the manufacturer built the hearing aid as requested, then a 90 dB SPL signal should not be uncomfortably loud for the patient.

In general, the verification protocol that we have provided is designed to present a "worst case scenario" for the patient (better that we do it at the time of the fitting while there is still an opportunity to correct the situation). Three factors are involved in creating this worst case listening situation.

1. Input stimulus. Some high gain–high output hearing aids will not be driven to saturation unless at least a 90 dB input signal is used (K-Amps generally require even higher levels to saturate). Many common environmental sounds experienced by the hearing aid user reach 90 dB SPL or greater.

2. High gain setting. In several types of hearing aids, in particular those that employ AGC-I, the output of the hearing aid is lowered when the VCW is lowered. It is important, therefore, to set the VCW at or above the level commonly used by the patient. A setting of 5 dB above prescriptive target should approximate a high VCW setting that the patient might use for quiet listening situations.[68] A VCW setting of "just-below-feedback" is also a reasonable method to ensure that a worst case situation has been accounted for.

3. *Type of Input Stimuli.* As discussed earlier, the type of input stimulus used to saturate the hearing aid will influence the SSPL90 setting; a pure-tone signal will create a higher maximum output, and consequently a lower hearing aid SSPL90 setting will result if a pure-tone signal is used. The difference in maximum output between a pure-tone and a broadband signal can be 15 dB or more. A narrowband signal has its energy concentrated at a specific point on the spectrum. In contrast, a broadband signal, such as speech, has its energy spread over a wide range of the spectrum, and the maximum energy at any one frequency is lower than the overall root mean square (RMS) level of the signal measured by a sound level meter. It is important to consider the different crest factors (the ratio of peak to RMS pressure or voltage) of different stimuli. For example, the crest factor of a pure tone is only 3 dB, whereas the crest factor of a broadband signal is generally much higher. Therefore, a broadband signal will saturate a hearing aid at a lower RMS level than will a pure tone.

While broadband signals such as speech might represent the most common loud sounds the patient will hear, some environment sounds (ringing telephones, sirens, whistles, and yapping dogs) have the potential to drive the hearing aid output to a level close to that which will be obtained for a pure tone. It is recommended, therefore, by a number of investigators that the safe, conservative approach to setting the SSPL90 is to evaluate an individual's loudness discomfort levels to pure tones, narrowband noise, or warble tones.[69–71] In so doing, tonal stimuli will remain below the level of discomfort and any wideband, complex signal would drive the hearing aid into saturation at or below this level as well.

As discussed, the most common, but perhaps least desirable, method of limiting the maximum output of hearing aid is the use of peak clipping. Although peak clipping does successfully limit the output of hearing aids to prevent discomfort, because it is a saturation phenomenon it creates additional harmonic and intermodulation distortion components that decrease the signal-to-noise ratio of signals processed by the hearing aid.[72] Given that compression can limit the output and prevent loudness discomfort as efficiently as peak clipping, there seems to be little reason not to use some form of compression for nearly all hearing aid fittings.[73–75]

When using hearing aids with adjustable compression knee-points, or adjustable compression ratios, the verification protocol outlined earlier can be modified. If the goal of the fitting is to use compression to limit the output prior to saturation, then the compression kneepoint or the compression ratio rather than the output trimmer can be adjusted during the behavioral testing to ensure that the maximum output is placed just below the "Uncomfortably Loud" category.

With AGC-I instruments it is important to remember that the maximum output decreases as a function of VCW rotation. To some extent, this provides forgiveness for the dispenser; if the output was set too high at the time of the fitting, the patient can correct this by lowering the hearing aid gain. Recall from the Introduction, however, that this is one of the maladaptive strategies that we want to prevent. We recommend adjusting the maximum output of AGC-I instruments with the VCW set 5 dB above the patient's normal use gain. This should account for those situations in which the patient has the gain of the instrument turned higher than normal for listening in quiet, yet not unnecessarily restrict the amplified dynamic range for average listening environments.

It is not uncommon for a patient's LDLs to increase following hearing aid use. It is important, therefore, to reverify the maximum output setting on repeat visits, and, if an increase in LDLs has occurred, the maximum output is raised accordingly. It is also possible that a new hearing aid user might select a use gain level significantly higher than indicated by the prescriptive method used. This could necessitate a downward adjustment of the compression knee-point for an AGC-I instrument. As pointed out by Skinner,[18] a patient's aided LDL can be affected by the spectral, temporal, and amplitude characteristics of the test signal, as well as the testing procedure and prior experience using hearing aids. It is recommended, therefore, that the output of the hearing aid be readjusted periodically following the initial fitting, as the user adjusts to the new amplification and experiences a variety of listening situations.

Table 3–3. Differences (in dB) Between Monaural and Binaural LDLs*

Subject	500 Hz	4000 Hz
1	1.5	3.0
2	0.5	5.0
3	−1.5	−7.0
4	1.0	−3.0
5	0.0	9.0
6	0.5	2.0
7	4.5	4.5
8	−0.5	−1.0
9	1.0	2.0
10	0.0	−1.0
11	0.0	0.5
12	2.5	−4.5
13	−2.5	1.0
Mean	0.5	0.8

* Positive numbers mean binaural LDL was lower than monaural LDL.

(From Hawkins.[77])

Selection and Validation Considerations

Binaural Fittings

To this point, we have primarily discussed the measurement of monaural LDLs, yet the majority of patients are fitted binaurally. It is reasonable to question, therefore, if it is necessary to conduct unaided binaural LDLs for individuals who will be fitted binaurally, or if the maximum output is adjusted differently when both ears are fitted with amplification. We know, for example, from loudness summation research, that for signals in the 100–110 dB SPL range there is a 6–10 dB binaural summation effect.[76] This might suggest that LDL values would be lowered by this amount when binaural fittings are employed.

There has been little research concerning binaural LDLs; however, at least one study had reported that there is no significant difference between binaural and monaural LDLs. Hawkins[77] compared binaural and monaural LDLs for 500 and 4000 Hz for 13 hearing impaired individuals. As shown in Table 3–3, mean differences were negligible. Even when individual data are examined, note that only two patients showed differences greater than 5 dB (and in one of these cases the *monaural* LDL was the lowest). Hawkins[77] concluded that when a loudness-matching paradigm is used summation is present, but when the task is couched in loudness-discomfort terms there does not appear to be a summation effect. The good news for clinicians is that when selecting SSPL90, binaural fittings simply can be treated as two separate monaural fittings. The good news for patients is that, although binaural summation will improve their thresholds, it does not lower their LDLs; the result is an expanded perceived-loudness dynamic range when they are fitted binaurally.

Method of Output Limiting

The hearing aid circuitry that is used to limit the maximum output of the instrument can influence the SSPL90 selection and maximum output setting. The development of the Class D amplifier has sparked interest in headroom (for a given input level and gain, the headroom is the decibel difference between the resulting output and the output at which the hearing aid reaches saturation). Manufacturers have been quick to advertise the Class D amplifier as less distorting. As discussed by Fabry,[78] however, the Class D amplifier, in and of itself, is not necessarily less distorting. Hearing aids using Class D amplifiers usually have a greater SSPL90, which creates more headroom, which might cause the patient to report that the instrument is less distorting. If the maximum output of the hearing aid is set too low, the amplitude peaks of speech will drive the hearing aid into saturation, and as a result the patient might lower his or her preferred listening level, which in turn will probably reduce hearing aid benefit. In general, therefore, headroom is considered good. It is not a simple matter, however, for if it were, we would simply fit everyone with outputs of 140 dB SPL.

The headroom issue relates to the fact that *perceptual* discomfort (caused by harmonic and intermodulation distortion of the hearing aid) will have some effect on the measure of *physical* discomfort.[4,79,80] That is, the less distortion of the amplified signal, the greater the output that will be accepted by the patient. Presumably, the closer that the amplified signal is to a reproduction of the signal delivered through the TDH-series or ER-3A earphones during the unaided testing, the greater the likelihood that agreement will be obtained between the selection and verification LDL measurements. For example, Fortune and Preves[4] found that aided LDLs conducted with hearing aids with HFA SSPL90 of 118–123 dB were only 2–3 dB below that of earphone LDLs and were 5 dB higher than LDLs conducted with hearing aids with HFA SSPL90 of 95–106 dB. In a related study, Cook et al.[81] investigated differences in LDLs when a speech signal was recorded unprocessed or processed by a peak clipping circuit and output limiting compression circuit in saturation. Mean LDLs for the unprocessed speech (recorded using ER-3A insert earphones) were approximately 5 dB higher than the compression processed speech and 7 dB higher than LDLs obtained with speech that was processed through a peak clipping instrument in saturation. This finding suggests that a compression instrument has the potential to extend an individual's aided dynamic range.

Multichannel Instruments

In the past 5 years there has been an introduction of several two or three channel hearing aids, the majority of which are programmable (digitally controlled analog circuits). Using multichannel hearing aids is a significant advantage to the audiologist concerned with adjustment of the hearing aid's maximum output. By altering the output potentiometer, compression kneepoints, or compression ratios, these instruments allow for independent adjustment of maximum output for the different channels. This means that the entire maximum output response, rather than just the peak, can be adjusted to match more closely the patient's LDLs across frequencies.

Consider a patient with a small dynamic range (e.g., 25–30 dB) fitted with a single channel instrument with a Class D amplifier. According to the verification procedure we have described, the RESR peak of the response at 3000 Hz would be adjusted to the patient's LDL at this frequency. Often, this will cause the RESR for other important frequencies (e.g., 1000–2000 Hz) to fall 10 dB or more below the patient's LDL. For patients with a small dynamic range, this could restrict amplification in an unacceptably large percentage of their useable auditory area. Using a two or three channel instrument, the compression knee points or compression ratios can be adjusted differently for different frequency regions. This allows for a much closer match between the RESR and the LDL, resulting in a substantial increase in the patient's overall aided dynamic range. As a rule of thumb, the smaller the unaided dynamic range, the greater the need for multichannel adjustable compression, and the closer that the RESR mimics the LDL function, the greater the chances that a successful fitting will result.

Summary

In this chapter, we emphasized the importance of output selection and verification when conducting hearing aid fittings. While many variables must be considered, it is possible to conduct both unaided and aided LDL measurements that are reliable and valid. The development of the ER-3A insert earphones have provided welcomed assistance for comparing clinical measurements to hearing aid specifications in 2 cc coupler values. The combined use of behavioral and probe-microphone measurements allows for a comprehensive verification protocol. Probe-microphone measurements of real-ear maximum output are especially important for young children, as overamplification always is a concern.

In conclusion, the selection and verification of the hearing aid's output is one of the most important components of the hearing aid fitting protocol. We believe, in fact, that within a few years, when digitally programmable hearing aids (employing various forms of adjustable compression) are the standard fitting, the shaping of the hearing aid's output function will be as routine as the shaping of the gain function is today.

References

1. Franks JR, Beckmann NJ: Rejection of hearing aids: Attitudes of a geriatric sample. *Ear Hear* 1982; 6:161–166.
2. Hawkins DB: Selection of a critical electroacoustic characteristic: SSPL 90. *Hear Instrum* 1984; 35:28–32.
3. Preves DA: Output Limiting and Speech Enhancement, in Studebaker GA, Bess FH, Beck LB (eds): *The Vanderbilt Hearing-Aid Report*. Parkton, MD: York Press, 1991, pp 35–51.
4. Fortune T, Preves D: Hearing aid saturation and aided loudness discomfort. *J Speech Hear Res* 1992; 35:175–185.
5. Watson LA: Certain fundamental principles in prescribing and fitting hearing aids. *Laryngoscope* 1944; 54:531–558.

6. Carhart R: Selection of hearing aids. *Arch Otolaryngol* 1946; 44:1–18.
7. Davis H, Hudgins CV, Marquis RJ, et al.: The selection of hearing aids. *Laryngoscope* 1946; 56:85–115, 135–163.
8. Hawkins D: Experts explore some practical issues in hearing aid selection and fitting. *Hear J* 1992; 45:18–26.
9. Hawkins DB: Loudness discomfort levels: A clinical procedure for hearing aid evaluations. *J Speech Hear Dis* 1980; 45:3–15.
10. McCandless GA: Hearing aids and loudness discomfort. Paper presented at Oticongress 3, Copenhagen, Denmark, 1973.
11. O'Neill J, Oyer H: *Applied Audiometry*. New York: Dodd, Mead, and Co., 1966.
12. Wallenfels HG: *Hearing Aids on Prescription*. Springfield, IL: Charles C. Thomas, 1967.
13. Beattie RC, Edgerton BJ, Gager DW: Effects of speech materials on the loudness discomfort level. *J Speech Hear Dis* 1979; 44:435–458.
14. Beattie RC, Svihovec DA, Carmen RE, et al.: Loudness discomfort level for speech: Comparison of two instructional sets for saturation sound pressure level selection. *Ear Hear* 1980; 1:197–205.
15. Morgan DE, Dirks DD: Loudness discomfort level under earphone and in the free field: The effects of calibration methods. *J Acoust Soc Am* 1974; 56:172–178.
16. Niemeyer W: Relations between the discomfort level and the reflex threshold of the middle ear muscles. *Audiology* 1971; 10:172–176.
17. Kawell M, Kopun J, Stelmachowicz P: Loudness discomfort levels in children. *Ear Hear* 1988; 9:133–136.
18. Skinner M: *Hearing Aid Evaluation*. Englewood Cliffs, NJ: Prentice-Hall, 1988.
19. Dirks D, Kamm C: Psychometric functions for loudness discomfort and most comfortable loudness level. *J Speech Hear Dis* 1976; 19:613–627.
20. Beattie RC, Boyd RL: Relationship between pure tone and speech loudness discomfort levels among hearing-impaired subjects. *J Speech Hear Disord* 1986; 51:120–124.
21. Hawkins DB: The effect of signal type on the loudness discomfort level. *Ear Hear* 1980; 1:38–41.
22. Zwicker A, Flottorp G, Stevens S: Critical bandwidth in loudness summation. *J Acoust Soc Am* 1957; 29:548–557.
23. Kamm C, Dirks DD, Mickey MR: Effect of sensorineural hearing loss on loudness discomfort level and most comfortable loudness judgments. *J Speech Hear Res* 1978; 21:688–691.
24. Scharf B, Hellman RP: Model of loudness summation applied to impaired ears. *J Acoust Soc Am* 1966; 40:71–78.
25. Bentler R, Pavlovic C: Comparison of discomfort levels obtained with pure tones and multitone complexes. *J Acoust Soc Am* 1989; 86:126–132.
26. Bentler, R: Relationship of perceived quality dimensions to threshold of discomfort, abstract. *Audiol Today* 1993; 5:40–41.
27. Filion PR, Margolis RH: Comparison of clinical and real-life judgments of loudness discomfort. *J Am Acad Audiol* 1992; 3:193–199.
28. Levitt H: Transformed up-down methods in psychoacoustics. *J Acoust Soc Am* 1971; 49:467–477.
29. Levitt H: Adaptive testing in audiology. *Scand Audiol* [suppl] 6:241–289.
30. Carhart R, Jerger J: Preferred method for clinical determination of pure tone thresholds. *J Speech Hear Dis* 1959; 24:330–345.
31. Beattie RC, Sheffler MC: Test–retest stability and effects of psychophysical methods on the speech loudness discomfort level. *Audiology* 1981; 20:143–156.
32. Cox R, Sherbecoe R: Effect of psychophysical method on the repeatibility of loudness discomfort levels. Paper presented at the American Speech-Language-Hearing Association Convention, Cincinnati, Ohio, 1983.
33. Hawkins D, Smith M: LDLs: Signal type, methodology and reliability. Paper presented at the American Speech-Language-Hearing Association Convention, Atlanta, Georgia, 1979.
34. Morgan DE, Wilson RH, Dirks DD: Loudness discomfort level: Selected methods and stimuli. *J Acoust Soc Am* 1974; 56:577–581.
35. Priede VM, Coles RRA: Factors influencing the loudness discomfort level. *Sound* 1971; 5:39–46.
36. Stephens SD, Anderson CM: Experimental studies on the uncomfortable loudness level. *J Speech Hear Res* 1971; 14:262–270.
37. Stephens SD: Studies on the uncomfortable loudness level. *Sound* 1970; 4:20–23.
38. Hawkins D, Walden B, Montgomery A, et al.: Description and validation of an LDL procedure designed to select SSPL90. *Ear Hear* 1987; 8:162–169.
39. Walker G, Dillon H, Byrne D, et al.: The use of loudness discomfort levels for selecting the maximum output of hearing aids. *Aust J Audiol* 1984; 6:23–32.
40. Sammeth CA, Birman M, Hecox KE: Variability of most comfortable and uncomfortable loudness levels to speech stimuli in the hearing impaired. *Ear Hear* 1989; 10:94–100.

41. Kallstrom L, Carstensen K: The perception of loudness and acoustic reflex. *Audiol Hear Educ* 1978; 3:36–38.
42. Kopra LL, Blosser D: Effects of method of measurement on most comfortable loudness level for speech. *J Speech Hear Res* 1968; 11:497–508.
43. Horning J: Tympanometry and hearing aid selection. *Hear Aid J* 1975; 8:50.
44. McCandless GA, Miller D: Loudness discomfort and hearing aids. *Natl Hear Aid J* 1972; 28:31.
45. Snow T, McCandless GA: The use of impedance measures. *Hear Aid J* 1976; 7:32–33.
46. Denenberg LJ, Altshuler MW: The clinical relationship between acoustic reflexes and loudness perception. *J Am Audiol Soc* 1976; 2:79–82.
47. Olson AE, Hipskind NM: The relation between levels of pure tones and speech which elicit the acoustic reflex and loudness discomfort. *J Audiol Res* 1973; 13:71–76.
48. Preves DA, Orton JF: Use of acoustic impedance measures in hearing aid fitting. *Hear Instrum* 1978; 29:22–24, 34–35.
49. Woodford CM, Holmes DW: Relationship between loudness discomfort level and acoustic reflex threshold in a clinical population. *Audiol Hear Educ* 1977; 2:9–10, 12.
50. Hawkins DA, Schum DJ: LDL measures: An efficient use of clinic time? *Am J Audiol* 1991; 1:8–10.
51. Kirkwood D: U.S. hearing aid sales summary. *Hear J* 1992; 45.
52. Hawkins D, Ball T, Beasley H, et al.: A comparison of SSPL90 selection procedures. *J Am Acad Audiol* 1992; 3:46–50.
53. Pascoe DP: Clinical measurements of the auditory dynamic range and their relation to formulas for hearing aid gain, in Jensen JH (ed): *Hearing Aid Fitting: Theoretical and Practical Views*. Copenhagen: Stouggaard Jensen, 1988, pp 129–154.
54. Cox RM: The MSU hearing instrument prescription procedure. *Hear Instrum* 1988; 39:6–10.
55. Seewald RC: The desired sensation level approach for children: Selection and verification. *Hear Instrum* 1988; 39:18–22.
56. Seewald RC: The desired sensation level method for fitting children: Version 3.0. *Hear J* 1992; 45:36–46.
57. Seewald RC, Ross M: Amplification for Young Hearing-Impaired Children, in Pollack M (ed): *Amplification for the Hearing Impaired*, ed 3. Orlando, FL: Grune & Stratton, 1988, pp 213–271.
58. Stuart A, Durieux-Smith A, Stenstrom R: Probe tube microphone measures of loudness discomfort levels in children. *Ear Hear* 1991; 12:140–143.
59. Cox R: Using LDLs to establish hearing aid limiting levels. *Hear Instrum* 1981; 5:16–20.
60. Libby ER: The LDL to SSPL90 conversion dilemma. *Hear Instrum* 1985; 36:15–16, 68.
61. Hawkins DB: Corrections and Transformations Relevant to Hearing Aid Selection, in Mueller HG, Hawkins DB, Northern JL: *Probe Microphone Measurements: Hearing Aid Selection and Assessment*. San Diego: Singular Publishing, 1992, pp 251–268.
62. Mueller HG: Terminology and Procedures, in Mueller HG, Hawkins DB, Northern JL: *Probe Microphone Measurements: Hearing Aid Selection and Assessment*. San Diego; Singular Publishing, 1992, pp 41–66.
63. Fikret-Pasa S, Revit L: Individualized correction factors in the pre-selection of hearing aids. *J Speech Hear Res* 1992; 35:384–400.
64. Zelisko DL, Seewald RC, Whiteside S: Comparing three procedures for predicting the ear canal SPL at LDL. Poster presented at the American Speech-Language-Hearing Association Convention, San Antonio, Texas, 1992.
65. Hawkins DB, Mueller HG: Test protocols for probe-microphone measurements, in Mueller HG, Hawkins DB, Northern JL (eds): *Probe Microphone Measurements: Hearing Aid Selection and Assessment*. San Diego: Singular Publishing, 1992, pp 269–278.
66. Feigin J, Kopun J, Stelmachowicz P, Gorga M: Probe-tube microphone measures of ear-canal sound pressure levels in infants and children. *Ear Hear* 1989; 10:254–258.
67. Hawkins DB, Northern JL: Probe-microphone measurements with children, in Mueller HG, Hawkins DB, Northern JL (eds): *Probe Microphone Measurements: Hearing Aid Selection and Assessment*. San Diego: Singular Publishing, 1992, pp 159–181.
68. Cox R, Alexander G: Preferred hearing aid gain in everyday environments. *Ear Hear* 1991; 12:123–127.
69. Hawkins DB: Selecting SSPL90 using probe-microphone measurements, in Mueller HG, Hawkins DB, Northern JL (eds): *Probe Microphone Measurements: Hearing Aid Selection and Assessment*. San Diego: Singular Publishing, 1992, pp 145–158.
70. Revit L: New tests for signal-processing and multichannel hearing instruments. *Hear J* 1991; 44:20–23.
71. Stelmachowicz P: Clinical issues related to hearing aid maximum output, in Studebaker G, Bess F, Beck L (eds): *The Vanderbilt Hearing-Aid Report II*. Parkton, MD: York Press, 1991, pp 141–148.

72. Preves DA: Output limiting and speech enhancement, in Studebaker G, Bess F, Beck L (eds): *The Vanderbilt Hearing-Aid Report II*. Parkton, MD: York Press, 1991, pp 35–51.

73. Mueller HG, Hawkins DB: Considerations in Hearing Aid Selection, in Sandlin R (ed): *Handbook of Hearing Aid Amplification, Volume II: Clinical Considerations and Fitting Practices*. San Diago: College-Hill Press, 1990, pp 31–60.

74. Mueller HG, Hawkins DB, Sedge R: Three important options in hearing aid selection. *Hear Instrum* 1984; 35:14–17.

75. Walker G, Dillon H: *Compression in Hearing Aids: An analysis, a Review and Some Recommendations*. National Acoustics Laboratories Report No. 90. Canberra: Australian Government Publishing Service, 1982.

76. Reynolds GS, Stevens SS: Binaural summation of loudness. *J Acoust Soc Am* 1960; 32:1337–1344.

77. Hawkins DB: Selection of SSPL90 for binaural hearing aid fittings. *Hear J* 1986; 39:23–24.

78. Fabry D: Experts explore some practical issues in hearing aid selection and fitting. *Hear J* 1992; 45:18–26.

79. Fortune T, Preves D, Woodruff B: Saturation-induced distortion and its effects on aided LDL. *Hear Instrum* 1991; 42:37–42.

80. Fortune T, Preves D: Hearing aid saturation, coherence, and aided loudness discomfort. *J Am Acad Audiol* 1992; 3:81–93.

81. Cook JAL, Hawkins DB, Leadbitter EM: The effect of peak clipping and compression output limiting on loudness discomfort levels, abstract. *Audiol Today* 1993; 5:42.

4

Using Coupler Tests in the Fitting of Hearing Aids

Lawrence J. Revit

Introduction

Coupler tests provide substantial information about the expected performance of a hearing aid. An important advantage of coupler tests is that they do not require the presence of the client. A dispenser can partially, or even fully, optimize the settings of a hearing aid before the client has ever worn the instrument. Other advantages of coupler tests are (1) an easily controlled test environment, (2) robust precision and repeatability, and (3) an array of special tests for answering specific questions about the expected performance of a hearing aid.

The range of information available from coupler tests far exceeds that of standard pure-tone tests[1] or even real-ear tests. Advanced coupler tests are especially effective in characterizing the performance of nonlinear hearing aids. *Without the client present*, a dispenser can pursue such questions as: How, if at all, does the tonal processing of a hearing aid change in response to changing input signals? What kinds of signals (speech, noise, or both) will cause non-linear processing to occur? Will the hearing aid produce unwanted audible effects, such as intermodulation distortion or the "pumping and breathing" of background noise? This chapter will discuss these and other applications of coupler tests in the fitting of hearing aids.

Relating the Coupler to the Real Ear

To obtain the maximum benefit from coupler tests, a dispenser should be aware of the acoustic differences between couplers and real ears. In brief, the differences are (1) the complex acoustic impedance of the occluded ear-canal and eardrum, versus the volume impedance of the 2 cc coupler; (2) the location of the hearing aid microphone at the head surface, in or near the ear, versus the effectively free-field location of the test position in a sound chamber;

(3) the tubing that connects the hearing aid to the ear, versus the tubing that connects the hearing aid to the coupler; (4) the venting and the unintentional leakage of sound into and out of the ear canal, versus the sealed condition of the coupler; and, finally, (5) the fact that when a hearing aid is worn, it replaces the natural amplifier provided by the open ear. A discussion of each of these acoustic conditions follows.

The Real-Ear-To-Coupler Level Difference (RECO)

When the output of a hearing aid couples to a comparatively small volume, the sound pressure level (SPL) in that volume will be relatively high. At low frequencies, the combined equivalent volume of the occluded ear canal and the eardrum is typically 1.3 cc versus the 2 cc volume of a standard coupler. Thus, the SPL in the ear canal at low frequencies is typically higher (approximately 3.5 dB) than in the coupler. As frequency increases, the acoustic impedance of the ear canal/eardrum increases relative to the 2 cc coupler. Accordingly,

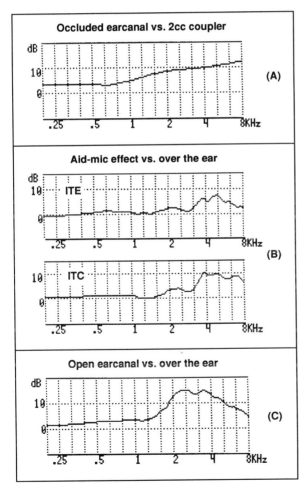

Figure 4–1. Factors affecting differences between coupler and real-ear measurements. (**A**) RECD—expected difference between the SPL in an occluded adult ear canal versus a 2 cc coupler. (**B**) SPL at the microphones of ITE and ITC instruments relative to the SPL at the OTE location. (**C**) REUR—open-ear response of the KEMAR manikin. (Note that the REUR curve has been graphically modified [smoothed] above 5 kHz.)

differences between the SPL in the ear canal and that in the 2 cc coupler are even greater at high frequencies than at low frequencies. Figure 4–1A shows the expected difference between the SPL in an occluded adult ear canal versus the SPL in a 2 cc coupler for an insert earphone having an output impedance similar to that of a hearing aid. (The examples in Fig. 4–1 were measured with a probe-tube microphone placed 17 mm into the ear canal. When a sound field was used, the loudspeaker was at an azimuth of 45°, and the sound-field reference point was just above the apex of the pinna.) This difference curve is called the *real-ear-to-coupler level difference* (RECD). The average-ear RECD in Figure 4–1A indicates that the real-ear aided response (REAR) of a typical hearing aid will be higher in overall level than the 2 cc coupler response (2CCR), with an additional rise in the higher frequencies. Children, who have higher ear canal/eardrum impedance than adults, have even larger RECDs.[2] Thus, the output of a hearing aid in a child's ear will be higher than what would be predicted by an average-adult RECD. Ears with abnormal impedance also have abnormal RECDs[3] and thus will have abnormal REARs compared with what is predicted from an average-adult RECD.

The Effect of the Location of the Hearing Aid Microphone

When a hearing aid is placed on the ear, the surfaces of the head and pinna reflect high frequency sound energy into the hearing aid microphone. These reflections increase the input level to the hearing aid at high frequencies as compared with a free-field condition. The extent of this high-frequency boost depends on how close the hearing aid microphone is to the opening of the ear canal. For a behind-the-ear (BTE) aid, the high-frequency boost is nearly negligible (3 dB or less).[4] For in-the-ear (ITE) and in-the-canal (ITC) aids, the high-frequency boost is significant.[3]

Figure 4–1B shows comparative estimates of the SPL at the microphones of ITE and ITC aids, relative to the SPL at the over-the-ear (OTE) location. As with the RECD, the effect of the location of a head-worn hearing aid microphone serves to increase the REAR relative to the 2CCR, especially at high frequencies.

The Relative Earmold Response

The relative earmold response affects hearing aids that have separate earpieces, mostly BTEs. When measuring an ITE or ITC, the tester uses an HA-1, direct-access coupler. *Direct access* means that the sound outlet of the hearing aid couples directly to the 2 cc volume of the coupler; there is no additional tubing. However, when measuring a BTE, the tester uses an HA-2 coupler, which has an earmold simulator as part of its construction. The HA-2 earmold simulator[1] is a 3 mm horn. Thus, an earmold having tubing other than a 3 mm horn of the same construction will alter the frequency response from what is measured in the HA-2 coupler. These alterations apply equally to both the 2CCR and the REAR. An earmold with constant-diameter No. 13 tubing, for example, will decrease the high-frequency gain by as much as 8 dB at 5 kHz compared with what would be predicted directly from the HA-2 response.

Table 4–1. Ear Mold Response Corrections (re: HA-2)

Earmold	Frequency (Hz)									
	250	*500*	*1k*	*1.5k*	*2k*	*3k*	*4k*	*5k*	*6k*	*8k*
Libby 4 mm	−1	−1	−2	0	0	2	3	0	0	7
Libby 3 mm	0	0	0	1	1	3	2	0	−4	−1
Macrae	−1	−1	−2	1	0	4	2	−3	−4	10
8CR	−1	−2	−3	−1	0	5	−3	−5	−2	8
6EF	0	0	0	0	0	2	2	−2	−3	−2
HA2	0	0	0	0	0	0	0	0	0	0
8B10	0	0	0	−1	−1	−2	−3	−4	−1	8
6R12	0	0	0	0	0	0	0	2	1	4
6B10	0	0	0	0	0	0	1	3	−5	−2
6B5	1	2	3	2	2	0	−1	−3	−2	2
6B0	0	1	1	0	0	−2	−5	−8	−7	−2
6C5	1	2	1	1	2	−5	−10	−13	−16	−10
6C10	1	3	0	−1	−3	−11	−17	−19	−22	−15
Cavity 1	−4	−2	1	−6	−15	−23	−30	−37	−35	−21
Cavity 2	−4	−3	−2	0	0	−12	−20	−28	−35	−21
Cavity 3	−2	−1	0	0	3	1	−11	−18	−24	−16

(Adapted from Dillor.[5])

When the client's earmold is available, the dispenser can test the hearing aid with the earmold attached, using a direct-access (HA-1) coupler. Testing with the earmold attached eliminates the need to correct for tubing factors when predicting the REAR from coupler measures.[5] When the earmold is not available, the reader can refer to Table 4–1, a catalog of expected earmold responses re the HA-2 simulator for several earmold types.

Venting Effects

As used here, the term *venting effects* refers to the effects of both intentional vents and unintentional leakage around the earmold or shell (slit leaks). Venting effects are complicated and can even be unpredictable, potentially affecting both the low-frequency response and the high-frequency response of a hearing aid. At low frequencies, venting lets sound energy "leak" from the ear canal. The complication is that venting also lets sound energy leak *into* the ear canal from the outside. Unfortunately, almost all the literature on venting completely neglects the "outside to in" path and reports only the low-frequency attenuation caused by the "inside to out" path. But when a vented hearing aid is worn, the two-way transmission of sound through the vent makes it relatively difficult to predict the real-ear gain at low-frequencies, variability depending on the dimensions of the vent, the properties of the ear canal, and the phase response of the hearing aid. The dispenser, therefore, is warned not to interpret either positive or negative low-frequency gain in sealed coupler responses as directly indicative of what to expect on the real ear when venting is used. The reader is referred to Lybarger,[6] Kates,[7] and Dillon[8] for detailed studies of the low frequency effects venting.

The high-frequency effects of venting are caused by feedback. At output levels below those for which feedback leads to oscillation (whistling), feedback can amplify and sharpen high-frequency resonant peaks. For example, what might be a rounded, 5 dB peak at 4 kHz in a coupler response could end up as a sharp, 15 dB peak in the REAR. The degree of such sharpening of resonant peaks from suboscillatory feedback depends on the dimensions of both the vent and the ear canal, as well as on the impedance of the ear. The combination of these factors can make the high-frequency effects of venting virtually unpredictable. The reader is referred to Cox[9] and Kates[7] for further study of the high-frequency effects of venting.

The Real-Ear Unaided Response

To this point, the discussion has dealt with factors affecting the relation between the 2CCR and the REAR. But dispensers are often interested in the real-ear insertion-gain response (REIR), which is the *net* difference in ear canal SPL achieved by placing a hearing aid in the ear. Without a hearing aid in place, the horn of the open ear provides a natural amplifier having about 15 dB of gain in the region of 2.5–5 kHz. This natural open-ear amplifier is known as the real-ear unaided response (REUR). The REIR is the difference between the REAR and the REUR. Figure 4–1C shows the simulated REUR of the KEMAR manikin, which is typical of real open ears. When the ear is occluded by a hearing aid, this open-ear amplifier disappears. The coupler response, therefore, must have an extra 15 dB of gain in the 2.5–5 kHz range, just to replace what is lost when the hearing aid is removed from the coupler and placed on the ear.

Once the dispenser understands the above properties that distinguish the real ear from the 2 cc coupler, one can *predict the real-ear response from the coupler response by* **adding** *to the coupler response what is* **gained** *by placing the hearing aid in the ear and by* **subtracting** *from the coupler response what is* lost *by placing the hearing aid in the ear.* Because the RECD increases the SPL in the ear canal over that in the coupler, one *adds the RECD* to the coupler response to predict the real-ear response. Because the location of a head-worn hearing aid microphone increases the input level over the effectively free-field condition of the coupler in the test box, one *adds the hearing aid microphone effect* to the coupler response to predict the real-ear response. Because the open-ear amplifier (REUR) is lost when the hearing aid is inserted into the ear, one *subtracts the REUR* from the coupler response to predict the REIR. Thus, for ITEs and ITCs (which do not have earmold tubing effects to consider), the combined conversion from a measured 2CCR to a predicted REIR is

Predicted REIR = Measured 2CCR + (RECD + Aid-Mic Effect − REUR)

(The conversion from a measured 2CCR to a predicted REAR is

Predicted REAR = Measured 2CCR + RECD + Aid-Mic Effect)

Taken together, the items RECD + Aid-Mic Effect − REUR have a funny sounding name: *GIFROC.* GIFROC is *CORFIG* spelled backwards. *CORFIG* was the original term;[10] it stands for *coupler response for flat insertion gain.* CORFIG and GIFROC are arithmetic inverses of each other.[11] The dispenser can predict an REIR from a coupler response by adding the GIFROC transformation to the measured 2CCR (as in the above equation). Likewise, the dispenser can *prescribe* a 2 cc coupler response by adding the CORFIG transformation to the prescribed insertion-gain response:

Prescribed 2CCR = Prescribed REIR + (REUR − RECD − Aid-Mic Effect)

(To prescribe a 2CCR from a prescribed RE<u>A</u>R:

Prescribed 2CCR = Prescribed REAR − RECD − Aid-Mic Effect)

The dispenser determines the prescribed REIR by applying a fitting formula to the client's audiogram (see Chs. 1 and 2). After adding the CORFIG transformation, the dispenser can either send the resulting 2CCR prescription to a custom manufacturer or use the 2CCR prescription to choose manufacturers' specifications when ordering or programming a hearing aid. Most dispensers add 10 dB of "reserve gain" to the prescribed 2CCR, so extra gain can be available to the user at the volume control. In this way, the prescribed 2CCR becomes a "full-on gain" specification. (Prescribing the 2 cc coupler SSPL90 is discussed in Ch. 3.)

In the absence of individual real-ear measurement data, the dispenser can use average-ear CORFIG and GIFROC data for prescribing and pre-adjusting the coupler response of a hearing aid prior to the initial fitting. Average-ear CORFIG and GIFROC transformation curves for ITE, ITC, and BTE instruments are shown in Figure 4–2. These transformation curves assume a completely sealed earpiece, a 45° azimuth, and an OTE sound field reference. (Loudspeaker azimuth and sound field reference can affect the insertion gain at high frequencies.[12] Average-ear CORFIG and GIFROC curves for 0° with a free-field reference were published by Bentler and Pavlovic.[13]) For vented hearing aids, the dispenser can add the average-case corrections given in Table 4–2 to the CORFIG transformation or can subtract them from the GIFROC transformation. When real-ear measurements are available, injecting real-ear data into these transformations can improve their accuracy considerably. In other words, the dispenser can build "customized" CORFIG or GIFROC transforma-

Table 4–2.   Average CORFIG Corrections for Low Frequency Venting Effects

	Frequency (Hz)				
	250	*500*	*750*	*1 k*	*1.5 k*
Tight seal	—	—	—	—	—
Slit leak	2	2	1	—	—
1 mm	1*	2*	1	—	—
2 mm	7*	1*	—	—	—
Long open	17*	10*	4*	1*	—
Short open	26*	21*	14*	10*	5*

* Use these values only if prescribed insertion gain is greater than 0 dB at that frequency. Otherwise, use no correction. Dashes indicate to use no correction. A slit leak is assumed for all vent conditions except "Tight Seal."

(Data from Dillon.[8])

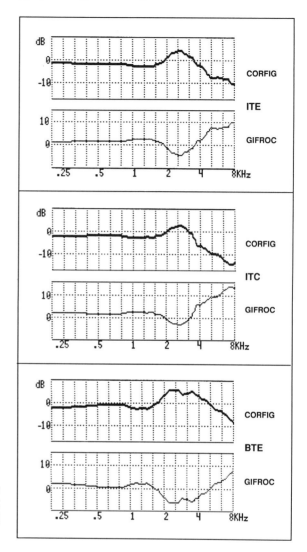

Figure 4–2. Average-ear CORFIG (bold) and GIFROC (thin) curves for ITE, ITC, and BTE instruments (45° azimuth).

tions by measuring the REUR and RECD individually on each ear to be fitted. These measurements (which require probe microphone equipment) are substituted for average data in the equations given earlier (for details on this technique, see Punch et al.,[14] Mueller,[15] and Killion and Revit[11]).

Types of Signals Used in Coupler Tests

As audiometric tests provide information about general hearing ability, coupler tests provide information about general hearing aid performance. As special diagnostic tests focus on particular aspects of auditory processing, special coupler tests focus on particular aspects of hearing aid signal processing. As the choice of test stimuli can influence the accuracy and specificity of an audiometric test, the choice of test signals has similar importance for coupler tests. When choosing an appropriate test signal for hearing aids, the basic rules are similar to those in audiometry: (1) choose a signal that best represents real-use conditions; and (2) choose a signal that exercises, as selectively as possible, a specific aspect of hearing aid performance.

Natural Speech

Natural speech (the term refers to speech sounds created by human talkers in the course of verbal communication) is the most important signal a hearing aid must process. Natural speech can also be a test signal for coupler tests, although such applications are rare. Nonetheless, a knowledge of some of the acoustic properties of natural speech can help the dispenser understand the applications and limitations of conventional test signals.

Natural speech consists of periodic (repeating) and aperiodic (nonrepeating) elements that vary widely in intensity and spectral content over time.[16] The periodic elements of speech are the voiced sounds. Voiced speech sounds, such as vowels, begin as a glottal "buzz" generated by the vocal chords. Glottal buzz is a harmonic composite of many frequencies. Each frequency (or "harmonic") is an integer multiple of the lowest, or "fundamental" frequency. The fundamental frequency determines the perceived "pitch" of a voice. Vocal fundamental frequencies range from about 100 Hz in adult males to about 400 Hz in small children. The upper harmonics of glottal buzz extend as high as about 6 kHz.

The physical elements of the vocal tract (the lips and the mouth cavity, for example) form a series of resonators that spectrally shape glottal buzz into a series of resonant peaks called *formants*. Formants create spectral patterns that a listener can recognize as vowels. By identifying the frequencies and relative amplitudes of formant peaks, a listener can distinguish one vowel from another.

The aperiodic elements of speech are the unvoiced sounds. Unvoiced speech sounds are generated by breath noise that has been filtered to varying degrees by the vocal tract. The frequency range of unvoiced sounds is extremely broad, extending from the very lowest frequencies to the region of 10 kHz. Averaged over long periods of conversational speech, the amplitude of unvoiced sounds is much lower than that of voiced sounds, partially because unvoiced sounds occur in relatively short, widely spaced bursts and thereby occupy less overall time than voiced sounds. But unvoiced speech sounds, too, *should be heard*, if at all possible. Several hearing aids are capable of amplifying the very-high-frequency components of unvoiced speech sounds. Unfortunately, because of the impedance properties of hearing aids and 2 cc couplers, coupler tests cannot measure these frequencies accurately. But the dispenser is cautioned not to ignore the very high frequencies just because they are difficult to measure.

Each speech sound, voiced or unvoiced, has a unique spectral pattern. Although the dominant energy in a given speech sound may span a one-or-two octave range, the distinguishing features of the spectral patterns of speech almost always span a broad frequency range—at least two octaves, but often several octaves. Thus, speech sounds are broadband signals. The auditory system discriminates one speech sound from another by identifying the distinguishing features within each broadband spectral pattern. An effective hearing aid, therefore, will preserve, or even enhance the spectral patterns of speech over a wide frequency range.

Spectral patterns are not the only elements of speech important for intelligibility. Rhythmic or temporal (time-related) patterns also contribute to speech intelligibility. The elements of temporal speech patterns vary in duration between tens, hundreds, and even thousands of milliseconds. Temporal patterns can provide important cues for listening in noisy situations, and they can be especially important for listeners learning speech for the first time. An effective hearing aid, therefore, will preserve or enhance the time-varying, rhythmic patterns of speech as well as the spectral patterns.

Speech-Shaped Random Noise

Random noise is an aperiodic broadband signal that has equal probability of containing any frequency in any phase. The long-term average spectrum of random ("white") noise contains equal amplitudes of all frequencies. But the averaging of many samples is required to obtain a smooth, flat spectrum.

Speech shaping, also called *weighting* or *coloring*, can adjust the average spectrum of random noise to match the average spectrum of natural speech. A speech-shaped spectrum has higher amplitudes in the low frequencies than in the high frequencies. But there are several important differences between speech-shaped random noise and natural speech. Among them are (1) Random noise is continuously random, while natural speech contains only brief moments during which random energy is dominant; for example, during frication and aspiration. (An example of frication is the *f* sound; an example of aspiration is the *h* sound.) (2) The relative phases of the frequency components of a random signal vary constantly; the relative phases of the frequency components of voiced speech vary far less. Consequently, interactions among frequency components (called *intermodulation distortion*) will likely be less apparent with averaged random signals than with voiced speech. (3) Because of the time required for spectral averaging, rapid, time-varying changes in hearing aid performance associated with the temporal patterns of natural speech cannot readily be tested using averaged samples of continuous random signals.

Speech-Shaped Composite

Similar to the glottal buzz of natural speech, a composite test signal is a broadband, periodic, harmonic tone complex having frequency elements at each integer multiple of the fundamental frequency. Like random noise, the spectrum of a composite signal can be shaped to match the long-term spectrum of natural speech. But unlike random noise, only one sample of the signal is required to achieve the desired spectrum. Thus, composite signals lend themselves to the rapid measurement speed required for real-time spectrum analysis. Another important feature of composite signals is that the frequency components are phase locked, meaning the relative phases of the frequencies do not change over time. Phase locking leads to two important advantages: (1) time–domain signal averaging can be used to significantly reduce the influence of extraneous noise on composite measurements, and (2) intermodulation distortion effects can be readily observed on composite frequency response curves.

Both speech-shaped random noise and speech-shaped composite signals are broadband signals, and, therefore, have the advantage of testing how a hearing aid processes several frequencies at once, over a wide frequency range. Because of this capability, broadband signals are more desirable than narrowband signals for assessing how well a hearing aid processes broadband speech sounds, although narrowband signals have important uses as well.

Narrowband Test Signals

Pure tones, warble tones, and narrowband noise are examples of narrowband test signals. The bandwidth of a pure tone is infinitely narrow; typical bandwidths of warble tones and narrowband noise are 1/10 octave and 1/3 octave, respectively.

The world is rich with narrowband signals (e.g., sirens, whistles, and beeps). Although narrowband test signals do not simulate natural speech, they have the advantage of being able to focus on a particular frequency band. Narrowband signals are, therefore, ideal for testing certain aspects of multichannel or frequency-specific signal processing. Also, narrowband signals provide a worst case scenario for assessing the maximum output of a hearing aid.

Advanced Coupler Tests

The concept of evaluating an aid solely according to the ANSI S3.22[1] standard has become outdated by the availability of advanced coupler tests and broadband signals. The ANSI S3.22 pure-tone test sequence satisfies the engineering purpose of providing a check of technical quality, but does not satisfy the broader purpose of characterizing the expected auditory effects of a hearing aid. The following discussion deals with advanced coupler tests using frequency response curves, input/output curves, and dynamic attack-and-release tests. The advanced forms of these tests use innovative test signals, both broadband and narrowband, and groups (or "families") of tests. After a brief description of each test, dispensers' anticipated questions will be posed and answered. Illustrated examples will demonstrate some of the acoustic effects of various types of signal processing.

Frequency Response Curves

Frequency response curves show the output or gain of a hearing aid in decibels as a function of frequency. Decibels are logarithmic units derived from comparisons of two sound pressures. For example, a measurement of "dB SPL" is actually a comparison of an observed sound pressure with a standard reference sound pressure (the reference pressure for 0 dB SPL is 20 μPa); a measurement of "dB gain" is actually a comparison of an observed output sound pressure with an observed input sound pressure. Decibels are plotted on a linear, vertical axis. Frequency (in Hertz) is plotted on a logarithmic, horizontal axis. The ratio of the scale of the vertical axis to the scale of the horizontal axis is called the *aspect ratio*. The standard aspect ratio[1] for hearing aid frequency response graphs is 50 dB per decade frequency. This means a change of 50 dB on the vertical scale is equal in length to a tenfold change in Hertz on the horizontal scale. Dispensers should be cautious when reading published articles showing hearing aid frequency responses: Sometimes the aspect ratio of published response graphs does not adhere to the standard, and results can be misleading. Commercial hearing aid specifications, on the other hand, are required by law to use the standard aspect ratio.

Frequency response curves for nonlinear hearing aids become especially useful when displayed as "families of curves." A family of curves is a group of curves of the same type, but with one parameter varied across curves. Consider that nonlinear signal processing involves a change in either the overall gain or the shape of the frequency response as a function of a change in the input signal. A good test, therefore, would vary the input signal and then display the resulting changes in response. The most common input parameter to vary with families of frequency response curves is the level of the input signal. In fact, a new ANSI publication[17] describes a standard protocol for obtaining families of curves using varied input levels of a broadband, speech-shaped test signal.

WHAT TYPE OF HEARING AID IS THIS? HOW WILL CHANGES IN THE ACOUSTIC ENVIRONMENT AFFECT THE FREQUENCY RESPONSE?

Families of frequency response curves can reveal the type of hearing aid being tested. Figures 4–3 and 4–4 show examples of families of frequency/gain curves. The curves were made using a broadband, speech-shaped composite

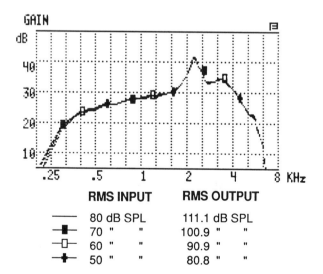

Figure 4–3. Family of frequency/gain curves for a linear, BTE hearing instrument.

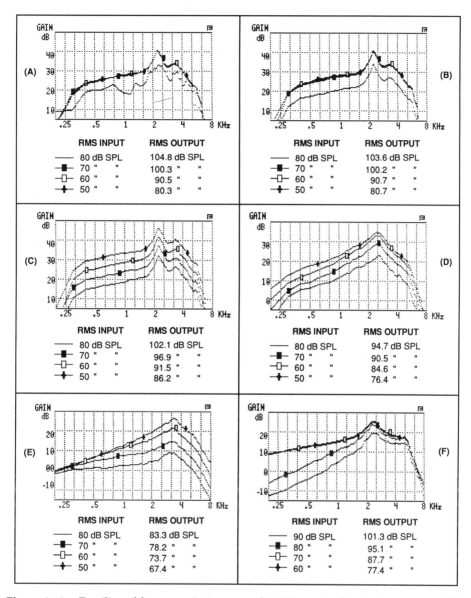

Figure 4–4. Families of frequency/gain curves for (**A**) a peak-clipping instrument; (**B**) a compression-limiting AGC-O instrument; (**C**) a dynamic-range compression AGC-I instrument; (**D**) a two channel-dynamic range compression instrument; (**E**) an adaptive high-frequency filter instrument; and (**F**) an adaptive low-frequency filter instrument.

signal that varied in overall root mean square (RMS) input level, in 10 dB increments, between 50 and 80 dB SPL (except when otherwise indicated). The curves display "dB gain" as a function of frequency, which means the input spectrum was subtracted from the output spectrum before display. The curves, therefore, do not show the SPL values of the output signal as a function of frequency; they show the net change, or *amplification*, of the signal as a function of frequency.

Figure 4–3 shows a family of curves for an uncommon hearing aid: one that is truly linear over a wide range of inputs. The shape of the frequency response is identical for each successive change in input level. As the RMS level of the input changed in 10 dB increments, the RMS level of the output changed by the same amount (shown below the graph). For the tests shown in Figure 4–3, the peak-clipping potentiometer of the hearing aid was adjusted to limit the maximum output at 132 dB SPL. This level was well above the highest level achieved in the family of curves. Thus, the output never reached the clipping point. This hearing aid contains no digital circuitry, but it could be called a programmable hearing aid because it has eight potentiometers that can be set for a wide variety of processing conditions. The same hearing aid was used to generate frequency response families (A, B and C in Fig. 4–4), but with different settings for each family.

Family A in Figure 4–4 shows a common problem. For this family, the peak-clipping potentiometer was adjusted to limit the output at 105 dB SPL. The frequency gain curves for RMS inputs of 50, 60, and 70 dB SPL are identical to those in Figure 4–3, indicating linear processing. But the curve for 80 dB SPL is jagged looking and shows reduced overall gain. The jaggedness of the response curve indicates severe intermodulation distortion; the reduced gain suggests that the distortion was caused by saturation. Saturation distortion at moderately high input levels is typical of peak-clipping instruments.

Family B in Figure 4–4 shows an alternate way of limiting maximum output. For this family of curves, the peak-clipping potentiometer was raised slightly, and an automatic gain control (AGC) potentiometer was adjusted to limit the maximum output at the same RMS level as for family A. For input levels of 50, 60, and 70 dB SPL, the overall gain and frequency response were identical to those of family A. For an input level of 80 dB SPL, however, the gain decreased (thus limiting the output), while the shape of the response curve remained unaltered by distortion. Saturation distortion was avoided because the AGC compression kneepoint (threshold) was adjusted to keep the output of the instrument below the peak-clipping level. With a properly adjusted AGC circuit, a dispenser can provide linear amplification over a wide range of inputs, while providing undistorted limiting of the maximum output.

Family C shows frequency responses of the same, single-channel hearing aid as in the previous examples. However, instead of using output-controlled compression (AGC-O) as before, the instrument was adjusted to provide input-controlled compression (AGC-I), with a compression ratio of 2:1. The 2:1 compression ratio is evident, because for each 10 dB increase in input level, the RMS output level (shown below the graph) increased by only 5 dB. This relatively low compression ratio is consistent with input-controlled, dynamic-range compression. The intent of this type of nonlinear processing is to fit a wide range of input levels into the reduced functional range of an impaired auditory sensory system. Observe that for each increase in signal level, the spacing between the curves remained constant. This means the gain decreased by the same amount at all frequencies, consistent with a broadband, single channel AGC circuit.

Compare the curves of family C with those of family D. The hearing aid of family D is not a single-channel instrument. It is a two-channel ITE hearing aid with independent AGC circuits for each channel. As the input level increased, gain decreased. But the spacing between the curves was slightly different for the low frequencies than for the high frequencies. The pattern indicates that the compression ratio was slightly different for the low-frequency channel than for the high-frequency channel. This type of nonlinear processing can be especially useful for fitting sloping hearing losses where the dynamic range of the impaired auditory system varies across frequency.

The automatic frequency response control (AFRC) exhibited by this two channel instrument is rather subtle. Families E and F show AFRC that is more dramatic. Family E shows frequency responses of a single-channel hearing aid with an adaptive high-frequency filter. As the level of the composite signal increased from 50 to 80 dB SPL, the gain in the high frequencies decreased by as much as 18 dB. Thus, input signals at lower amplitudes produced more "treble boost" than did higher-level signals. The intent of this type of nonlinear processing is to provide more high-frequency gain for soft sounds than for loud sounds.

Family F shows frequency responses of a hearing aid with an adaptive low-frequency filter. RMS levels of 60–90 dB SPL were used for this test. As the level of the speech-shaped composite signal increased from 60 to 90 dB SPL, the gain in the low frequencies decreased by as much as 21 dB. Thus, higher level signals produced more "bass cut" than did lower-level signals. The primary intent of this type of nonlinear processing is to reduce the masking of high-frequency cues by interfering low-frequency signals. The reader may note that two channel AGC can combine the advantages of both adaptive high-frequency filtering and adaptive low-frequency filtering into one hearing aid.

WHAT ARE THE OUTPUT LEVELS PRODUCED BY A SPEECH-SHAPED
SIGNAL? WILL LOUD SPEECH SIGNALS BECOME DISTORTED?

The previous examples displayed frequency response in terms of gain (in dB). Another way of displaying frequency response is in terms of output (in dB SPL). Family A in Figure 4–5 shows output curves for the same instrument as used for the gain curves of family A of Figure 4–4. These output curves present a different view of signal processing. The output curves do not show the rising slope as apparent in the gain curves. This is because for the output curves, the speech shaping of the input spectrum was not removed from the display as it was for the gain curves. The output curves, therefore, reflect the high frequency roll-off of the test signal as well as the signal processing done by the hearing aid.

For family A of Figure 4–5, each 10-dB increase in RMS input level between 50 and 70 dB SPL resulted in a 10 dB increase in the RMS output level. There was also no change in the shape of the curves for these moderate input levels. These two results together indicate linear processing. However, once the maximum output of the hearing aid was approached, peak-clipping (saturation)

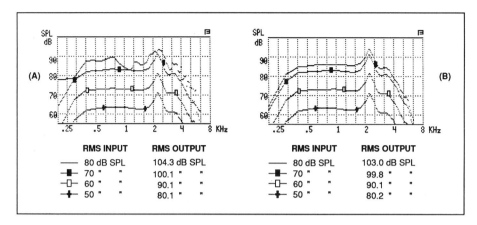

Figure 4–5.   Families of frequency–output curves for **(A)** a peak-clipping instrument and **(B)** a compression-limiting AGC-O instrument.

distortion caused the response curve to become jagged. To the hearing aid wearer, speech inputs of 80 dB SPL or higher will likely sound garbled or harsh when processed through this hearing aid. Typically, a hearing aid wearer's own voice often exceeds 80 dB SPL at ear level. Also, speech peaks in noisy or close listening situations often exceed 80 dB SPL. Thus saturation distortion can be a real problem. Fortunately, the output family B in Figure 4–5 shows, once more, that saturation distortion can be avoided with the use of an AGC-O limiter. While the RMS maximum output in family B was nearly the same level as in family A, no distortion was evident in the high level test of family B.

It is important to note that frequency/response curves using random-noise and pure-tone signals will not reveal the same degree of jaggedness as seen in the composite curves of family A (Figs. 4–4 and 4–5), even though saturation distortion may be present. Because natural speech always has a random component, absent from phase-locked composite signals, the observation of jaggedness as a test for intermodulation distortion using phase-locked composite signals should be considered a stringent test. Nonetheless, in the experience of this author (who has a moderate to severe hearing loss), when jaggedness is visible on a response curve obtained with a speech-shaped composite signal, the hearing aid sounds distorted.

Input/Output Curves

An input/output (I/O) curve shows the output level of a hearing aid as a function of the input level. Output level, in dB SPL, is plotted on the vertical axis. Input level, also in dB SPL, is plotted on the horizontal axis. The standard aspect ratio[1] is one to one, meaning that a 1 dB change on the vertical axis corresponds to a 1 dB change on the horizontal axis. The test signal for I/O curves can be broadband or narrowband, although it is not clear whether a broadband I/O test provides new information over what is available from a family of broadband frequency/response curves. Narrowband I/O tests, however, emphasize a single frequency, and thus can focus on a specific region where signal processing is likely to take place.

AT WHAT I/O LEVELS IS THE HEARING AID LINEAR OR NONLINEAR?

Because of the one to one aspect ratio of I/O graphs, linear processing appears as a straight line sloping upward at a 45° angle. For example, graph A of Figure 4–6 shows an I/O curve of a linear instrument. Anything other than a straight line sloping upward at a 45° angle would indicate nonlinear processing. Graph B is an I/O curve of a peak-clipping instrument. The output for a 2000 Hz pure-tone input was limited at 108.5 dB SPL. All input levels above 75 dB SPL resulted in the same output. Graph C is an I/O curve of a compression-limiting instrument. The output limiting appears similar to that of I/O curve B. Indeed, the nearly identical shapes of the two I/O curves prevent the observer from determining the mechanism that limited the maximum output. Thus, although I/O curves can reveal the presence of nonlinear processing, they cannot necessarily reveal the nature of that processing.

IS THE NONLINEAR PROCESSING INPUT-CONTROLLED OR OUTPUT-CONTROLLED?

A single I/O curve can reveal whether nonlinear processing is present, but a *pair* of I/O curve can reveal whether a nonlinear circuit is input-controlled or output-controlled (such as with AGC-I and AGC-O). The first step in obtaining an I/O curve is to decide on a test frequency. The best choice is the test frequency specified by the manufacturer of the hearing aid. When the manufacturer's specifications are not available, a family of frequency/response curves can reveal a frequency at which nonlinear processing is evident. The tester can then choose a frequency in the region of nonlinear activity. As an example, family F of Figure 4–4 shows frequency–response curves for a hearing aid having an adaptive low-frequency filter. This family of curves confirms that nonlinear processing takes place in the low frequencies. A low-frequency signal would thus be a good choice when generating an I/O curve for this hearing aid.

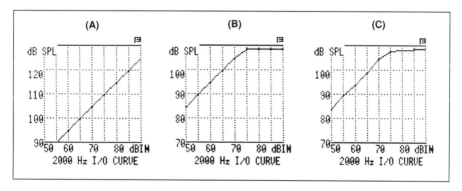

Figure 4–6.   Input/output curves for (**A**) a linear instrument, (**B**) a peak-clipping instrument, and (**C**) a compression-limiting instrument.

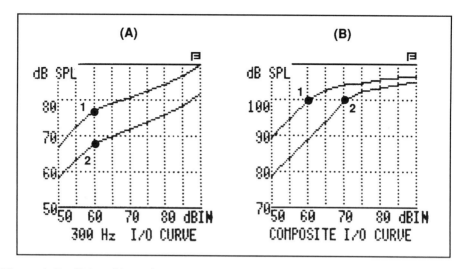

Figure 4–7. Pairs of input/output curves. In each graph, volume control was full-on for curve No. 1; volume control was approximately −10 dB for curve 2. **(A)** An input-controlled adaptive low-frequency filter circuit. **(B)** An output-controlled AGC circuit.

Graph A of Figure 4–7 shows two I/O curves for this instrument. The frequency of the pure-tone test signal was 300 Hz. Curve 1 was generated with the volume control set to full-on. Curve 2 was generated with the volume control set to reduce the gain by about 10 dB. The graph shows that the knee points for both curves occurred at the same input level, independently of the setting of the volume control. The kneepoint, therefore, was determined entirely by the input level. Almost all adaptive low-frequency filters are input controlled, as in this case, because they are designed to respond to changes in the environmental noise level at the input of the hearing aid.

Graph B of Figure 4–7 shows a pair of I/O curves for a compression-limiting AGC-O instrument. A speech-shaped composite signal was used to test this broadband, single channel device. As in graph A, the volume control was adjusted to produce about 10 dB less gain for curve 2 than for curve 1. In this case, however, the kneepoints occurred at different input levels, but at the same output level for both curves. In other words, the kneepoint was determined entirely by the output level.[18] This output-controlled type of AGC is often preferred for output-limiting compression because the maximum output will remain fixed, regardless of how the user adjusts the volume control.

Attack-and-Release Tests

As an eliciting stimulus is presented and then removed, attack-and-release tests measure the time required for a signal-processing circuit to take effect and then return to its original state. Figure 4–8 shows how an attack-and-release test progresses. A signal is first presented at a low SPL and then abruptly raised to a higher level. With the abrupt change, the signal-processing circuit reacts by adjusting the gain. This reaction takes some time. According to

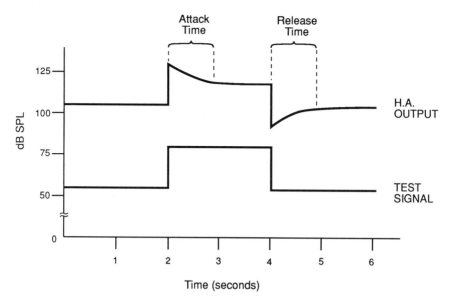

Figure 4–8. Schematic diagram of an attack-and-release test. Input signal changes abruptly from 55 dB SPL to 80 dB SPL and then to 55 dB SPL. Test measures the time to reach within 2 dB of the steady-state value after each abrupt change in input level.

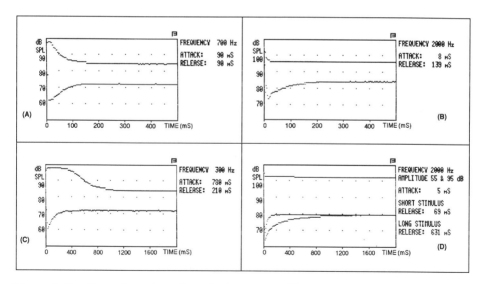

Figure 4–9. Examples of attack-and-release tests. Upper trace, attack; lower trace(s), release. (**A**) Adaptive low frequency filter with moderate attack time. (**B**) Broadband, compression-limiting AGC-O. (**C**) Adaptive low frequency filter with very long attack time. (**D**) Adaptive release time; dual-trace release test indicates that release time varied according to the stimulus duration.

ANSI S3.22[1] the attack test measures the time required for the output to reach within 2 dB of the steady-state adjusted value. (The criteria for attack and release time may change in future revisions of ANSI S3.22.) Then, the input signal is abruptly reduced to its original level. The signal-processing circuit reacts by returning the gain to its original value; but this adjustment also takes time. The release test measures the time required for the output to return to within 2 dB of the original steady-state value.

As with I/O curves, the test signal for attack-and-release tests can be either broadband or narrowband. But narrowband signals emphasize a single frequency, thereby focusing on the specific region where signal processing is likely to occur. Graph A of Figure 4–9 shows an example of an attack-and-release test. Note that the horizontal axis is not frequency but time, in milliseconds. The vertical axis is output, in dB SPL. The upper trace shows the attack, and the lower trace shows the release. For the attack, 0 ms represents the moment the signal abruptly changed from 55 to 80 dB SPL. For the release, 0 ms represents the moment the signal abruptly changed from 80 dB SPL to 55.[1] The numerical attack and release times at the right of the graph indicate the elapsed time between the moment the signal level changed abruptly and the moment the output level reached within 2 dB of the steady-state value.

WHAT TYPES OF SIGNALS WILL CAUSE PROCESSING TO OCCUR?

Because differing signals have differing temporal patterns, the attack time of a nonlinear circuit can, in part, determine which signals will or will not cause nonlinear processing to occur. For example, the conversational speech of a single talker is a pulsing signal, alternating between sounds and gaps, with each sound segment normally lasting from tens to hundreds of milliseconds. Background noise, such as multitalker babble, does not pulsate nearly as much; the gaps of one talker's speech are filled in by the sounds of another's. In contrast, transient signals, such as the clanking of a plate, last only a few milliseconds. A circuit with a short attack time will react to all signals, whereas a circuit with a long attack time may effectively "ignore" transient signals or pulsing speech signals, reacting only to ongoing background noise. A short attack time, therefore, is desirable for output limiting, to protect the hearing aid wearer from the adverse effects of all high-level signals, including transients. A long attack time, however, may be more desirable for adaptive low-frequency filtering, because the circuit, then, will not react to the pulses of speech—but only to the ongoing din of background noise.

Graph B of Figure 4–9 shows an attack-and-release test for a hearing aid having output-limiting AGC. A 2 kHz pure-tone signal was used for this broadband, single-channel circuit. (Two kHz is the frequency specified by ANSI S3.22[1] for testing broadband AGC devices. Almost any test frequency would be acceptable. At 2 kHz, gain is sufficiently strong to ensure that the test will be relatively noise free.) The attack time was so short (8 ms) that the downward part of the upper trace (at the left edge) is barely visible. With this rapid an attack, the output will be limited for nearly any high-amplitude input signal. In contrast, graph C of Figure 4–9 shows an attack-and-release test of a hearing aid having an adaptive low-frequency filter. This adaptive circuit "waits" several hundred milliseconds before reacting to changing input levels. This circuit will thus respond only to steady, ongoing signals (such as continuous background noise).

WILL THE LISTENER EXPERIENCE ACOUSTIC SIDE EFFECTS, SUCH AS DROPOUTS OR PUMPING AND BREATHING?

As discussed above, a short attack time is desirable in output-limiting AGC; but a short attack time can be associated with audible "side effects." The nature of these side effects depends, in part, on the release time. Consider the following scenario: A listener wearing a hearing aid is having lunch with a friend in a noisy restraurant. The friend is talking, and the listener is struggling to hear. Suddenly a nearby waiter "clanks" one plate against another. An effective output-limiting AGC circuit will protect the listener by reducing the gain. But the friend keeps talking, not knowing that the gain of the listener's hearing aid has momentarily been reduced. If the gain does not return to its normal level soon after the "clank," subsequent parts of the conversation may be missed. A relatively short release time, therefore, may be required to avoid such "dropouts" in conversation associated with transient stimuli.

Now take the scenario a step further: In this noisy environment, not only transient "clanks" and "plinks" but even the friend's voice may be loud enough to activate the AGC circuit. Thus, gain may be reduced throughout the conversation. The reduced gain may be acceptable, because the listener would likely have adjusted the volume control accordingly. But if the release time is very short (as it must be to avoid "dropouts"), the gain will rapidly increase during gaps in the friend's speech, allowing amplified background noise to "fill in" the gaps between speech sounds. Background noise will go up and down in level, depending on whether there are sounds or gaps in the friend's speech. This phenomenon is known as "pumping and breathing." At best, pumping and breathing can be audible and annoying, especially to new hearing aid users. At worst, rhythmic patterns of conversational speech can be masked, in an already difficult listening environment. Fortunately, pumping and breathing can be avoided if the release time is sufficiently long.

Thus a dilemma exists: Avoiding dropouts may require a short release time, whereas avoiding pumping and breathing may require a long release time. A solution would be a circuit that adapts the release time according to the duration of the stimulus. With an adaptive-release circuit, the release time is relatively short for transient stimuli (e.g., plates clanking) and relatively long for longer stimuli (e.g., conversational speech segments). Graph D of Figure 4–9 shows a triple-trace attack-and-release test of a hearing aid having an adaptive-release circuit. The attack time (upper trace) was tested in the normal way, except that the upper amplitude was 95 dB SPL instead of 80 dB SPL. The observed attack time was very fast (5 ms). The release time (lower traces) was tested twice: once using a short stimulus (0.1 seconds), and again using a long stimulus (2.0 seconds). The results show that the release time for the short stimulus was relatively short (69 ms), while the release time for the long stimulus was relatively long (631 ms). Because of the adaptive release time, this AGC hearing aid will likely cause less annoyance from dropouts and pumping and breathing than will an AGC aid having a fixed release time.

Caveat Regarding Signal Duration for Automated Test Sequences

Before leaving this discussion of advanced coupler tests, the reader should be aware of the relation of attack and release times to automated test sequences using varying input levels. The following caution applies both to I/O tests and to families of frequency/response tests. With tests performed at multiple input levels, the results can be erroneous if the duration of the input signal at a particular level is not sufficiently long to permit the hearing aid to reach its steady state before the measurement is taken. For example, Figure 4–10 shows I/O curves using a computerized sequence that automatically raised the level of a 300 Hz pure-tone test signal in 5 dB steps. For curve A, the tone was presented for 0.1 seconds at each input level before the hearing aid output was measured. In 0.1 seconds, this hearing aid did not have sufficient time to reach its steady state. In contrast, curve B shows an accurate low-frequency I/O curve for this hearing aid. At each input level, there was a 2.0 second delay between the onset of the tone and the acquisition of the measurement. The 2.0 second delay allowed sufficient settling time for steady-state accuracy. As a rule of thumb, automated test sequences should allow at least twice the ANSI[1] release time between the onset of the stimulus and the acquisition of the measurement at each input level.[19]

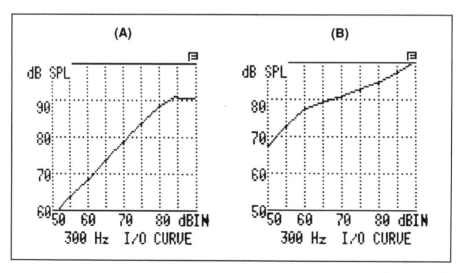

Figure 4–10. Low-frequency input/output curves for an adaptive low-frequency filter having a long attack time (0.78 second). Curve A is not accurate because short signal duration (0.1 second) did not allow the circuit to reach steady state for each input level. Curve B used a longer signal duration (2.0 seconds); curve B is accurate because the circuit reached steady state at each input level.

ANSI S3.22 Test Sequence

The ANSI S3.22[1] tests for hearing aid performance have a limited, but important role in the fitting of hearing aids. In every fitting, it is a good idea for the dispenser to run the S3.22 pure-tone test sequence at least twice: once when the hearing aid is delivered, to verify that the instrument is performing to the manufacturer's specifications; and again after all modifications have been performed, to check for unexpected anomalies in the performance that could occur following changes in programming or trimmer settings. Fabry[18] reported once fitting a patient with an aid that achieved a very good match between real-ear performance and target performance. Surprisingly, the patient soon returned dissatisfied. A diagnostic ANSI S3.22 test sequence revealed that the adjustments made during the fitting session caused the equivalent input noise to increase to 44 dB SPL. This unacceptable result would have been discovered earlier had the ANSI puretone sequence been run before the conclusion of the initial fitting session.

Maximum Output Test

One last point should be made concerning pure-tone versus broadband signals as related to a "worst case" test for maximum output. With a swept pure tone, only one frequency is presented at a time. Therefore, a hearing aid can produce its total maximum output power at each individual test frequency (barring distortion components). With a broadband signal, many frequencies are presented at a time, and thus the maximum output power is distributed across a range of frequencies. Because of this distribution of power with broadband signals, the observed output level at individual frequencies will always be less than the total RMS output (see Fig. 4–5). For a given RMS input level, the total

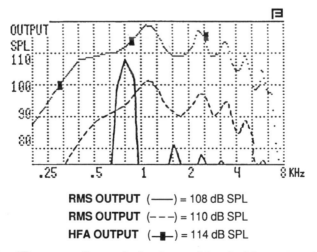

RMS OUTPUT (——) = 108 dB SPL

RMS OUTPUT (– – –) = 110 dB SPL

HFA OUTPUT (—■—) = 114 dB SPL

Figure 4–11. "Boo-oo-oop" sound of a fax machine (solid trace) and maximum output curves using swept pure-tone (filled boxes) and flat-weighted broadband signal (dashes), both test signals at 90 dB SPL RMS. All curves recorded through a BTE hearing aid on an HA-2 2 cc coupler. (From Revit.[20])

RMS output for a broadband signal may be similar to the *average* output for a swept pure-tone signal (see Fig. 4–11); but the output levels at individual frequencies will be less than for a swept pure-tone signal.

As an example, the solid trace in Figure 4–11 is the spectrum of the "boo-oo-oop" signal of a fax machine recorded through a hearing aid attached to a 2 cc coupler 3 ft from the fax machine. Except for the upper harmonics that are about 30 dB down, this signal is essentially a narrowband signal centered at 800 Hz, having an RMS level of 108 dB SPL. The upper trace (filled boxes) is an output frequency response obtained for the same hearing aid using a swept pure-tone signal at 90 dB SPL (akin to an ANSI[1] SSPL-90 curve). The lower trace (dashes) is an output frequency response obtained for the same instrument, but using a flat-weighted, broadband composite signal, also at 90 dB SPL (total RMS). The RMS level of the broadband output response was 110 dB SPL, close to the 108 dB SPL of the narrowband fax signal. But the point on the broadband curve at 800 Hz was only 94 dB SPL, greatly underestimating the output for the narrowband fax signal. The point at 800 Hz on the pure-tone curve, in contrast, slightly overestimated the output level of the fax signal. The swept pure-tone signal presented a "worst case" scenario by concentrating the total power of the test signal at one frequency at a time. A swept pure-tone would, therefore, seem preferable to a broadband signal for testing maximum output power at individual frequencies.

This is not to say that a broadband signal provides little information about the output capabilities of a hearing aid; only that a broadband test signal provides the best information about other broadband signals (like speech), whereas a pure-tone test signal provides the best information about high amplitude narrowband signals that could be encountered in daily life.

Future Issues: Signal and Environment

Recent reports (see Chs. 13 and 14) indicate that future fitting strategies will be based not on insertion gain, but on the SPL values of an amplified speech spectrum as measured in the ear canal. Such strategies, while having a high degree of face validity, raise important questions regarding test signals. If a broadband, speech-shaped signal is used, what is the "ideal" shape? Many researchers advocate using the long-term average spectrum of speech as a model for determining the frequency response of a hearing aid. But a long-term average spectrum includes both sounds and silences. The task of selecting the frequency response of a hearing aid would seem to have little to do with silences. Perhaps a better speech-spectrum model would consider the average of sounds, while ignoring silences. But can any single spectrum suffice for all tests? Does not the spectrum of speech change with changing communication conditions? Even if one ideal speech-shaped signal could be identified, could any such *steady-state* signal simulate the changing rhythms and dynamics of natural speech? These issues of test signal must be addressed before future fitting strategies can reach their maximum utility.

Another issue is that hearing aids are used in environments other than test boxes and test rooms. With the advent of hearing instruments designed to change the way they perform in changing acoustic environments, work is needed on (1) effectively simulating the listening environments hearing aid wearers are likely to encounter and (2) designing tests that assess the communicative abilities of hearing aid wearers in those environments.

References

1. ANSI S3.22-1987: *American National Standard: Specification of Hearing Aid Characteristics.* New York, Acoustical Society of America, 1987.
2. Feigin JA, Kopun JG, Stelmachowicz PG, Gorga MP: Probe-tube microphone measures of ear-canal sound pressure levels in infants and children. *Ear Hear* 1989; 10:254–258.
3. Fikret-Pasa S, Revit LJ: Individualized correction factors in the preselection of hearing aids. *J Speech Hear Res* 1992; 35:384–400.
4. Madaffari PL: Pressure response about the ear. Paper presented at the 88th Meeting of the Acoustical Society of America, St. Louis, MO, 1974.
5. Dillon H: Earmolds and high frequency response modification. *Hear Instrum* December 1985, 36:8–12.
6. Lybarger SF: Earmolds. In Katz J (ed): *Handbook of Clinical Audiology*, ed 3. Baltimore: Williams & Wilkins, 1985.
7. Kates JM: Acoustic effects in in-the-ear hearing aid response: Results from a computer simulation. *Ear Hear* 1988; 9:119–131.
8. Dillon H: Allowing for real ear venting effects when selecting the coupler gain of hearing aids. *Ear Hear* 1991; 12:406–416.
9. Cox RM: Combined effects of earmold vents and suboscillatory feedback on hearing aid frequency response. *Ear Hear* 1982; 3:12–17.
10. Killion MC, Monser EL: CORFIG: Coupler Response for Flat Insertion Gain (Chapter 8), in Studebaker GA, Hochberg I (eds): *Acoustic Factors Affecting Hearing Aid Performance*, ed 1. Baltimore, University Park Press, 1980.
11. Killion MC, Revit LJ: CORFIG and GIFROC: Real Ear to Coupler and Back (Chapter 5), in Studebaker GA, Hochberg I (eds): *Acoustic Factors Affecting Hearing Aid Performance*, ed 2. Boston: Allyn and Bacon, 1993.
12. Ickes M, Hawkins D, Cooper W: Effect of loudspeaker azimuth and reference microphone location on ear canal probe tube microphone measurements. *J Am Acad Audiol* 1991; 2:156–163.
13. Bentler R, Pavlovic CV: Transfer functions and correction factors used in hearing aid evaluation and research. *Ear Hear* 1989; 10:58–63.
14. Punch J, Chi C, Patterson J: A recommended protocol for prescriptive use of target gain rules. *Hear Instrum* 1990; 41:12–19.
15. Mueller HG: Individualizing the ordering of custom hearing aids (Chapter 9), in Mueller HG, Hawkins DB, Northern JL (eds): *Probe Microphone Measurements: Hearing Aid Selection and Assessment.* San Diego: Singular Publishing Group, Inc., 1992.
16. Borden GJ, Harris KS. *Speech Science Primer: Physiology, Acoustics, and Perception of Speech.* Baltimore: Williams & Wilkins, 1983.
17. ANSI S3.42-1992: *American National Standard: Testing Hearing Aids With a Broad-Band Noise Signal.* New York: Acoustical Society of America, 1992.
18. Fabry DA: *Recent Advances in Hearing Aid Design: Clinical Implications.* Short course presented at California Speech-Language-Hearing Association, 40th Annual State Conference, San Francisco, 1992.
19. Revit LJ: Testing ASP instruments with low-frequency input/gain and input/output curves. *Hear J* 1989; 42(6).
20. Revit L: New tests for signal-processing and multichannel hearing instruments. *Hear J* 1991; 44:20–23.

5

Use of Real-Ear Measurements To Verify Hearing Aid Fittings

John E. Tecca

Introduction

The development of real-ear measurements (REMs) represents one of the most important advances for clinical measurement of hearing aid performance. REMs have contributed to our understanding of the role of the outer and middle ear in influencing hearing aid performance. In addition, we now have a much better understanding of the intrasubject and intersubject variabilities that occur in fitting hearing aids.

Broadly stated, the term real-ear measurement can be applied to probe tube measurements of sound pressure levels developed within the ear canal or changes in behavioral threshold (i.e., functional gain) that occur when a hearing aid is worn. This chapter emphasizes the use of probe tube measurements, primarily insertion gain, to verify hearing aid performance with adults. Although much of the material discussed applies to children, it is beyond the scope of this chapter to provide extensive information on pediatric applications.

Real-ear insertion gain (REIG) is the term used to describe the difference between sound pressure levels measured at a given frequency in the ear canal with and without a hearing aid in place. Real-ear insertion response (REIR) refers to the difference between sound pressure levels measured across a range of frequencies in the ear canal with and without a hearing aid in place. REIG and REIR represent the physical changes in sound pressure level caused by the presence of a hearing aid. Changes in the audibility of sound may be reasonably inferred from this measurement, but REIG and REIR measurements should never be considered direct measurements of hearing.

Over the past 10–15 years an extensive body of literature has demonstrated the validity, reliability, and utility of REMs.[1–24] Results of a recent survey indicated that 65%–70% of audiologists make use of REM equipment in their practice.[25] Instrumentation has become so user friendly and affordable that there is little justification for not having it available in every office that provides hearing aid services.

Although the use of REM equipment has become increasingly popular, there still is no standard for its routine use recommended by the American National Standards Institute (ANSI) or the American Speech-Language-Hearing Association (ASHA). This should not be surprising, given the relatively recent introduction of REMs. Currently, ANSI S3.80 Committee on Probe Microphone Measurements of Hearing Aid Performance is developing a standard for REMs, and recommendations have been introduced for terminology to be used in discussing the most common measurements (e.g., real-ear unaided response [REUR], real-ear aided response [REAR], and REIR).[26] This chapter offers a practical discussion of procedures used in making REMs based on available research and clinical experience. A section of the chapter is devoted to pitfalls that may be encountered in routine practice. Additionally, a number of examples are included to demonstrate measurement procedures and illustrate fitting problems.

Why Verify?

The title of this chapter suggests that there is reason to verify real-ear hearing aid performance. While this may seem intuitive to many, Bratt and Sammeth[27] described a survey by Hedges that indicated that, at best, only about two-thirds of the 138 respondents from within the Veterans Administration audiology program routinely perform REMs. It is likely that these results from a sample including only audiologists are better than would be obtained from a sample of all dispensers, including both audiologists and nonaudiologist hearing aid specialists. There are at least five reasons that argue for routine verification of hearing aid performance with REMs.

The primary justification for the use of REMs is that the performance of a hearing aid on any given ear is not well predicted from average group data.[10,24,28,29] Several transfer functions have been developed for predicting real-ear hearing aid gain based on coupler data.[30–32] These methods work very well when the subject has an "average ear" such as KEMAR or when group data are used. Predictions for a "typical" subject are likely to deviate from the "average ear" by an unpredictable amount.

Figure 5–1 shows the mean and range of REIG for a group of ten subjects fitted with very similar linear full-shell in-the-ear (ITE) hearing aids in the office of the author. The range of 2 cc coupler gain for this group of hearing aids did not exceed 4 dB at the octave test frequencies between 250 and 4000 Hz. The REIG data were obtained at the time that the hearing aids were fitted by one audiologist (J.E.T.) using the protocol described in the next section. In analyzing the results, the REIG data were normalized at 2000 Hz in order to account for differences due to volume control setting. Despite this adjustment, the range of REIG among subjects was 8–13 dB, depending on test frequency. It is apparent that predictions of real-ear performance based on any transfer function developed from average group data would have resulted in large errors. Clearly, these data argue strongly for real-ear verification of hearing aid

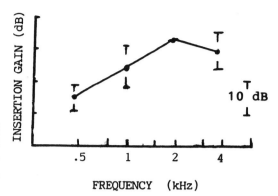

Figure 5–1. Mean and range of REIG for ten linear full-shell ITE hearing aids having equivalent electroacoustic characteristics when measured in a 2 cc coupler.

performance. When it is necessary to predict real-ear hearing aid performance, a transfer function specific to the subject's own ear should be used.[33–36]

The second reason to use REMs to verify hearing aid performance is that it provides information essential for evaluating and/or improving a hearing aid fitting. It makes little sense to perform a test if the results simply confirm that which is already known. It also is of little benefit to verify performance if the dispenser has no means to improve the fitting if necessary. The pattern of the real-ear frequency response provides essential information for the dispenser to use in modifying a fitting. REIG measurements should be used in conjunction with prescriptive targets (discussed in Chs. 1 and 2) as an initial fitting goal.

Figure 5–2 shows REIR curves measured at a 45° azimuth toward the better ear for a patient fitted with a wireless BICROS hearing aid. She had moderate mixed hearing loss at all frequencies except 2000 Hz at which a mild sensorineural hearing loss was present for the right ear. The left ear had profound sensorineural hearing loss. A hearing loss of this nature presents a real challenge for effective fitting due to the availability of only one aidable ear and the audiometric configuration of the hearing loss in that ear.

The initial REIR curve (Fig. 5–2A) was obtained using a standard earhook coupled to a vented earmold. A large, undesirable peak in the response is observed in the 2–4 kHz region. The standard earhook was replaced with a 680 ohm damped earhook. This resulted in minimal smoothing of the REIR (Fig. 5–2B). A 2 kHz notch earhook was then used. This very effectively nulled the gain at 2 kHz, but a sharp peak was still present between 3 and 4 kHz (Fig. 5–2C).

The final modification was accomplished with a low pass earhook. This essentially eliminated gain from 2 kHz through the higher frequencies. Interestingly, the patient found the sound quality of the low pass modification to be pleasant, while the other modifications produced a harsh sound quality. Note that, although this final modification produced a reasonably good match between the REIR and the NAL-R target for the frequencies up to about 2000 Hz, inadequate gain was provided in the higher frequencies.

In many cases it will not be feasible to match a target exactly, and compromises will need to be made (discussed in greater detail in the next para-

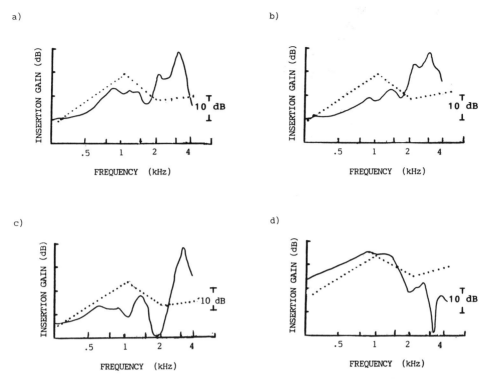

Figure 5–2. REIR curves (solid line) and NAL-R target curves (dotted line) for a patient fitted with a wireless BICROS hearing aid using four different earhooks. (**a**) Standard earhook. (**b**) 680 ohm earhook. (**c**) 2 kHz notch filter earhook. (**d**) Low pass earhook.

graph). Sound quality preferences of the hearing aid wearer should be considered in reaching the final hearing aid setting.

Certainly, there are technologic limitations that can make it impossible to achieve a given prescriptive target. Bratt and Sammeth[27] investigated the ability of a manufacturer to build custom-made ITE hearing aids (n = 89) to achieve a prescribed REIR. To achieve only a 50% acceptance rate, they found that a tolerance in excess of 10 dB REIG was required at one or more frequencies within the 250–4000 Hz range. This finding occurred despite the fact that their experimental design permitted manipulation of volume controls, potentiometers, and vents in order to achieve a best fit to the prescriptive targets.

The inability to achieve a prescribed real-ear target with a given instrument does not preclude the possibility of circuit revision at the factory or changing instruments. Many of the problems encountered in reaching target insertion gain are being reduced by increased flexibility in the potentiometer adjustments available on some recently introduced analog hearing aids and with digitally programmable hearing aids. Pragmatically, there will probably always be instances when dispensers must abandon their insertion gain targets, either because it is simply not technically feasible to reach them or because the hearing aid wearer objects to the perceived sound quality. This issue becomes further complicated when one considers the fact that prescriptive formulas were developed for linear circuits and there is increasing use of nonlinear circuits. Dispensers should not allow themselves to be so bound to prescriptive targets that they fail to give weight to other important issues.

The third reason to use REMs to verify hearing aid performance is that they provide baseline documentation for future revisions to a fitting, if necessary. After all necessary modifications have been made to a hearing aid to achieve the prescribed real-ear response, the hearing aid should be tested in the 2 cc coupler without changing the settings of the volume control or any potentiometers. This provides an individualized real ear to 2 cc coupler transfer function for each ear. The value of this process is to allow accurate prediction of real-ear performance from 2 cc coupler measurements in future visits if revisions need to be made. That is, the subject's own real-ear to 2 cc coupler transfer function is available instead of an average transfer function, as discussed earlier. While it is desirable routinely to verify every modification with REMs, it is not always practical or feasible.

Two applications of this individualized transfer function are described. In fitting high frequency hearing loss, an ITE hearing aid with IROS venting is often used. While the frequency potentiometer on this instrument allows flexible response modifications, it is often very sensitive and nonlinear. That is, minor adjustments of the potentiometer may provide large changes in the frequency response, but these changes are not consistent throughout the range of adjustment. The 2 cc reference to the real ear response allows the dispenser to return the settings to the desired position after service or to make minor modifications to the response without reevaluating the subject. The second example is with fitting patients confined to nursing care facilities. They may be reasonably healthy at the time a hearing aid is initially fitted. However, there are frequent instrument malfunctions and loss of hearing aids in nursing care facilities. In the event that it is necessary to repair or replace a hearing aid at a time when REIG measurements could not be reliably repeated on a patient, the initial data will allow a very close approximation for resetting the hearing aid.

A fourth reason to use REMs is that they can provide an excellent educational or counseling tool. Due to the speed of real-ear tests, students can obtain immediate feedback as they learn the effects of electronic or acoustic modification of hearing aids and earmolds. Additionally, many clients are extremely interested in the display of their test results on the computer monitor. The visual image often simplifies discussions regarding either benefits or limitations of a given hearing aid fitting.

A fifth and final reason to use REMs to verify hearing aid performance is that it is a means of demonstrating to professionals from other disciplines that audiology is an accountable profession. Increasingly, accrediting bodies and third-party insurers are requiring ongoing quality improvement documentation.[37] Documentation of real-ear hearing aid performance is one important means of demonstrating that audiologists are achieving clinical goals or formulating methods to improve hearing aid fittings.

Test Protocol

Probe tube measurements currently offer the most reliable and comprehensive means of measuring real-ear hearing aid performance. Yet there are numerous factors that can adversely influence the results. Most of the important factors affecting test reliability have been described elsewhere in professional journals[2–4,7–9,11–13,16–19,21–24] or textbooks.[38–40] The purpose of this section is not to review the literature, but to integrate it into a method for routine clinical use when making REIG measurements.

The specific procedures that are used depend on the type of hearing aid being evaluated, the instrumentation being used, the environment, and the type of measurement (i.e., REUR, REAR, or REIR) being made. The following procedure is appropriate for the majority of fittings that are encountered clinically. That is, more than 80% of the fittings that are done today involve ITE or ITC hearing aids.[25] The majority of these instruments are mild to moderate gain linear nondirectional hearing aids. The procedures described here are a modification of the method described previously by Tecca.[38] Specific procedures appropriate with other types of fittings are delineated later in this chapter.

Otoscopic Observation

Before initiating probe tube measurements the ear canal should be inspected otoscopically. The primary objective is to determine if the canal is free of cerumen or other debris. If it appears that the canal is significantly occluded or if cerumen is situated at a point where it may interfere with placement of the probe tube, it should be removed prior to testing.[41,42] The otoscopic examination also allows determination of the course of the ear canal. This will make it much easier to guide the probe tube to its resting position.

Insertion of Probe Tube

The probe tube should be inserted to a depth within about 6–8 mm from the tympanic membrane.[2] The length of the average adult ear canal is 25 mm. Since the typical distance from the ear canal opening to the intertragal notch is about 10 mm, the total distance from intertragal notch to tympanic membrane is about 35 mm. Inserting the tip of the probe tube 27–30 mm past the intertragal notch should cause it to reach the desired distance from the tympanic membrane. Measurements made a distance of 6–8 mm from the tympanic membrane should be equivalent to those obtained at the tympanic membrane for the frequency range of interest.[2] This method has been used for several years rather than measuring from the length of the hearing aid or earmold. It is quick, consistent, and has never caused an injury to the tympanic membrane. Placing a small piece of a tacky adhesive putty, such as that used to seal hearing aids in an HA-1 coupler, on the tube and pressing it against the intertragal notch will usually hold it securely.

Although the focus of this chapter is on REIG measurements with adults, most of the principles and procedures are equally appropriate with children.

The issue of probe tube insertion depth for children requires special consideration because of their smaller ear canal dimensions. Inserting a probe tube 27–30 mm beyond the intertragal notch may reach the tympanic membrane of young children. Kruger[43] demonstrated that the effective ear canal length and the REUR will usually reach adult values before 2 years of age. Data from Bentler[44] subsequently showed that adult REUR values for resonant frequency and amplitude are reached before 3 years of age. However, there was considerable variability among subjects in these studies, and both authors address the problem of variability related to probe tube insertion depth. Kruger[43] and Bentler[44] estimated insertion depth using otoscopic visualization. This can be quite a challenging maneuver on a young child, especially one who is active or uncooperative.

It has been effective to use the earmold as a guide in setting probe tube insertion depth, as was previously recommended for adults.[38] This is accomplished by placing the probe tube along the inferior edge of the earmold or hearing aid. Mark the probe tube at a point that will allow its medial tip to extend into the ear canal about 5 mm beyond the medial tip of the earmold or hearing aid. It is important to identify a landmark in the concha region where the lateral edge of the earmold or hearing aid terminates. This location is used as the reference point to align the mark on the probe tube during insertion into the ear canal. The sound pressure levels (SPL's) measured with this technique may be somewhat different than at the tympanic membrane.[2] However, the errors should be small at frequencies below about 4000 Hz, and accurate REIG measurements can be made. Furthermore, this technique minimizes the risk of causing discomfort to the child.

Equalization

While several methods of sound field equalization may be used,[11–13] the modified comparison method is usually preferred because it provides greater control over variations in signal level at the test location. This method requires that a reference microphone be located along the side of the head. The reference microphone monitors the test signal and causes the sound pressure level to be adjusted as necessary to maintain a constant SPL at the reference point.

The modified comparison method may be used with either an "on-line" reference microphone, which results in real-time corrections to the signal level, or an "off-line" method, which uses a reference stored in memory to make adjustments to the measured response. Ideally, corrections are made in real time. There is evidence that the precise position of the reference microphone may exert an effect on test reliability.[3,8,16]

The reference microphone should be next to the hearing aid microphone or at about the same position that would be occupied by a behind-the-ear (BTE) hearing aid. Unfortunately, it is not always possible to vary the position of the reference microphone due to the design of different models of REM equipment. If the reference microphone is consistently located at the same position and it is adequately secured, test reliability should not be unduly influenced.

Loudspeaker Location

The loudspeaker is situated 12–18 inches from the patients head using an azimuth of 45°. This location minimizes the contribution of reverberant energy and ambient noise, and the patient usually does not feel that the speaker is too close. REIG measurements have been made at distances from 12 inches to 1 m[19,38] at azimuths from 0° to 45° with good reliability and at an azimuth of 90° with significantly poorer reliability.[8,9]

Again, the exact distance and azimuth are not as important as consistency. However, it should be noted that with certain types of hearing aids, REIG results will differ according to the azimuth of the loudspeaker, and this must be considered in interpretation of results.[9,45]

Signal Level

A signal level of 60–70 dB SPL is typically used. This level is great enough to minimize the likelihood of contamination by ambient noise without being strong enough to drive the hearing aid into saturation. A lower level may be used in a very quiet room, or a stronger level may be necessary in a room with greater ambient noise levels. If there is concern about contamination from ambient noise, repeat the REUR with a higher test signal level. If there is concern about hearing aid saturation, repeat the REAR with a lower test signal level. In either case, the curves will be parallel if the initial level was adequate.

Signal Type

In general, the broadest band signal available on the probe tube system should be used.[14,18] In an optimal test environment, comparable results will be obtained with either broadband or pure-tone stimuli.[21] However, the type of test signal will influence the REIG results if a hearing aid is operating nonlinearly. This point is discussed in detail below (see Nonlinear Hearing Aids). It should also be noted that significantly greater output levels will be measured with pure-tone than with broadband test signals. Consequently, it has been suggested that measures of the saturation response of a hearing aid should be made with pure-tone stimuli.[18]

REUR

After instructing the patient not to move, measure the REUR. This measure determines the sound pressure levels present in the open-ear canal prior to placement of the hearing aid. This measure is affected by the equalization method, the location of the reference microphone, and the status of the subject's outer and middle ear. The REUR serves as the referent for determining the REIR of the hearing aid.

REAR

Next, place the hearing aid or earmold in the ear canal without moving the probe tube. Adjust the volume of the hearing aid to produce the desired gain or, alternatively, adjust the volume control to the wearer's preferred setting. Another efficient method is to allow the patient to adjust the volume control to a comfortable level while listening to speech or a broadband noise presented at 65–70 dB SPL. Measure the REAR of the hearing aid. This measure is affected by all factors mentioned above for the REUR plus the characteristics of the hearing aid.

REIR

The REIR is the difference between the REUR and the REAR curves. The measured REIG values are compared with the prescribed REIG target values. If a satisfactory match is obtained, testing is complete. If the results are unacceptable, any necessary modifications are made and the aided measure is repeated. This process is repeated until the prescribed target is met or the dispenser determines that no further improvement can be produced.

It is a common practice to look at the REIR without considering the REUR and REAR. Displaying the REUR and REAR curves can be very helpful in evaluating the adequacy of a fitting. For example, in many cases the REIR does not match the prescriptive target for the frequencies above 2,000 Hz. The probem may be due to the frequency response of the hearing aid or to the person's external ear characteristics. Examining the REUR and REAR can pinpoint the source of the problem and help to determine if further improvements are feasible.

There are a number of other real-ear procedures that can be helpful in prescribing a hearing aid or verifying its performance. These include the real-ear occluded response (REOR), the real-ear saturation response (RESR), and the real-ear coupler difference (RECD). Some of these have been discussed at length in Chapter 3, the focus of this chapter is on the REUR, REAR, and REIR.

Several illustrative cases are described that include probe tube measurements made according to the protocol described above. Figure 5–3A shows a commonly encountered real-ear response for a patient fitted with a full-shell ITE hearing aid for a mild to moderate sensorineural hearing loss. The REUR has a rather common shape, with a maximum peak of about 20 dB. The REAR rises above the unaided response just below 1000 Hz and continues to demonstrate significant gain beyond 4000 Hz. The shape of the REIR is fairly smooth, although minor peaks and valleys are present. Note that the REIR and NAL-R target curves are close to each other except for the region between 500 and 1000 Hz, where obtained gain is less than the target. In this case, the gain was decreased by adjusting a low frequency tone potentiometer due to the sound quality preference of the hearing aid wearer.

Figure 5–3B shows the REMs for a patient fitted with a full-shell ITE hearing aid for a moderate to severe sensorineural hearing loss. The REUR is marked by a very sharp resonance peak exceeding 30 dB. The REAR is reasonably smooth and reaches a peak very near the peak of the REUR, with an abrupt decline in the higher frequencies. The REIR is reasonably close to the NAL-R target curve for the frequencies below about 2000 Hz. The REIR then abruptly declines below the target for frequencies above 2000 Hz. The external ear

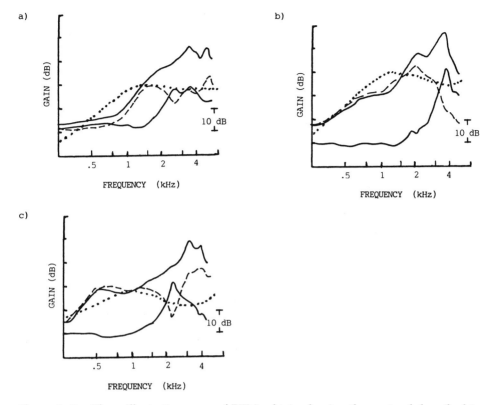

Figure 5–3. Three illustrative cases of REMs obtained using the protocol described in the text. (**a**) A "typical" patient fitted with a full-shell ITE hearing aid for a mild to moderate sensorineural hearing loss. (**b**) A patient fitted with a full-shell ITE hearing aid for a moderate to severe sensorineural hearing loss. Note the strong influence of the sharp resonance in the REUR on the REIR. (**c**) A patient fitted with a full-shell ITE hearing aid on an ear with an enlarged mastoid cavity. Note the influence of the lower resonance frequency in the REUR on the REIR. Upper solid line, REAR; lower solid line, REUR; broken line, REIR; dotted line, NAL-R target.

characteristics of this patient largely negate the high frequency amplification noted in the REAR, making it unlikely that effective high frequency amplification can be provided.

The REMs for a patient with an enlarged mastoid cavity and moderate conductive hearing loss are shown in Figure 5–3C. The REUR is markedly abnormal, with a sharply rising resonance peak just above 2000 Hz and gradually falling in the higher frequencies. The REAR is not unusual, showing significant gain throughout most of the frequency range without marked peaks or valleys. The REIR is marked by a valley in the response just above 2000 Hz and a sharp increase in gain for the higher frequencies due to the influence of the external ear characteristics. As in Figure 5–3B, providing a smooth REIR that matches the prescriptive target is complex and perhaps not feasible with conventional amplification or most programmable hearing aids.

Variations in Protocol

There are fittings that require modifications to the previously described protocol in order to obtain valid results. The following sections discuss four of the variations that may be necessary. If not specifically discussed, all other aspects of the protocol remain unchanged.

High Gain Hearing Aids

High gain hearing aids introduce several important factors that should be considered when making REMs. First, in most cases, significant low frequency gain is desired when fitting high gain hearing aids. Second, high gain hearing aids produce, by definition, high gain. A tight fitting earmold is required to prevent feedback and to preserve low frequency amplification. Inserting a probe tube between the hearing aid or earmold and the ear canal wall creates a slit leak. This vent reduces gain to the very low frequencies and reduces the usable gain before the point where feedback occurs. In these cases, it is desirable to have earmolds prepared with a channel drilled parallel to the sound bore for insertion of the probe tube. The hole is plugged following probe measurements. Methods have been described elsewhere for combining real-ear and coupler methods when feedback is a problem.[38,46] As mentioned earlier, whenever possible it is desirable to obtain the REIG results through direct measurement rather than by inference from 2 cc coupler measurements.

Figure 5–4 presents an example of variations in the REAR of a high gain BTE hearing aid related to probe tube insertion. The greatest gain across the frequency range is measured with the probe tube inserted through a channel in the earmold (dotted curve). Care is required while inserting the earmold, or the probe tube may be inadvertently folded over. Similarly, during an attempt to insert the probe tube between the earmold and the ear canal wall, the tube was compressed too tightly, resulting in about a 40 dB reduction in the measured gain (bottom solid curve). When the tube was repositioned and

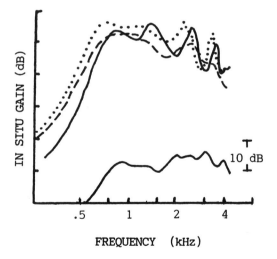

Figure 5–4. Variations in REAR measurements obtained with different placements of the probe tube for a patient fitted with a high gain BTE hearing aid. Dotted line, probe tube inserted through a channel in the earmold; dashed line, probe tube inserted between the earmold and the ear canal wall; upper solid line, probe tube inserted between the earmold and the ear canal wall with improperly seated earmold; lower solid line, probe tube compressed between the earmold and the ear canal wall.

the earmold reseated, an REAR similar to the one obtained with the probe tube inserted through the probe channel of the earmold was obtained (dashed curve). However, less overall gain and some low frequency vent effects are oberved. In the final curve the earmold was not seated quite properly (top solid curve). Although the volume control setting was the same as for the previous measurements, suboscillatory feedback occurred, causing undesirable peaks in the response and even greater low frequency venting.

A third consideration in measuring the performance of high gain hearing aids is the input level of the test signal. A high gain hearing aid may be driven into saturation (input level plus gain exceeds the output limits of the hearing aid) with input levels of 65–70 dB SPL or less. An evaluation of the REAR obtained with a hearing aid in saturation will inaccurately portray the gain and frequency response of the instrument. The lowest input signal level that will not be contaminated by ambient noise should be used. As an additional consideration, some probe tube systems have a mechanism that terminates the test if the output of the hearing aid exceeds a predetermined level. The default setting of the system must be adjusted to a higher level to allow measurement of the anticipated output levels.

A final consideration in verifying the performance of high gain hearing aids relates to the auditory capabilities of the subject.[17] REIG measurements are valuable only to the extent that they allow valid predictions of the audibility of sound. Some individuals using high gain hearing aids may have very limited auditory function and respond to the feeling of low frequency sound vibrations rather than actually hearing. In these instances. REIG results may suggest greater improvement in audibility than actually occurs. Functional gain measurements will probably yield more valid results in such cases.

Nonlinear Hearing Aids

Results obtained with nonlinear hearing aids may be affected by the type of signal and by the input level of the signal. If the signal level is below the compression kneepoint (the level at which the hearing aid compression circuitry is activated), similar REIG will be measured with either a pure-tone or a broadband test signal. However, at levels above the compression kneepoint, use of a pure tone may cause a "blooming" or exaggeration in the low frequency response of the hearing aid.[14,18,47] This occurs because the swept tone is held at a constant level, and hearing aids typically have greater compression thresholds for the low frequencies than the high frequencies. Therefore, the swept tone allows the hearing aid to behave linearly in the low frequency regions but activates the compression circuitry in the high frequency regions. A broadband stimulus is the signal of choice in testing compression hearing aids, since it will not cause the "blooming" effect.

It is desirable to measure the response of compression hearing aids with several signal input levels in order to verify the function of the compressor and to adjust its kneepoint when necessary. An example is presented in Figure 5–5A. The response of an ITE hearing aid with input compression (AGC-I) was initially measured with the compression kneepoint set to its highest setting,

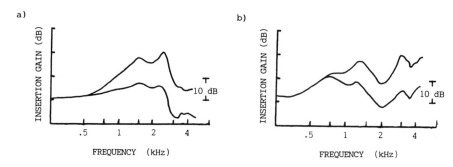

Figure 5–5. REIR measurements for two types of nonlinear hearing aids. **(a)** An ITE hearing aid having AGC-I circuitry. Input levels were 65 dB sound pressure level for the upper curve and 80 dB sound pressure level for the lower curve. **(b)** An ITE hearing aid having K-Amp circuitry. Input levels were 50 dB sound pressure level for the upper curve and 80 dB sound pressure level for the lower curve.

thereby allowing the instrument to function essentially as a linear instrument. Necessary frequency–response modifications were made to the hearing aid before adjusting the compression threshold. Without changing the volume control setting, the level of the test signal was increased 5 dB. The AGC-I threshold was then decreased until the compressor was activated (i.e., decrease in gain). Finally, the level of the test signal was gradually increased to 80 dB to verify that adequate attenuation occurred to prevent discomfort. Unrelated to the effect of the AGC-I circuitry, it is also noteworthy that the REIR rolls off abruptly in the region of 3000 Hz where a large external ear resonance occurs.

The results for a patient fitted with an ITE hearing aid containing K-Amp circuitry is shown in Figure 5–5B. K-Amp hearing aids have very low compression thresholds, and their frequency response gradually flattens as the signal level increases beyond the kneepoint. The REIRs were obtained with input levels of 50 and 80 dB SPL. Note the gradually rising pattern of amplification extending to the upper frequency limits of the equipment for an input level of 50 dB SPL. When the input is increased to 80 dB SPL the REIR drops below 10 dB. The results verify that the K-Amp circuitry is effectively modifying the amount of gain and the shape of the frequency response as input level is changed. Note the rise in the two REIR curves up to about 1200 Hz with declining gain to about 2000 Hz. This pattern of response is less than optimal and can be related to the interaction of the 3 mm vent and the overall gain of the hearing aid.

Contralateral Routing of the Signal Variations

Contralateral routing of the signal (CROS) hearing aids (discussed in detail in Ch. 11) present an interesting variation of the protocol used to evaluate most instruments. The added variables are hearing aid microphone location, reference microphone location, and loudspeaker location. For a CROS fitting the hearing aid microphone is located at the "bad" ear and the receiver is located at the "good" ear. For a BICROS fitting the hearing aid has a microphone at each ear while the receiver is located at the "better" ear. In either case, the probe tube microphone must be located in the ear canal of the "better" ear.

The loudspeaker may be located nearly anywhere within a range of ±90° relative to the subject's nose. If the dispenser wishes to obtain a conventional REIR measurement, the most straightforward approach is to place the loudspeaker at 0° azimuth. The reference microphone is located next to one of the hearing aid microphones, or, if desired, two measurements can be made with the reference microphone on each side of the head. The comparison of one or both aided measures to the unaided measure indicates the REIR.

The dispenser may wish to assess the head shadow effect. In this case the REUR should be measured with the loudspeaker initially located 45° to the side of the head, where the hearing aid receiver will be located. This demonstrates the optimal path for sound reaching the "better" ear. A second REUR should be measured with the loudspeaker 45° to the side of the head, where the hearing aid microphone will be located. The reference microphone should be located on the same side as the loudspeaker. If the reference microphone cannot be separated from the measuring microphone, it should be deactivated and a substitution method should be used. The difference between the two REUR curves demonstrates the head shadow effect. This comparison is very useful in explaining why a patient has difficulty hearing when sound originates from the "bad" side.

Finally, an REAR is measured with the loudspeaker on the side of the head where the hearing aid microphone is located. This curve may be referenced to both unaided curves. Comparing the REAR to the REUR from the "bad" side demonstrates elimination of head shadow and the benefit derived from having a CROS microphone. Comparing the aided response to the unaided response from the "good" side is more representative of the amount of amplification that is provided and should be the guiding curve relative to prescriptive targets. It is this relationship that must be carefully monitored so that excessive amplification is not provided. Overamplification of sound to the "good" ear is a primary reason for failure of CROS fittings.

The situation is only slightly more complicated when a BICROS fitting is accomplished. In addition to the three curves that are made for the CROS fitting, an REAR is measured from the "better" side. The unaided reference is the REUR for the "better" ear.

Pitfalls in Verifying Real-Ear Performance

There are numerous factors that can compromise REMs. Use of an appropriate test protocol can minimize the risk of obtaining spurious test results. Potential problems are more likely avoided if the tester has a set of expectations as to how the real-ear results should look. While it is true that real-ear results are not precisely predicted from coupler data, they generally will be close. When obtained results differ significantly from expected results, the tester should look for possible explanations. The following sections provide some of the common pitfalls that can be encountered clinically.

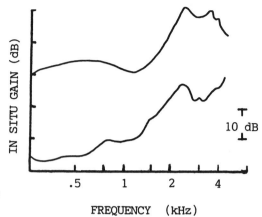

Figure 5–6. REUR measurements for a patient before and after cerumen removal. The upper curve was obtained after cerumen was removed and the lower curve with the tip of the tube embedded in the cerumen.

Cerumen

Cerumen can affect either the REUR or the REAR. Occlusive cerumen can result in measurement of inaccurate sound pressure levels and aberrations to the frequency response if the obstruction is located beyond the probe tip. Commonly the probe tip will reach the cerumen, resulting in total occlusion of the tube. There should be no mistaking this situation, as the measured sound pressure levels may be greater than 20 dB different than the equalization levels. There are some probe systems that will suggest that the probe tube may be blocked when an inordinately low SPL is measured.

Occasionally, cerumen may only partially occlude the probe tube. This situation is more difficult to identify from the test results. It may cause only slight reduction in the overall SPL while causing significant reduction in the high frequency response. The situation is further complicated when the probe tube does not reach the cerumen during the unaided measure, but is pushed into the cerumen by the hearing aid or ear mold during the REAR measurement. The audiologist should make every effort to have the ear cleared of cerumen or other debris before completing REMs.

Figure 5–6 shows the REUR measured for a subject with the ear canal about 30% occluded by soft wax. The probe tube was placed against the cerumen for the first measure. The cerumen was then removed and the measure repeated with the probe tube at the same location. The levels measured before the cerumen was removed were less than the levels at the reference microphone. The two measurements differed by more than 20 dB.

Test Position

Testing should be completed with the subject at least 5 ft from the nearest wall. Closer distances can result in REMs being contaminated by reflections of the loudspeaker off of the walls. Depending on the acoustics of the room, it may be quite apparent from the test results that there is an error condition. The artifact may also be very subtle, affecting only a portion of the REIR curve.

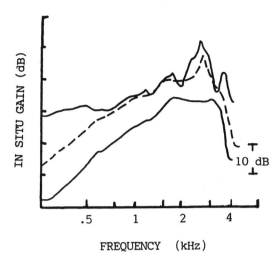

Figure 5-7. Effect of acoustic feedback on REMs. Upper solid line, volume control set just beyond the point of audible feedback; dashed line, volume control set just below the point of audible feedback; lower solid line, volume control set to a comfortable listening level.

Feedback

It can be frustrating to find that leakage created by a probe tube is sufficient to cause a hearing aid to feed back at the user's preferred volume setting. Audible feedback is easily detected by its sound or by the distortion products that it contributes to the probe tube measure (Fig. 5-7). Suboscillatory feedback is not as easily noted since squealing is absent. Attempts to reduce the hearing aid gain just below the point of audible feedback often leave the hearing aid unstable. The wearer of the hearing aid may notice that the sound quality is harsh while the presence of sharp peaks in the probe measure is confirmation (Fig. 5-7). If one or more spikes are noted in the response, the hearing aid volume should be reduced and the measurement repeated. The presence of oscillatory acoustic feedback will cause severe aberrations of the REAR and should be readily apparent under this condition. In either case, feedback renders the test results invalid.

Head Movement

Any movement of the subject during REMs can invalidate the results. Yet many individuals have difficulty remaining still for the brief period when the stimulus is presented. Tecca[39] described several types of subject movements that are encountered clinically. It is essential that the tester visually monitor subjects during testing to ensure that they remain still. While errors will occur with any equalization method, these errors can be minimized if an "on-line" reference microphone is used. Since the reference microphone is constantly making real-time adjustments for changes in the sound pressure level, it can compensate for minor movements.

Earmold Placement

Failure to seat the earmold or hearing aid shell adequately in the subject's ear will result in decreased low frequency gain due to unintentional venting (Fig.

5–4). This problem often occurs when an inexperienced tester is afraid that inserting the earmold or shell will drag the probe tube too deeply into the ear canal and touch the eardrum. It may also occur with a very tight earmold or hearing aid shell that is difficult to insert. In either case, the result is an invalid probe tube measure. The tester should always insert the earmold prior to testing so that a feel can be obtained for the way it inserts and how it appears when properly seated. It is then much easier to judge the adequacy of the earmold placement when it is inserted on top of the probe tube.

Probe Tube Insertion Depth

The probe tube should be inserted to a depth that is at least equal to the length of the hearing aid–earmold canal plus an additional 5 mm.[48] Artifacts may be present in the measured response if the tip of the probe tube is closer to the sound outlet of the hearing aid. It is equally important that the probe tube remain in the same position for REUR and REAR measurements. Hawkins and Mueller[7] presented very convincing data on the large errors that are observed when the probe tube position varies significantly between tests. Furthermore, Dirks and Kincaid[2] showed that the most accurate and stable results are obtained when the tip of the probe tube is located within 6–8 mm of the tympanic membrane when making probe tube measurements between 250 and 6000 Hz.

Conclusion

Probe tube measurements offer a powerful and versatile method for verifying hearing aid performance. Properly used, they enable a dispenser to assess accurately the adequacy of most any hearing aid fitting. Improperly used, they lead to significant clinical error.

An exercise to demonstrate the magnitude of clinical error has been used by the author during inservice training of audiologists. Each member of a group is instructed to measure the REIR of a hearing aid on the same ear of the same subject. The audiologists are instructed to make the measure in the manner routinely used clinically. Variations occur in nearly every conceivable test parameter with the expected large variation in REIR. It seems incredible that such variability really can occur for tests performed on the same ear with the same hearing aid. Even greater variation would be expected if the measurements were made at different facilities with different equipment.

The important message of this exercise is not that there is only one correct way to make REMs. Rather, it is that a consistent method should be used in order to make meaningful interpretations of the data. As noted previously, there is currently an ANSI working group developing a standard for probe tube measurements. However, until this is available it is essential that audiologists consistently use a protocol such as described in this chapter. Additionally, it is important to document variations in the "standard" protocol necessary in specific cases.

It is equally important that the hearing aid control settings be documented for each test. These include the volume setting, the settings of all potentiometers, and the vent characteristics. Future adjustments of the hearing aid are greatly facilitated by careful documentation.

This chapter has focused on use of REIG measurements. It is important to recognize that this is only one type of real ear response. Probe tube measurements may be used in verifying the output of hearing aids[5,38,46] or in measuring the response characteristics of assistive listening devices.[5,6,38] It is encouraging that probe tube measurements offer an extremely flexible technique that should continue to be appropriate for future generations of hearing aids.

Acknowledgments

I sincerely thank Martie Ormsby and G.N. Danavox, Inc., for providing financial support essential to completing this manuscript. It would not have been possible to take the time away from my practice to write this chapter without their assistance. I am grateful to Kelly Wenzler for helping to identify suitable case studies and for preparing all of the figures and to Susan Duly for editing and modifying the figures. I also thank Michael Valente, Ph.D., Daniel Orchik, Ph.D., and an anonymous reviewer for the time they spent reading this chapter and the many helpful suggestions they offered.

References

1. Dillon H, Murray N: Accuracy of twelve methods for estimating the real ear gain of hearing aids. *Ear Hear* 1987; 8:2–11.
2. Dirks DD, Kincaid GE: Basic acoustic considerations of ear canal probe measurements. *Ear Hear* 1987; 8:60–67.
3. Feigin JA, Nelson-Barlow NL, Stelmachowicz PG: The effect of reference microphone placement on sound pressure levels at an ear level hearing aid microphone. *Ear Hear* 1990; 11:321–326.
4. Harford ER: A new clinical technique for verification of hearing aid response. *Arch Otolaryngol* 1981; 107:461–468.
5. Hawkins DB: Clinical ear canal probe tube measurements. *Ear Hear* 1987; 8:74–81.
6. Hawkins DB: Assessment of FM systems with an ear canal probe tube microphone system. *Ear Hear* 1987; 8:301–303.
7. Hawkins DB, Mueller HG: Some variables affecting the accuracy of probe tube microphone measurements. *Hear Instrum* 1986; 37(1):8–12, 49.
8. Ickes MA, Hawkins DB, Cooper WA: Effect of reference microphone location and loudspeaker azimuth on probe tube microphone measurements. *J Am Acad Audiol* 1991; 2:156–163.
9. Killion MC, Revit LJ: Insertion gain repeatability versus loudspeaker location: You want me to put my loudspeaker W-H-E-R-E? *Ear Hear* 1987; 8:68-73.
10. Mason D, Popelka GR: Comparison of hearing-aid gain using functional, coupler, and probe-tube measurements. *J Speech Hear Res* 1986; 29:218–226.
11. Moskal NL, Goldstein DP: Probe tube systems: Effects of equalization on real ear insertion and aided gain. *Ear Hear* 1992; 13:46–54.
12. Preves DA: Some issues in utilizing probe tube microphone systems. *Ear Hear* 1987; 8:82–88.
13. Preves DA, Sullivan RF: Methods of sound field equalization for real ear measurements with probe microphones. *Hear Instrum* 1987; 38(1):16–20.
14. Preves DA, Beck LB, Burnett ED, et al.: Input stimuli for obtaining frequency responses of automatic gain control hearing aids. *J Speech Hear Res* 1989; 32:189–194.
15. Ringdahl A, Leijon A: The reliability of insertion gain measurements using probe microphones in the ear canal. *Scand Audiol* 1984; 13:173–178.

16. Shotland LI, Hecox KE: The effect of probe tube reference placement on sound pressure level variability. *Ear Hear* 1990; 11:306–309.
17. Stelmachowicz PG, Lewis DE: Some theoretical considerations concerning the relationship between functional gain and insertion gain. *J Speech Hear Res* 1988; 31:491–496.
18. Stelmachowicz PG, Lewis DE, Seewald RC, et al.: Complex and pure-tone signals in the evaluation of hearing-aid characteristics. *J Speech Hear Res* 1990; 33:380–385.
19. Tecca JE: Insertion gain measures in nonstandard rooms. Presentation at the annual convention of the American Speech-Language-Hearing Association, 1987, New Orleans, LA.
20. Tecca JE, Woodford CM: A comparison of functional gain and insertion gain in clinical practice. *Hear J* 1987; 40(6):23–27.
21. Tecca JE, Woodford CM, Kee DK: Variability of insertion-gain measurements. *Hear J* 1987; 40(2):18–20.
22. Valente M, Valente M, Goebel J: Reliability and intersubject variability of the real ear unaided response. *Ear Hear* 1991; 12:216–220.
23. Valente M, Meister M, Smith P, et al.: Intratester test–retest reliability of insertion gain measures. *Ear Hear* 1990; 11:181–184.
24. Zemplenyi J, Dirks D, Gilman S: Probe-determined hearing-aid gain compared to functional and coupler gains. *J Speech Hear Res* 1985; 28:394–404.
25. Cranmer KS: 1992 Hearing Instruments dispenser survey results. *Hear Instrum* 1992; 43(6):8–9, 12–15.
26. Schweitzer HC, Sullivan RF, Beck L, et al.: Developing a consensus for "real ear" hearing instrument terms. *Hear Instrum* 1990; 41(2):28, 46.
27. Bratt GW, Sammeth CA: Clinical implications of prescriptive formulas for hearing aid selection, in Studebaker GA, Bess FH, Beck LB (eds): *Vanderbilt Hearing-Aid Report II*. Parkton, MD: York Press, 1991, pp 23–33.
28. Hawkins DB, Haskell GB: A comparison of functional gain and 2 cc coupler gain. *J Speech Hear Disord* 1982; 47:71–76.
29. Schum DJ: Inter-subject variability effects on coupler to real ear correction curves. *Hear Instrum* 1986; 37(3):25–26.
30. Bentler RA, Pavlovic CV: Transer functions and correction factors used in hearing aid evaluation and research. *Ear Hear* 1989; 10:58–63.
31. Burnett ED, Beck LB: A correction for converting 2 cm^3 coupler responses to insertion responses for custom in-the-ear nondirectional hearing aids. *Ear Hear* 1987; 8:89–94.
32. Lybarger SF, Teder H: 2 cc coupler curves to insertion gain curves: Calculated and experimental results. *Hear Instrum* 1986; 37(11):36–37, 40.
33. Mueller HG: Individualizing the order of custom hearing aids. *Hear Instrum* 1989; 40(2):18–22.
34. Punch J, Chi C, Patterson J: A recommended protocol for prescriptive use of target gain rules. *Hear Instrum* 1990; 41(4):12–19.
35. Tecca JE: *Precision Prescription*. Stowe, OH: Audiotechnica, 1989.
36. Valente M, Valente M, Vass W: Selecting an appropriate matrix for ITE/ITC hearing instruments. *Hear Instrum* 1990; 41(4):20–24.
37. Frattali CM: Quality assurance today: Learning the basics. *ASHA* 1990; 32:39–40.
38. Tecca JE: Clinical application of real-ear probe tube measurement, in Sandlin RE (ed): *Handbook of Hearing Aid Amplification, Volume II, Clinical Considerations and Fitting Practices*. Boston: College-Hill Press, 1990, pp 225–255.
39. Tecca JE: Reliability of insertion gain measures. *Semin Hear* 1991; 12:15–25.
40. Hawkins DB, Mueller HG: Procedural considerations in probe-microphone measurements, in Mueller HG, Hawkins DB, Northern JL (eds): *Probe Microphone Measurements Hearing Aid Selection and Assessment*. San Diego, CA: Singular Publishing Group, Inc., 1992, pp 67–90.
41. American Speech-Language-Hearing Association Ad Hoc Committee on Advances in Clinical Practice: External auditory canal examination and cerumen management. *ASHA* 1992; 34:22–24.
42. Roeser RJ, Adams RM, Rosland P, et al.: A safe and effective procedure for cerumen management. *Audiol Today* 1992; 4(3):26–30.
43. Kruger B: An update on the external ear resonance in infants and young children. *Ear Hear* 1987; 8:333–336.
44. Bentler RA: External ear resonance characteristics in children. *J Speech Hear Dis* 1989; 54:264–268.
45. Killion MC, Monser EL: CORFIG: Coupler response for flat insertion gain, in Studebaker GA, Hochberg I (eds): *Acoustical Factors Affecting Hearing Aid Performance*. Baltimore: University Park Press, 1980, pp 147–168.
46. Sullivan RF: Aided SSPL90 response in the real ear: A safe estimate. *Hear Instrum* 1987; 38:36.

47. Heide J: Testing electroacoustic performance of ASP and nonlinear hearing aids. *Hear J* 1987; 41(4):33–35.
48. Burkhard MD, Sachs RM: Sound pressure in insert earphone couplers and real ears. *J Speech Hear Res* 1977; 20:799–807.

6

Use of Paired Comparisons in Hearing Aid Fittings

FRANCIS K. KUK

The Need to Go beyond Prescriptive Formulae

The use of prescriptive formulae to specify frequency-gain characteristics of a hearing aid simplifies hearing aid selection. Satisfaction is assumed when the measured gain of the hearing aid matches the gain prescribed by the formula. Knowledge of individual preference and psychophysical skills are not required or needed when using this selection process. An implicit requirement for the use of prescriptive formulae is that audiological indices (e.g., thresholds, most comfortable listening levels [MCL], and loudness discomfort levels [LDL]) can be measured reliably and accurately. Furthermore, when predicting 2 cc coupler frequency-gain characteristics, the formulae require that the individual wearer has ear canal characteristics that resemble those of the average wearer.

Unfortunately, neither of these requirements can be met all the time. For example, several investigators have shown that auditory thresholds could vary from 4 to 9 dB upon retest.[1,2] Suprathreshold loudness judgments (i.e., MCLs, LDLs) can be even more variable depending on instructions, stimulus type, and psychophysical method employed to measure such indices.[2,3] Fluctuations in the listener's internal criteria could also affect the reliability of such indices. Additionally, the presence of a fluctuating loss (e.g., Ménière's disease) or of an ear with atypical middle ear resonance and impedance characteristics may result in the prescribed frequency-gain response as being inappropriate for the hearing aid wearer.[4] These observations suggest that, unless one can control the intra- and intersubject variability seen in audiological measurements and account for the individual differences when specifying frequency-gain response, there is the potential that the prescribed frequency-gain response may be inappropriate for the wearer.

Assuming that audiologic indices can be defined accurately and that target gain may be achieved, individual frequency-gain responses specified by group data (as in the prescriptive approach) may not be satisfactory to all hearing aid wearers. For example, Neuman et al.[5] showed that seven of eight hearing aid wearers preferred frequency-gain responses that were different from those prescribed when using an MCL approach.[6] Kuk and Pape[7] reported that 18 of 20 subjects selected frequency-gain responses that deviated from National Acoustic Laboratories' (NAL) prescription.[8] On the other hand, Byrne and Cotton[9] reported that only 10%–20% of their hearing aid wearers selected a frequency-gain response that deviated significantly from the NAL prescription. These observations suggest that additional measures are needed to verify the appropriateness of the prescribed frequency-gain responses in order to ensure maximum wearer satisfaction.

Alternative methods to select frequency-gain response on a hearing aid may be necessary. There is increasing evidence that hearing aid wearers prefer unique frequency-gain responses from their hearing aids when they listen in various acoustic environments and/or when they use different criteria to select preferred frequency-gain responses.

For example, Byrne[10] revealed that preferred frequency-gain response that was selected with a criterion of "pleasantness" was different from that selected based on the judgment of "intelligibility." Kuk[11] demonstrated that the preferred insertion gain for listening to one's own vocalization is different from listening to externally presented stimuli. Tecca and Goldstein[12] showed that hearing impaired listeners preferred less low frequency gain from a hearing aid as the stimulus level was increased. Presently, no guidelines are available to specify how these frequency-gain responses should be prescribed. The concerned clinician needs to ensure that the measured frequency-gain response provides optimal performance under these special listening situations or that the frequency-gain response can be modified to accommodate the needs in these situations.

Advances in technology improve the sophistication of current hearing aids. The newer compression hearing aids and those using digital signal processing techniques promise new and better ways to serve individuals with hearing impairment. Unlike linear hearing aids with which there are at least several generally accepted approaches for their fitting, there are only a few manufacturers of nonlinear hearing aids that provide guidelines to clinicians on fitting these devices. Unfortunately, methods to evaluate the adequacy of the manufacturers' guidelines or of the performance of these devices are lacking. As in traditional linear hearing aids, verification of optimal settings on these devices is necessary to ensure success with the special circuits. One approach that can help to verify the appropriateness of the selected hearing aid settings and can potentially be an alternative approach for hearing aid selection is the paired comparison technique.

What Is Paired Comparison?

The method of paired comparison was attributed to Fechner as a data collection technique for the study of sensory perception.[13] In this method, an experimental subject makes binary decisions on a number of stimuli that are presented in pairs. The criteria of judgment are usually set by the experimenter. The

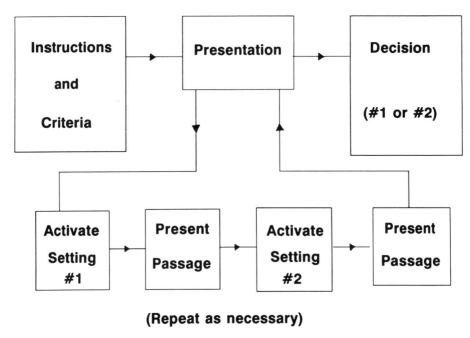

Figure 6-1. Sequence of events in a single paired comparison trial.

subject's task is to indicate which one of the two comparison stimulus intervals meets the experimenter's criterion. In hearing aid research, the results of the comparison may show the relative "perceptual" distances among a list of items being compared,[14] or the comparison may show the relative ranking of the comparison hearing aids [15] Moreover, the comparison may result in a recommendation of the best hearing aid.[16] Finally, a combination of settings on a programmable hearing aid may be recommended based on the results of this process.[5,7,17]

Figure 6-1 is a block diagram representation of the sequence of events involved in a paired comparison trial. Two settings (e.g., different low frequency gain) on a programmable hearing aid are compared. There are three important components in a single paired comparison trial. They include the Instructions, the Presentation, and the Decision. In the Instructional stage, the clinician explains the task and specifies the criterion for judgment to the listener. For example, one may use the following instructions for selection of hearing aid setting that maximizes speech intelligibility.

> You will listen to a short passage played back twice, each time with a different hearing aid. As the passage is played back, I will indicate to you which is hearing aid No. 1 and which is hearing aid No. 2. After you have listened through both hearing aids, you must indicate which hearing aid (1 or 2) yields more intelligible speech. By that I mean the hearing aid with which you can understand more of the spoken passage. You must indicate one preference even though you may find these two hearing aids to sound very similar. I will gladly repeat the presentation if you so desire. Do you have any question?

During the Presentation stage, the clinician adjusts the hearing aid to the appropriate settings for comparison. These two combinations of settings are stored in the temporary memory of the programmable hearing aid. The clinician activates one memory of the hearing aid, alerts the listener of hearing aid No. 1, and plays back the stimulus. Typically, short (between 10 and 20 seconds) discourse passages can be used as stimulus for comparison. Afterwards, the clinician sets the hearing aid to the other memory, announces hearing aid No. 2, and plays back the same passage for comparison. This process is repeated until the listener is ready to make a decision on the hearing aid.

The listener must make a preference judgment on the two hearing aid settings in the Decision stage. He or she must decide if hearing aid No. 1 or hearing aid No. 2 meets the criterion of better speech intelligibility regardless of the similarity or dissimilarity between the two comparison hearing aids. Responses like "no difference" and "they both sound good/bad" are not acceptable. If such were the response, the listener will be reinstructed, and the same stimulus will be presented again.

Although the performance of hearing aids selected using paired comparison procedures has been favorable, absolute performance is not measured and thus its performance is not guaranteed. The hearing aid settings that are selected using paired comparisons only reflect the listener's relative judgment for the settings available for comparison. Maximum satisfaction is guaranteed only if at least one of the available combinations results in maximum satisfaction. Direct measurement of listener satisfaction with the selected hearing aid settings may be needed in order to determine absolute performance.

History of the Use of Paired Comparison in Hearing Aid Selection

A requirement for using paired comparison to evaluate hearing aids in the clinic is the ability to switch rapidly among various electroacoustic settings (or hearing aids) for comparison. This was impossible using conventional hearing aids without undue delay during the switching process. Zerlin[18] is credited for first proposing a manageable way of performing paired comparison.

In this method, speech was recorded through two hearing aids each coupled to separate couplers. Output from the couplers was recorded on two separate tracks of a magnetic tape. Different pairs of hearing aids were connected to the couplers, and processed speech was recorded in the sequence in which they would be presented during the evaluation. The output from the tape recordings was presented to the listeners through earphones. Listeners switched between the two tracks of the tape and indicated preferences for one of the two taped-speech segments. This was used to indicate their preference for the hearing aid that was used to process the speech signal. Figure 6–2 shows a schematic diagram of how stimuli were recorded and played back in the earlier paired comparison trials. This approach of recording and then playing back the stimuli was improved by subsequent investigators. For example, a manikin (KEMAR) with a Zwislocki coupler was used to record in the sound field in order to approximate the acoustic effects associated with the head and body

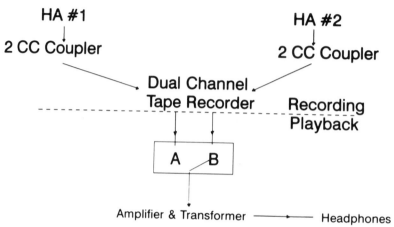

Figure 6–2.   Instrumentations involved in original paired comparison trials.

baffle and ear canal response.[15] Hearing aid receivers and/or earmolds were used as output transducers in more recent studies.[19]

Although this approach allows rapid comparison between speech processed by different hearing aid settings, this is impractical for clinical use because of the labor involved in the recording process, the limitations in the number and variations of hearing aid settings that can be compared, the time involved in clinical comparison, and the difficulty of transferring the results of the paired comparison to commercial hearing aid use. Paired comparison was primarily used as a research tool.

Clinical pairwise quality judgments have been made with a master hearing aid.[20,21] Using this approach, the clinician adjusts the settings on a master hearing aid (the size of a portable audiometer), and speech (taped or live) is delivered through headphones to the listeners, who then indicate their preference as the settings are adjusted and presented in pairs. The setting that is preferred will be recommended. Although the labor involved in recording speech stimuli is eliminated, accurate simulation of true hearing aid performance in commercial hearing aids is still a major difficulty with the master hearing aid approach. Guidelines to vary the settings systematically were also lacking.

Levitt et al.[17] were the first to vary the frequency-gain responses systematically on a wearable master hearing aid using an adaptive procedure (the simplex procedure). In this procedure, listeners identified nonsense syllables while wearing a master hearing aid that was adjusted to various settings.

Through selective testing of choice electroacoustic settings, the simplex procedure converges at a combination of settings on the master hearing aid that yields a maximum speech understanding score. Although the method had significant appeal, it was not adopted for clinical use because of its complexity, inefficiency, and dependence on a computer. Several hours were needed to select a frequency-gain response using the simplex procedure.

Neuman et al.[5] modified the simplex procedure to incorporate the use of pairwise comparison. Rather than comparing speech recognition scores among the selected settings, the modified simplex procedure used subjective judgment of relative intelligibility as a criterion and allowed systematic pairwise comparison of settings. These modifications substantially reduced the time to select a frequency-gain response.

The advent of digitally programmable hearing aids facilitates the use of paired comparisons in a clinical environment. Four features of programmable hearing aids contributed significantly in this regard. The readers are warned that not all programmable hearing aids share all four features. The wide range of electroacoustic adjustments on some programmable hearing aids allows them to be viewed as stand alone wearable master hearing aids and be used for a wide range of listening conditions and for a wide range of hearing loss configurations.

In several programmable hearing aids, switching of settings can be performed rapidly through the use of a programming cord or via a remote control device using frequency-modulated (radio frequency and ultrasonic) signals. This allows rapid switching between comparison settings. The availability of multiple memories in some programmable hearing aids also facilitates comparison of frequency-gain responses in the clinic and in everyday listening situations. Although not widely available, some manufacturers of programmable hearing aids can interface their units directly to external computers so that paired comparison can be performed in an automatic manner. The computer controls for stimulus delivery, tracks responses, and adjusts settings on the hearing aid according to defined rules and algorithms. This could significantly reduce the time involved in the comparison and improve the reliability in which comparisons are made. Indeed, Kuk[22] demonstrated the feasibility of adapting the use of the modified simplex procedure to select frequency-gain responses for a commercially available programmable multimemory hearing aid.

Paired Comparison Techniques

Although paired comparison only involves binary decisions on pairs of stimuli, stimulus pairing (i.e., the manner in which the different settings are paired and compared) affects the information available from the comparison. The different strategies in which this technique has been used in hearing aid research include the round-robin tournament, single- and double-elimination tournaments, simple up–down procedure, and the modified simplex procedure. Although these strategies can be performed manually, the use of a computer (with custom software) could greatly facilitate comparison.

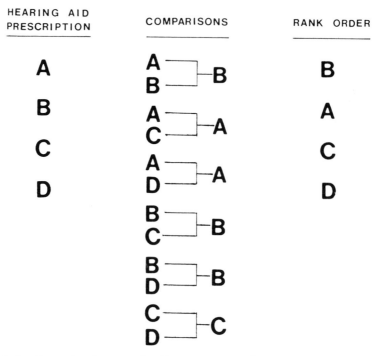

Figure 6–3.   Example of a round-robin tournament. Letters A–D represent four different hearing aids each fit using specific prescriptive formulae.

ROUND-ROBIN TOURNAMENT

The object of a round-robin tournament is to rank order the available hearing aids or different settings within a hearing aid based on some defined criteria. In this approach, every hearing aid (or combinations of settings) is paired and compared with every other hearing aid (or settings). For N hearing aids or combinations of settings, a round-robin tournament involves $N(N − 1)/2$ pairs of comparisons. As a result, hearing aids are ranked according to the frequency in which they are chosen. Figure 6–3 illustrates the manner in which hearing aids containing the necessary settings appropriate to achieve one of four prescriptive formulae (i.e., A, B, C, and D) are compared in a round-robin tournament. Subjects may be asked to judge which one of two hearing aid settings provides clearer speech or better intelligibility (or any other criteria) as they listen to discourse passages presented in a noise background. The result is a rank order of hearing aid prescriptions based on subject preference.

The advantage of the round-robin tournament is its ability to rank order hearing aids. In addition to selecting the best hearing aid (or setting) among the comparisons, the round-robin tournament also allows the study of relationships among electroacoustic parameters and their relative contribution to the perceptual process. For example, Punch et al.[14] used this approach to study factors governing subjective preference for hearing aid processed speech.

From a clinical standpoint, the round-robin tournament may be practical only if (1) specific ranking information is needed among the comparison hearing aids and (2) the number of comparison hearing aids (or settings) is small (e.g., under four). Other methods may be more efficient to verify the appropriateness of a selected frequency-gain response. For example, Neuman et al.[5] reported that it required an average of 83.8 minutes to complete a round-robin tournament, but only 8 minutes to complete a modified simplex procedure when the same combinations of settings (total of 25) are compared.

SINGLE-ELIMINATION TOURNAMENT

The object of an elimination tournament is to determine which one of several hearing aids (or combinations of settings within a hearing aid) is more preferable than the others. In this approach, each hearing aid is first compared with one other hearing aid. Winners of each pair of comparison are further compared several times to result in an overall winner. For N hearing aids where N is an integer power of 2, there will be N − 1 pair of comparison hearing aids.

An example of a single-elimination tournament is shown in Figure 6–4. Numbers identify the hearing aids in the comparison. A hearing aid will be eliminated if it loses any comparison. However, a hearing aid can only become the winner when it has won M rounds of comparison where 2^M equals N, the total number of hearing aids. For example, in Figure 6–4, three rounds of comparisons are needed to determine a winner when $8(2^3)$ hearing aids are

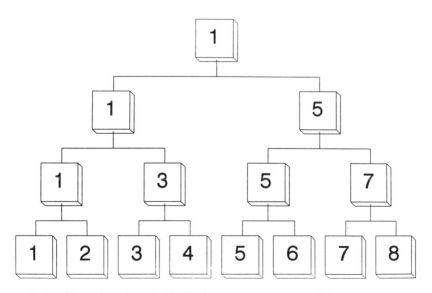

Figure 6–4. Example of a single-elimination tournament. Numbers 1–8 represent eight different hearing aids for comparison.

compared. No ranking information is available from the results of an elimination tournament.

The manner in which hearing aids are paired in a single-elimination tournament is important. Comparison hearing aids can be paired either by random assignment or according to some seeding rules. A good seeding rule is to pair hearing aids with greater difference in their frequency-gain characteristics. Variability in the selection will be increased if hearing aids with similar electroacoustic characteristics are paired.[23,24]

DOUBLE-ELIMINATION TOURNAMENT

When two hearing aids with relatively similar characteristics are compared, it is possible that the "better" hearing aid is eliminated because of random error. To safeguard a "good" hearing aid from being eliminated in the early rounds of comparison, Studebaker and his colleagues[19,25] proposed the use of a double-elimination tournament as a means to compare hearing aids (or combinations of settings within a single hearing aid). Instead of being eliminated after only one loss, each hearing aid has to lose twice before it is eliminated from the tournament. Higher test–retest reliability was reported with the double-elimination tournament than with the single-elimination tournament.[25]

Figure 6–5 illustrates a double-elimination tournament. Assume again that the same eight hearing aids are compared. Winners of each round of comparison will be further compared within the Winners' bracket. On the other hand, losers in the Winners' bracket are compared with winners in the Losers'

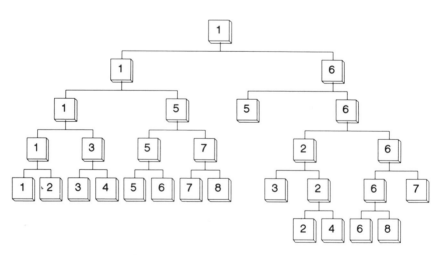

Winners' Bracket   **Losers' Bracket**

Figure 6–5. Example of a double-elimination tournament. Numbers 1–8 represent eight different hearing aids for comparison.

bracket. The winner in each bracket is compared one last time to determine the overall winner (i.e., hearing aid No. 1). There are 2(N − 1) pairs of comparisons for N hearing aids, where N is an integer power of 2.

SIMPLE UP–DOWN PROCEDURE

The "goodness" of the verified settings using a round-robin or an elimination tournament depends on the "goodness" of all settings selected for comparison. One may need to compare with a large number of settings in order to ensure that a recommended setting is indeed the best setting available on the hearing aid. Because of potentially large numbers of settings that need to be compared and the time constraints in a clinical setting, the use of round-robin and elimination tournaments may not be practical.

An adaptive procedure is an estimation procedure in which a listener's response on a test trial dictates the direction of stimulus change in the next trial. This helps to focus comparisons to only those settings contributing to the estimation and allows one to fine tune a selected setting without testing a large number of settings. As in all estimation procedures, one assumes the existence of only one combination of hearing aid settings that will optimize listener preference. The goal of the adaptive procedure is to estimate "that setting" in the shortest amount of time while satisfying the clinician's and/or the hearing aid wearer's criteria.

The simple up–down procedure is an adaptive procedure that allows verification (and fine tuning) of settings in one dimension. In using this procedure, the clinician first estimates the initial hearing aid setting that the listener may find most satisfactory. This initial setting is the *initial estimate*. This initial setting can be based on any prescriptive formula, on manufacturer recommendations, or on clinician intuition. When the method of paired comparison is used, this initial estimate is compared with another setting that differs from the initial estimate on the same adjustable parameter of the hearing aid. A selected criterion (e.g., relative intelligibility) is used for comparison between two settings. Any acoustic stimuli can be used for judgment (e.g., discourse presented in noise). Comparisons continue with different settings that are varied in a systematic manner until the criterion to terminate comparisons is met.

Figure 6–6 is an illustration of a simple up–down procedure to determine optimal low frequency setting on a hearing aid. Assume that the initial estimate corresponds to a low frequency setting at interval 3. The listener compares this setting with interval 4. The direction of comparison during the first trial is arbitrary. The change in adjustment between these settings is termed a *step*, and the magnitude of such change is termed the *step size*. Assume that the listener prefers the setting with more low frequency gain (i.e., interval 4). This indicates that the direction of the next comparison should be in the direction of more low frequency gain (i.e., intervals 4 and 5 will be compared). A comparison in the same direction is termed a *run* (trials 1 and 2). If during the second trial the listener prefers less low frequency gain (i.e., interval 4 over

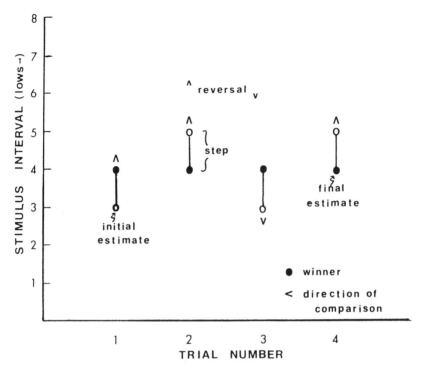

Figure 6–6. Example of a simple up–down procedure to verify or select optimal low frequency setting on a hearing aid.

interval 5), a *reversal* (in the direction of preference) has occurred. In Figure 6–6, reversals occurred after trials 2, 3, and 4. Although one can continue the comparison indefinitely, comparison is terminated after the third reversal, with interval 4 being the listener's preferred low frequency setting on the hearing aid. This preferred setting is termed the *final estimate*. In this case, the initial estimation of optimal low frequency gain differs from the listener's preference by one interval.

The simple up–down procedure differs from the round-robin and elimination tournaments in the manner in which settings are selected for comparison and the number of comparisons. Assume that eight intervals on the low frequency dimension are compared. The round-robin tournament requires all eight intervals to be compared with each other to result in 28 pairs of comparisons. Seven pairs of comparison are needed in the single-elimination tournament- and 14 pairs are needed in the double-elimination tournament. In the simple up–down procedure illustrated previously, only four comparisons were needed to estimate the preferred low frequency gain.

It is important to note that whereas all intervals are compared in the round-robin and elimination tournaments, only the intervals near the final estimate are compared several times in the simple up–down procedure. Intervals 1, 2, 6, 7, and 8 were not compared. This observation, however, is only true when the initial estimate is close to the final estimate and when the listener is consistent in his or her judgments. More comparisons will be needed if these assumptions are not met.

Because not all settings are evaluated in the simple up–down procedure, an occasional listener not showing strong preference for a particular setting may reveal random preference during the evaluation and lead to errors in the estimation procedure. The round-robin and elimination tournaments, because of their sampling of all comparison settings, will not be as affected by homogeneous preference.

There are several issues to consider when using a simple up–down procedure. These issues are fully discussed by Levitt[26–28] but will be briefly reviewed for completeness.

Choice of Initial Estimate.   In theory, the initial estimate should be as similar to the final estimate as possible in order to ensure maximum efficiency. The disadvantage of a dissimilar initial estimate is that it will require more comparisons in order to reach the final estimate. The advantage, however, is that these estimates may enable listeners to discriminate better the differences between stimulus intervals and to be better familiarized with the test routine. Levitt[26–28] recommended that data obtained from the first run should not be analyzed in order to minimize bias resulting from an inappropriate initial estimate.

Different approaches have been attempted to determine the best initial estimate. For example, Neuman et al.[5] used a frequency-gain response that placed the average speech spectrum at the user's MCL as the initial estimate. Kuk and Pape[7] used the frequency-gain response recommended by NAL-R as the initial estimate. However, both studies showed that the final estimates deviated from the initial estimates for a majority of subjects. Furthermore, the listening conditions, types of stimuli, and criteria used to make the comparison can alter the final estimate. In other words, there may not be one fixed optimal initial estimate for all test conditions. Clinicians who use this technique for the first time may consider following the approach of Leijon et al.[29] and Kuk and Pape[7] by using frequency-gain response recommended by NAL-R as the initial estimate. After trying this on a few listeners (perhaps 10–20), it should become possible for clinicians to choose initial estimates based on their knowledge of the final estimates obtained under the same listening condition.

An alternative approach is to compare several distinct settings (less than four) on the hearing aid using a tournament strategy. The winner of the comparisons may be used as the initial estimate for selecting the best setting available on the hearing aid.

Step Size.   The ideal step size for statistical efficiency depends on the consistency of the listener's response and the accuracy of the preceding estimates. Theoretically, a small step size should be used if the listener is consistent in his or her response and if the estimate is close to the final estimate. When using small step sizes, the precision of the estimation is increased, but at the expense of increasing evaluation time. A large step size allows one to converge at the final estimate quickly, but at the expense of losing estimation precision. In practice, one would not know how consistent a listener is until after the comparison has started. This suggests that the use of a fixed step size may not be the most efficient.

Robbins and Monro[30] recommended starting with a large step size (arriving at the vicinity of the final estimate sooner) and gradually reducing the step size as comparison continues. Mathematically, the step size on run N is d/N, where d is the step size used on the first run. For example, the step size for the third run may be reduced to one interval if the step size for the first run was set at three intervals. In practice, this rule may be difficult to implement on commercial hearing aids because most can vary only in limited, discrete intervals on each parameter. A compromise may be to start the first run with a step size of two intervals and reduce it to one interval after the first reversal.

Termination Rule.   Rules to terminate an adaptive procedure are necessary after the clinician is reasonably certain that the final estimate reflects the listener's preference. In the example provided earlier, three reversals were required to terminate the comparison. In theory, one can terminate a comparison after the first reversal. However, the accuracy of the estimation may not be acceptable. Precision and reliability in estimation improve as the number of reversals are increased. However, the time involved in the estimation will be increased also. In practice, three reversals can be used with fair reliability.[5,7]

The simple up–down procedure, in its various forms, has been used to estimate thresholds, to estimate most comfortable listening level,[31] and to select and verify low frequency gain on a noise reduction hearing aid.[32]

MODIFIED SIMPLEX PROCEDURE

The simplex procedure was originally proposed by Box[33] as a means to optimize productivity. It was adapted by Levitt et al.[17] and later modified by Neuman et al.[5] as an alternative to select the optimal settings on more than one parameter on a wearable master hearing aid. Like the simple up–down procedure, the modified simplex procedure assumes the existence of one and only one combination of settings on a hearing aid that optimizes listening under a specific condition.

Like the simple up–down procedure, the process starts with an estimation of the listener's preferred settings on the hearing aid (prescriptive phase to determine initial estimate). This combination is compared with other combinations of settings in a systematic manner (adaptive phase to determine final estimate) until the termination rules are met. The goal of the comparison is to select a combination of settings that reflects the listener's preference for the listening condition.

Figure 6–7 shows the hypothetical coupler frequency-gain responses of a programmable hearing aid (Fig. 6–7A) and its matrix representation (Fig. 6–7B). The high and low frequency parameters can be represented as different dimensions on the two-dimensional matrix. Each cell on the matrix represents a unique combination of high and low frequency gain. For example, in Figure 6–7, cell (2L, 2H) represents the frequency response with a low frequency

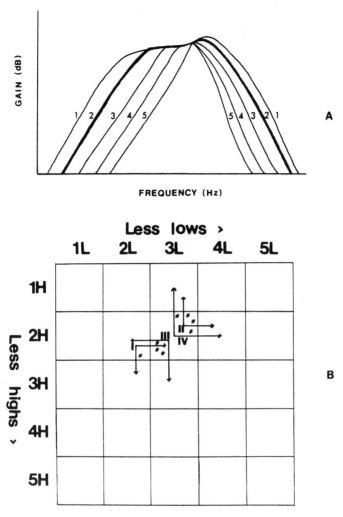

Figure 6–7. Example of a modified simplex procedure to verify or select optimal low and high frequency settings on a hearing aid. (**a**) Hypothetical coupler responses; (**b**) a matrix representation of the comparison.

setting of 2 and a high frequency setting of 2 (darkened curve). A total of 5 × 5 or 25 combinations of electroacoustic settings are available for comparison.

Assume that cell (2L, 2H) represents the initial estimate. Comparisons will be performed in the low and high frequency dimensions with the initial estimate as the vertex of the comparison. The direction of the first comparison can be arbitrary (i.e., cells with more or less gain can be chosen for comparison). In this example, we choose cells with less gain. In the low frequency region, one compares (2L, 2H) with (3L, 2H), and in the high frequency region one compares (2L, 2H) with (2L, 3H). Assume that the listener prefers less low frequency gain and more high frequency gain. That is, cell (3L, 2H) is preferred over cell (2L, 2H), and cell (2L, 2H) is preferred over cell (2L, 3H). The winning cells are indicated by a number sign (#).

The vertex of the next comparison will be formed by coordinates of the winning cells. Because "3L" and "2H" are the winning intervals in the low and high frequency regions, respectively, cell (3L, 2H) becomes the new vertex. The direction of the new comparison is with cells with even less low frequency gain (i.e., 4L) and greater high frequency gain (i.e., 1H). The comparison cells will be (4L, 2H) and (3L, 1H). Assuming that the listener selects cell (3L, 2H) over cell (4L, 2H) and cell (3L, 2H) over cell (3L, 1H), the new vertex is again formed at cell (3L, 2H). However, the direction of the next comparison is reversed to cells with more low frequency gain and less high frequency gain. This is recorded as the first reversal.

As illustrated in Figure 6–7, the second reversal is encountered after the third comparison when cell (3L, 2H) is compared with cell (2L, 2H) in the low frequency region and cell (3L, 3H) in the high frequency region. The third reversal is encountered after the fourth comparison when cell (3L, 2H) is compared with cell (4L, 2H) in the low frequency region and cell (3L, 1H) in the high frequency region. If the termination rule is set at three reversals, the new vertex formed at cell (3L, 2H) will become the final estimate or preferred frequency-gain response for the listener.

This example shows a case in which all the comparison settings are within the range of values available on the specific instrument. For listeners who may prefer a parametric value that is beyond the range available on the instrument, Levitt[27] recommended that testing proceed with a value within the available range as if a reversal had occurred.

Issues that are important to consider in the simple up–down procedure are also important to consider in the modified simplex procedure. These issues include initial estimate, step size, and termination rules. An additional consideration in the modified simplex procedure is the optimal number of parameters to include in the comparison. Increasing the number of parameters to compare will increase the number of unique combinations of settings dramatically. In general, the number of combinations is given by N^m, where N is the number of stimulus intervals within a dimension and m is the number of dimensions. For example, if three dimensions each with five intervals are compared, a total of 125 (5^3) settings will be available for comparison. Although not all combinations are compared, it is inevitable that more comparisons are necessary as the number of dimensions are increased. To keep the number of comparisons manageable, a rule of thumb is to compare only those parameters whose optimal settings one cannot easily predict.

Similar to the simple up–down procedure, listeners who do not show a strong preference for only one combination of settings (i.e., multiple preferences or same preference for all settings) may exhibit random preference judgments during paired comparisons and lead to errors in the estimation process. A sampling of the listener's preference prior to using the modified simplex procedure may be helpful. Despite this potential limitation, Neuman et al.[5] and Kuk and Pape[7] failed to find any of their subjects (N = 8 and N = 20, respectively) who showed multiple preferences in their studies.

The modified simplex procedure yields a final estimate that agrees remarkably well with those selected with round-robin and double-elimination tournaments. Neuman et al.[5] showed that four of eight subjects participating in their study chose the same setting as the final estimate using the three procedures. The remaining subjects chose an adjacent cell as the final setting. Furthermore, an average of 8 minutes was required to complete a modified simplex procedure, but 36.3 minutes was necessary to complete a double-elimination tournament, and 83.8 minutes was necessary to complete a round-robin tournament. Based on the results of these studies, the modified simplex procedure may be the most efficient of the three procedures.

Advantages of the Paired Comparison Technique

The use of the paired comparison as a clinical tool to select hearing aid settings has been reported over the past 15 years.[14–16,19,25,34,35] It is generally agreed that this method provides a viable alternative with which to verify and select frequency-gain characteristics of hearing aids. Some of the advantages of paired comparison technique in relation to conventional methods are discussed in the following sections.

Greater Sensitivity

The most frequently cited advantage of paired comparison is its sensitivity over speech recognition tests in differentiating the improvements provided by settings of different amplification systems even when such differences are not apparent when using speech recognition tests.[12,15,16,18,34,36–38]

Studebaker et al.[19] compared the number of times a hearing aid was correctly selected in a paired comparison task with the absolute difference in word recognition scores between two comparison hearing aids. They reported that correct identification increased exponentially as the difference in mean word recognition scores between the two comparison hearing aids increased. For example, at a 0 dB signal-to-noise ratio (S/N), hearing impaired subjects required an 8% difference in word recognition scores between two comparison hearing aids in order to correctly select the one with better intelligibility in 75% of the comparisons. Normal hearing subjects require only a 3% difference in word recognition scores to achieve the same level of selection.

Byrne and colleagues[10,39,40] evaluated the sensitivity of paired comparison to differentiate frequency-gain responses that are more homogeneous in electroacoustic characteristics than those reported in earlier studies. Despite the homogeneity, these authors reported that 70%–80% of the comparisons showed a significant preference for one frequency-gain response, whereas few significant differences were observed when using speech recognition testing.

Equal or Greater Reliability

The reliability of the method of paired comparison, or the consistency with which subjects select a preferred hearing aid, is reportedly high. Zerlin[18] showed that 7 of 11 subjects ranked the same hearing aid first in both test and retest trials when using a paired comparison procedure. Studebaker et al.[16] revealed correlations (R) in excess of 0.70 for paired comparison data obtained across different subject populations and in different laboratory settings. For the same subjects, significantly lower correlations were obtained (between −0.40 to 0.70) on word recognition tests. This illustrates the relative consistency with which reliability data on paired comparison were obtained in different laboratories. Punch and Beck[41] and Punch and Parker[42] also showed higher reliability when using pairwise quality judgments in comparison with word recognition testing.

The reliability of paired comparison judgment may be affected by test conditions and choice of judgment criteria. For example, Punch[15] found that subjects were most reliable when male speech was used as the stimulus, whereas music yielded the least reliable selection. Punch and Howard[34] showed higher reliability when using clarity judgments of connected discourse presented in quiet than with intelligibility judgments of discourse presented in noise. Studebaker et al.[43] demonstrated higher reliability in intelligibility rankings at a 0 dB S/N ratio than at an S/N of +7. Kuk and Pape[7] reported similar findings.

Individuals with a hearing impairment may not be as reliable during paired comparison testing as normal hearing listeners. Studebaker et al.[19] compared the reliability of pairwise judgment of relative intelligibility and word recognition score (NU-6) between normal hearing and hearing impaired subjects. When paired comparison data were analyzed, 83% of normal hearing subjects and 54% of hearing impaired subjects ranked the same hearing aid first in both test and retest sessions. When data from word recognition tests were analyzed, 42% of normal hearing subjects and 49% of hearing impaired subjects ranked the same hearing aid first in both sessions. Schwartz et al.[44] also obtained similar findings. These data suggest that the reliability of paired comparison is as good as, if not better than, speech recognition.

Kuk and Pape[7] evaluated the within-session and between-session reliabilities in which elderly hearing aid wearers (N = 20) selected their preferred frequency-gain response using pairwise clarity judgment of discourse passages as the criterion. An average of 80% of all subjects showed less than 5 dB variation in their frequency-gain response selection upon retest. A similar consistency was seen when between-session and within-session data were examined. This reflects minimal learning effects and suggests that this method can be expected to yield reliable results when clear instructions are provided and discourse passages (read by a male speaker) are used to elicit judgments.

Valid Predictor of Hearing Aid Performance

Two approaches to validate the results of paired comparison include correlation with speech recognition scores and "real-world" evaluation of the selected settings. Results of correlations between paired comparison judgments and speech recognition scores varied according to the criteria and test conditions used in the paired judgment. Punch and Howard[34] reported low correlation (R

= −0.46, to 0.34) between results of paired comparison of relative intelligibility and sentence scores on the CID Sentence Test. On the other hand, Studebaker et al.[16] using the same criterion, found excellent correlation (R = 0.98) between results of paired comparison and scores on the SPIN test.

Studebaker et al.[19] demonstrated the validity of paired comparison judgment of intelligibility by reporting that almost 73% of hearing aids chosen as the best during paired comparison judgment also received the highest mean speech recognition score, whereas only 63% of the hearing aids that obtained the best individual scores also had the highest mean speech recognition score. Neuman et al.[5] also showed that six of eight subjects obtained equal or higher individual speech recognition scores with hearing aids selected using paired comparison than those selected using an MCL approach.[6]

On the other hand, pairwise judgment of speech quality may not yield a high correlation when evaluating intelligibility. For example, Punch and Parker[42] reported negligible correlations between subjective judgments of speech quality and speech recognition scores despite significant correlation (R = 0.70) between relative intelligibility judgment and speech recognition scores. Albeit the low correlation between speech quality judgment and measured speech intelligibility, Punch and Parker[42] did not observe poorer measured speech intelligibility for hearing aids selected on the basis of quality. A later study[45] confirmed the low correlation between speech quality judgments and speech intelligibility scores. On the other hand, Studebaker and Sherbecoe[37] found that hearing aids selected on the basis of speech quality provided better measured speech intelligibility than hearing aids selected with magnitude estimation of speech intelligibility. This points to the potential difference between hearing aids selected with paired comparison and those with magnitude estimation.

Hearing aid settings that are selected with paired comparison may result in increased user satisfaction than those selected using a prescriptive method. Kuk and Pape[46] evaluated listeners' everyday satisfaction with hearing aids selected with the NAL-R formula and those selected with pairwise clarity judgment of discourse passages read by a male speaker and mixed in a babble noise (S/N = +5). Listeners completed a questionnaire to indicate their satisfaction with the hearing aid in 22 listening situations. Subjects with a sloping hearing loss (N = 10) showed similar preference for hearing aids fit with either approaches. Of the nine subjects who have a relatively flat hearing loss, seven showed significantly higher satisfaction for hearing aids selected with the pairwise approach, and only one showed higher satisfaction for a hearing aid selected with the NAL-R formula. Four of the seven subjects selected more low frequency gain than NAL-R recommendation, while the remaining three subjects selected less low frequency gain than NAL-R specifcation.

The results of this study[46] and those reported by Neuman et al.[5] show that hearing aids selected with the paired comparison technique are just as effective as, if not more effective than, those selected with a prescriptive method. This suggests that the use of paired comparison to verify hearing aid fitting may further enhance the fitting of hearing aids for some wearers.

Ability to Judge Several Subjective Attributes

The method of paired comparison has been used with different criteria. This includes "overall quality,"[15,29,32,38,41,47–49] "intelligibility,"[18,36,39,49] and "pleasantness" or "naturalness."[9,10,29,40] Other scales, e.g., "hollowness,"[32] "noise interference,"[50] and "amount of distortion," although not used with paired comparison, could potentially be useful as criteria for paired comparison judgment. Kuk and Tyler[51] demonstrated that listeners with hearing impairment could differentiate among various subjective criteria. These criteria could potentially be useful in evaluating nonlinear and other types of signal processing hearing aids.

Ability to be Performed Under More Listening Conditions

Byrne[52] indicated that speech testing performed in quiet or in conditions of poor S/N ratios (e.g., $<-10\,dB$) does not help to differentiate amplification systems and restricts the test conditions for which speech recognition tests can be performed. He further indicated that paired comparison judgments are less susceptible to the ceiling effect than are speech recognition tests. Consequently, paired comparison may be used in more test conditions (e.g., different S/N ratios, different types of noise backgrounds) than speech recognition tests in order to verify the appropriateness of settings selected for a programmable hearing aid.

Reduced Testing Time

The reliability of clinical speech recognition test is related to the number of items on the test. For example, Studebaker[53] calculated that a 10% difference between two speech scores is considered significant at the 5% probability level if 135 test items are presented. At least 3,381 test items must be presented if the same level of confidence is desired for only a 2% difference between test scores. Consequently, the time required to obtain a reliable result may be substantial.

Paired comparison procedures can be completed in substantially reduced time. Yet the results can be equally satisfactory, if not providing greater satisfaction than the settings that are selected using speech recognition tests. For example, an average of only 8 minutes is required to select the low and high frequency gain settings on a master hearing aid.[5] This makes paired comparison technique an ideal clinical tool with which to examine a large number of hearing aid settings under different listening conditions.

Minimal Involvement of Auditory Memory

In the method of paired comparison, acoustic stimuli processed by two hearing aid settings are presented sequentially with minimal time delay between presentations. This reduces any memory factor that may affect the sensitivity of the judgment. Studebaker[53] suggested that judgment of small differences between stimuli is easier when performed in a comparative mode of minimal delay than in an isolated mode.

Simple Instructions and Easy Task

Listeners are instructed to choose one of two stimulus intervals that meets the set criterion (e.g., better sound quality). A verbal or manual response (i.e., press one of two response buttons) is usually accepted. The task can be performed by listeners of all ages. For example, Eisenberg and Levitt[54] reported that almost all hearing impaired chidren are capable of performing paired comparison tasks by 6.5 years of age. The oldest subject (88 years old) in a study by Kuk and Pape[7] reported no difficulty completing the paired comparison task.

Wide Applications

The method of paired comparison has been used to study sound quality perception of hearing aids,[14] selection of MCL,[31] adjustment of noise reduction hearing aids,[32] comparison of frequency-gain responses selected by different prescriptive formulae,[49] selection of frequency-gain responses for different listening situations,[7,11] and selection of gain for monaural and binaural hearing aid fittings.[35,55] As digitally programmable hearing aids gain wider acceptance, it is conceivable that this technique will find even greater applications (e.g., selection of compression settings).

Individualized Fitting

The method of paired comparison not only verifies if the selected settings are appropriate for the individual listener but also specifies new settings if alternative settings are preferred. The result of paired comparison procedures can lead to a more appropriate combination of settings tailored to the individual's preference and psychophysical limitations. Furthermore, there is the psychological advantage to the listeners that they are actually involved in the hearing aid evaluation process. Unlike information provided by prescriptive formulas, final settings recommended by paired comparison procedures may not be restricted to frequency-gain response only. Potentially, other electroacoustic parameters, such as compression settings (e.g., release time, compression ratios) or different types of signal-processing techniques may also be examined using this technique.

Clinical Applications

While the technique of paired comparison shows the promise to be a powerful clinical and research tool, its potential may not be realized unless it is implemented properly in the clinic. This section will discuss the clinical implementation of this technique.

Timing for Paired Comparison

An important issue to consider is when and for whom paired comparison should be used. While it has been demonstrated that individuals from 6.5 to 88 years of age can reliably perform the task,[7,54] it is unclear if inexperienced hearing aid wearers are as reliable in their judgments as experienced hearing aid wearers, especially, if the judgments are to be made during the initial visit. Furthermore, the time needed to carry out the procedure will necessarily limit the time that can be available for other activities during the initial visit, e.g., counseling, real-ear measurements, and so on. For these reasons, it may be strategically desirable to delay the use of the paired comparison technique with first time hearing aid wearers to 2–3 weeks after they are initially fit with their hearing aids. Frequency-gain responses that are selected with a prescriptive formula may be adequate for the interim. This 2–3 week delay gives the wearers an opportunity to become acquainted with the amplified sound. In addition, it gives the wearers an opportunity to identify problem areas with the use of the hearing aids, as well as the listening situations in which use of the selected frequency-gain response is less than satisfactory. Such information may form the basis for selecting stimulus materials to use during subsequent paired comparisons. Because experienced hearing aid wearers are typically more accustomed to amplified sound and to the operation of hearing aids, it may not be necessary to introduce this "warm-up" period before performing paired comparison.

Clinical Implementation of Paired Comparison Technique

PAIRED COMPARISON AS A VERIFICATION TOOL

Paired comparison technique can be used as a verification tool or as a selection tool. The purpose of paired comparison when used as a verification tool is to ensure that the selected frequency-gain response of a hearing aid is more preferrable than a selected number of alternative frequency-gain responses. For example, one may want to ascertain that frequency-gain response selected by NAL-R is indeed more preferrable than variants of the NAL-R response (e.g., more low frequency gain, less high frequency gain) or that it is more preferrable than those selected with other prescriptive formulas. Typically, one would compare this frequency-gain response with only a limited number of alternative frequency-gain responses (less than four). It is not necessary that these frequency-gain responses be systematically related to each other. Indeed, it may be worthwhile to choose alternative settings that are sufficiently different from the prescribed frequency-gain response in order to ensure maximum notable differences between comparison frequency-gain responses. The small number of comparison settings and the potential lack of systematic relationship among comparison settings suggest that the use of tournament strategies like the round-robin and single- and double-eliminations would be appropriate. Additional measures (i.e., fine tuning) may be necessary if a comparison setting is more preferrable than the selected frequency-gain response.

Paired comparison procedure (as a verification tool) can be implemented easily in the clinic with today's programmable hearing aids. Although a computer may facilitate comparisons among the selected settings, the few number of comparison settings suggests that one may accomplish the goal of verification manually with only the programmable hearing aid and a playback device (e.g., a cassette player). The absolute requirement is the presence of two or more memories (temporary or permanent) on the programmable hearing aid for efficient switching between comparison settings. Because less than four settings are typically compared in a verification task, a programmable hearing aid with four memories that are easily accessible would be ideal for this purpose. Each comparison setting (and the prescribed setting) will be stored in separate memories for retrieval and comparison.

For example, one will illustrate how a round-robin tournament can be implemented on the Widex Quattro hearing aid, which has four permanent memories located on a remote control device. Assume that one wants to verify that the frequency-gain response selected by NAL-R (arbitrarily labeled as A) is more preferrable than three other frequency-gain responses: NAL-R but with 8 dB less gain at 4,000 Hz (labeled as B); NAL-R but with 8 dB less gain at 500 Hz (labeled as C); and NAL-R but with 5 dB less gain at 500 Hz and 5 dB more gain at 4,000 Hz (labeled as D). These four hearing aid settings can be stored in the four memories with setting A in memory No. 1, setting B in memory No. 2, and so on.

The clinician will perform paired comparison in the manner described on page 110. Switching of hearing aid settings is accomplished by simply pressing the appropriate memory button. It is important to realize that hearing aid designation (i.e., Nos. 1 and 2) has no bearing to the label of each memory. That is, memories 1, 3, or 4 can all be labeled as hearing aid 2 in the instructions. The clinician will record the listener's preference manually before a new pair of memories are compared. This will continue until all memories are compared with each other (in a round-robin). Figure 6–3 summarizes the order in which the memories are compared and the results of the comparison. In this case, memory B, the setting with 8 dB less high frequency gain than NAL-R specification, is preferred over NAL-R gain. This setting may be recommended in lieu of the originally selected frequency-gain response. Alternatively, this setting may be used as the initial estimate to determine further the optimal setting on the hearing aid for the listener. The selected setting (i.e., NAL-R in memory A) will be recommended if no preference is seen for any memory during the comparison trials. Such is the case if all four memories are preferred an equal number of times.

PAIRED COMPARISON AS A SELECTION TOOL

The purpose of selection is to determine, among the large number of potential settings on the hearing aid, the one that is most preferrable for the specific listening condition. Use of paired comparison for this purpose is especially meaningful when the clinician desires to seek alternative frequency-gain responses for the hearing aid wearer. Such may be the case when the result of verification suggests the need for an alternative frequency-gain response than the prescribed one; when the listener expresses dissatisfaction for a selected frequency-gain response; when the listener expresses the desire for better hearing in atypical listening situations (e.g., listening to music); or when the clinician desires to select several frequency-gain responses for improved hearing in different acoustic environments.

While both verification and selection may result in a "winner" frequency-gain response, the result of selection is fine tuned to the individual's preference. Such a guarantee cannot be made with the result of verification. Additionally, verification assumes that a prescribed frequency-gain response is optimal before paired comparison while selection makes no assumption on the appropriateness of any selected frequency-gain response. Any combination of settings (or frequency-gain responses) available on the programmable hearing aid may be equally effective or ineffective.

Because of the potentially large number of settings that can be compared in a selection process, an adaptive strategy would probably be more efficient than a tournament strategy in selecting the preferred frequency-gain response. As discussed in earlier sections, a simple up–down strategy would be desirable for selection on one electroacoustic dimension, while a modified simplex procedure would be required for selection of settings on more than one dimension.

Two requirements must be satisfied in order to implement adaptive paired comparison strategies on commercial programmable hearing aids. One requirement is that the electroacoustic dimension(s) under comparison must have fixed intervals so that comparisons can proceed in discrete steps. Almost all commercial programmable hearing aids satisfy this requirement. The second requirement is that the unit must have at least $(N + 1)$ temporary or permanent memories to allow paired comparison in N dimensions, i.e., two memories for one dimension, three memories for two dimensions, and so on. An alternative to the second requirement is the use of programmable devices that can be interfaced to a computer with which adjustment of settings can be accomplished by software written in order to eliminate the need for storage of settings for comparison.

Let us examine how a modified simplex procedure can be implemented on a commercial programmable hearing aid (e.g., Starkey Trilogy II) for manual selection of optimal high and low frequency settings on the device. Because settings on two electroacoustic dimensions are compared (i.e., $N = 2$), all three memories (i.e., $N + 1$) of the hearing aid (via a remote control device) will be utilized to facilitate comparison. A matrix representation of the combinations of settings similar to that illustrated in Figure 6–7 must be prepared prior to the comparison so that one can manually track listener responses and update memory content accurately.

Assume that one follows the same sequence of comparisons shown in Figure 6–7. In the first round of comparison, one may store the frequency-gain setting represented by cell (2L, 2H) into memory No. 1. Frequency-gain responses represented by cells (3L, 2H) and (2L, 3H) can be stored in memories 2 and 3, respectively. Memory assignment is arbitrary. The same sequence of comparison illustrated in Figure 6–1 can be followed. It is extremely important to indicate on the matrix the winner of each pair of comparison so that settings for the next round of comparison can be easily determined. In the example illustrated in Figure 6–7, settings represented by cells (3L, 2H), (3L, 1H), and (4L, 2H) are stored in each memory of the hearing aid for the second round of comparison. In this way, memory update is only necessary after every round of comparison.

Table 6–1. Comparison of Paired Comparison Technique Used as a Verification Tool and as a Selection Tool

Parameter	Verification	Selection
Purpose	To establish that prescribed frequency-gain response is preferred over other alternatives	To select the best frequency-gain response available on the hearing aid
Assumptions	Prescribed frequency-gain response is most preferred	No assumption is made on preference
# comparison settings	Typically less than four	Varies depending on number of settings on hearing aid and strategy used
Strategy	Nonadaptive; round-robin and eliminations	Adaptive; simple up–down and modified simplex
Implementation	Best if automated; can be without computer; need four memories on HA; memory update not needed	Automation desirable; can be without computer; need N + 1 memories on HA where N is the number of dimensions; memory update necessary
Initial estimate	Frequency-gain response selected by dispenser favorite prescriptive approach	Arbitrary; typically selected with prior knowledge of optimal final estimate
Comparison settings	May not vary systematically from initial estimate	Varies in systematic manner from initial estimate
Final estimate	Reflects if prescribed setting is preferred over selections; does not guarantee best selection or setting on hearing aid	Guarantees to be the best setting available on the hearing aid for the specific listening environment

Table 6–1 summarizes the differences between paired comparison used as a verification tool and as a selection tool.

Based on this analysis, an efficient use of paired comparison technique is to use it as a verification tool first with a few selected frequency-gain responses. If the results of verification show that the prescribed setting is preferred, such a setting may be recommended to the wearer. If one of the comparison settings is preferred over the prescribed setting, the winner of the comparison may be used as an initial estimate in a more in-depth search for optimal setting using adaptive paired comparison technique. A block diagram showing a model of how paired comparison can be used in the clinic is shown in Figure 6–8.

Stimulus/Test Conditions

An advantage of paired comparison is the potentially infinite number of test conditions in which one can compare selected hearing aid settings. In theory, one could compare hearing aid settings in listening conditions that are identified as difficult by the hearing aid wearers. The task for the clinician is to have replications (i.e., on cassette tape or compact disc) of these listening conditions available and to evaluate the wearers using these acoustic materials. This,

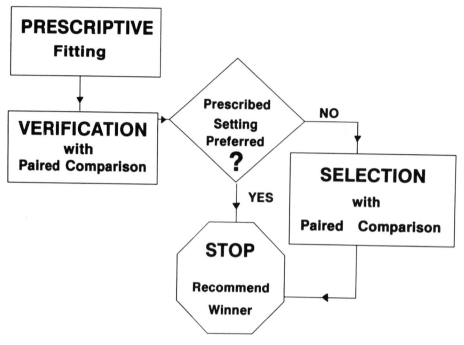

Figure 6–8.   Model showing how paired comparison can be integrated in the hearing aid evaluation procedure.

however, may be clinically impractical because no two wearers' listening environments are identical. Furthermore, there is the difficulty of physically recreating the various listening environments in a clinical setting. A compromise may be the use of some standardized listening conditions for general use and have available a few representative sound effects that would provide the listening situations frequently encountered by the population of hearing aid wearers who are served in the community.

In our clinic, we find the use of discourse-in-noise a good stimulus to verify and select hearing aid settings for typical daily use. It is important to realize that the level of the stimulus used and the S/N ratios employed in the comparison could affect the appropriateness of the selected frequency-gain response. Specifically, our experience indicates that frequency-gain responses selected with discourse passages presented at 62 dB sound pressure level (root mean square [RMS], A-scale) in the presence of babble noise and at a favorable S/N ratio (>+5) are most preferrable for typical listening situations. The same speech stimuli, presented at 72 dB sound pressure level A and at a less favorable S/N (e.g., <0) yield frequency-gain responses that are preferrable in a loud, noisy situation. These two test conditions can be marked for general use with paired comparison. Cox and Alexander[56] and Pearsons, et al.,[57] also offered some speech and noise levels that can be used in different listening conditions. Sound effects that may be useful for selection of frequency-gain responses in specific listening situations include those of, but are not exclusive to, wind noise, music (orchestral and individual instruments), office noise (typewriter noise, computer fan noise), restaurant noise, and traffic noise. Additionally, one may perform paired comparison in an empty office or a large hall in order to verify or select frequency-gain response for listening in reverberant environments. The levels at which these sound effects may be presented need further investigation.

The criterion that one uses to verify or select a frequency-gain response is dependent on the needs of the hearing aid wearer for the frequency-gain response. If the intent is to maximize speech understanding ability, such criterion must be specified. If the intent is to search for a "natural" sounding hearing aid, such criterion must be indicated. An earlier section summarizes some of the criteria that were used (and may be used) during paired comparison. It is important to remember that the criterion used will affect the outcome of the comparison.[10,11] A criterion of "clarity" is recommended for general use because it is the criterion by which most hearing aid wearers judge their hearing aids.[58]

Integration with Other Measures

The paired comparison technique is a relative measure. The result of the comparison does not guarantee that the particular programmable hearing aid includes the best frequency-gain response for the specific hearing aid wearer or if the programmable hearing aid is appropriate for the wearer. Although a potential limitation of this technique, one can easily overcome this limitation with the use of additional measures to ensure wearer satisfaction for the selected frequency-gain response. For example, the use of real-ear measures after paired comparison could ensure that the wearer is actually using some amplification from the hearing aid and not responding to "phantom attributes" during paired comparison. Frequently, direct questioning of wearer satisfaction with the selected or verified frequency-gain response will yield valuable information on the appropriateness of the selected device. Regular follow-up examinations (and readjustment of settings, if necessary) may also enhance the wearer's satisfaction with the hearing aid.

The technique of paired comparison is an important tool that can enhance the success of a hearing aid fitting. It should be regarded as part of an evaluation battery and not as a stand-alone test. Integration of results on more than one measure is necessary to ensure maximum wearer satisfaction with the selected hearing aid.

References

1. Byrne D, Dillon H: Comparative reliability of warble tone thresholds under earphones and in sound field. *Aust J Audiol* 1981; 3:12–14.
2. Skinner M, Miller J: Amplification bandwidth and intelligibility of speech in quiet and noise for listeners with sensorineural hearing loss. *Audiology* 1983; 22:253–279.
3. Cox R, Bisset J: Prediction of aided preferred listening levels for hearing aid gain prescription. *Ear Hear* 1982; 3:66–71.
4. Gilman S, Dirks D, Stern R: The effects of occluded ear impedance on the eardrum SPL produced by hearing aids. *J Acoust Soc Am* 1981; 70:370–386.
5. Neuman A, Levitt H, Mills R, et al.: An evaluation of three adaptive hearing aid selection strategies. *J Acoust Soc Am* 1987; 82:1967–1976.

6. Pascoe D: An approach to hearing aid selection. *Hear Instrum* 1978; 29(6):12–16, 36.
7. Kuk F, Pape N: The reliability of a modified simplex procedure in hearing aid frequency response selection. *J Speech Hear Res* 1992; 35:418–429.
8. Byrne D, Dillon H: The National Acoustic Laboratories' (NAL) new procedure for selecting the gain and frequency response of a hearing aid. *Ear Hear* 1986; 7:257–265.
9. Byrne D, Cotton S: Evaluation of the National Acoustic Laboratories' new hearing aid selection procedure. *J Speech Hear Res* 1988; 31:178–186.
10. Byrne D: Effects of frequency response characteristics on speech discrimination and perceived intelligibility and pleasantness of speech for hearing-impaired listeners. *J Acoust Soc Am* 1986; 80:494–504.
11. Kuk F: Preferred insertion gain of hearing aids in listening and reading-aloud situations. *J Speech Hear Res* 1990; 33:520–529.
12. Tecca J, Goldstein D: Effect of low frequency hearing aid response on four measures of speech perception. *Ear Hear* 1984; 5:22–29.
13. Thurstone L: A law of comparative judgment. *Psychoacoust Rev* 1927; 34:273–286.
14. Punch J, Montgomery A, Schwartz D, et al.: Multidimensional scaling of quality judgments of speech signals processed by hearing aids. *J Acoust Soc Am* 1980; 68:458–466.
15. Punch J: Quality judgments of hearing aid processed speech and music by normal and otopathologic listeners. *J Am Audiol Soc* 1978; 3:179–188.
16. Studebaker G, White R, Hoffnung S: Evaluation of a paired comparison technique for selecting hearing aid characteristics. Paper presented at the meeting of the American Speech Language and Hearing Association, 1978, San Francisco, CA.
17. Levitt H, Collins J, Dubno J, et al.: *Development of a Protocol for the Prescriptive Fitting of a Wearable Master Hearing Aid.* CSL Research Report No. 11, National Institute of Neurological and Communicative Disease and Stroke. New York: City University of New York, 1978.
18. Zerlin S: A new approach to hearing aid selection. *J Speech Hear Res* 1962; 5:370–376.
19. Studebaker G, Bisset J, Van Ort D: Paired comparison judgments of relative speech intelligibility. Paper presented at the meeting of the Acoustical Society of America, 1980, Los Angeles, CA.
20. Watson N, Knudsen V: Selective amplification in hearing aids. *J Acoust Soc Am* 1940; 11:406–419.
21. Pascoe D: Frequency responses of hearing aids and their effects on the speech perception of hearing-impaired subjects. *Ann Otol Rhinol Laryngol Suppl* 1975; 23:1–40.
22. Kuk F: Evaluation of the efficacy of a multimemory hearing aid. *J Am Acad Audiol* 1992; 3:338–348.
23. Montgomery A, Schwartz D, Punch J: Tournament strategies in hearing aid selection. *J Speech Hear Dis* 1982; 47:363–372.
24. White R, Studebaker G: An evaluation of elimination tournament strategies for hearing aid selection. Paper presented at the meeting of the *American Speech Language and Hearing Association,* 1978, San Francisco, CA.
25. Studebaker G, White R, Hoffnung S: Evaluation of a paired comparison elimination paradigm as a method of selecting hearing aids. Paper presented at the meeting of the *Acoustical Society of America,* 1979, Cambridge, MA.
26. Levitt H: Transformed up–down methods in psychoacoustics. *J Acoust Soc Am* 1970; 49:467–477.
27. Levitt H: Adaptive testing in audiology. *Scand Audiol Suppl* 1978; 6:241–291.
28. Levitt H: Adaptive procedures for hearing aid prescription and other audiological applications. *J Am Acad Audiol* 1992; 3:119–131.
29. Leijon A, Lindkvist A, Ringdahl A, et al.: Sound quality and speech reception for prescribed hearing aid frequency responses. *Ear Hear* 1991; 12:251–260.
30. Robbins H, Monro S: A stochastic approximation method. *Ann Math Stat* 1951; 22:400–407.
31. Wall L, Gans R: Test–retest reliability of a forced-choice procedure for determining the most comfortable loudness level of speech. *Ear Hear* 1984; 5:118–122.
32. Kuk F, Plager A, Pape, N: Hollowness perception in noise reduction hearing aids. *J Am Acad Audiol* 1992; 3:39–45.
33. Box G: Evolutionary operation: A method for increasing industrial productivity. *Appl Stat* 1957; 26:679–685.
34. Punch J, Howard M: Listener-assessed intelligibility of hearing aid-processed speech. *J Am Audiol Soc* 1978; 4:69–76.
35. Punch J, Jenison R, Allan J, et al.: Evaluation of three strategies for fitting hearing aids binaurally. *Ear Hear* 1991; 12:205–215.
36. Studebaker G, Bisset J, Van Ort D, et al.: Paired comparison judgments of relative intelligibility in noise. *J Acoust Soc Am* 1982; 72:80–92.
37. Studebaker G, Sherbecoe R: Magnitude estimation of the intelligibility and quality of speech in noise. *Ear Hear* 1988; 9:259–267.

38. Witter H, Goldstein D: Quality judgments of hearing aid transduced speech. *J Speech Hear Res* 1971; 14:312–322.
39. Byrne D, Parkinson A, Newall, P: Hearing aid gain and frequency response requirements for the severely/profoundly hearing-impaired. *Ear Hear* 1990; 11:40–49.
40. Murray N, Byrne D: Performance of hearing-impaired and normal hearing listeners with various high-frequency cut-offs in hearing aids. *Aust J Audiol* 1986; 8:21–28.
41. Punch J, Beck E: Low frequency response of hearing aids and judgments of aided speech quality. *J Speech Hear Dis* 1980; 45:325–335.
42. Punch J, Parker C: Pairwise listener preferences in hearing aid evaluation. *J Speech Hear Res* 1981; 24:366–374.
43. Studebaker G, White R, Hoffnung S, et al.: Studies of a paired comparison hearing aid selection procedure. Paper presented at the meeting of the American Speech Language and Hearing Association, 1979, Atlanta, GA.
44. Schwartz D, Walden B, Prosek R: Electroacoustic correlates of hearing aid quality judgments. Paper presented at the meeting of the American Speech Language and Hearing Association, 1979, Atlanta, GA.
45. Punch J, Beck L: Relative effects of low frequency amplification on syllable recognition and speech quality. *Ear Hear* 1986; 7:57–62.
46. Kuk F, Pape N: Relative satisfaction for frequency responses selected with a simplex procedure in different listening conditions. *J Speech Hear Res* 1993;36:168–177.
47. Harris R, Goldstein D: Effects of room reverberation upon hearing aid quality judgments. *Audiology* 1979; 18:253–262.
48. Jeffers J: Quality judgments in hearing aid selection. *J Speech Hear Dis* 1960; 25:259–266.
49. Sullivan J, Levitt H, Hwang J, et al.: An experimental comparison of four hearing aid prescription methods. *Ear Hear* 1988; 9:22–32.
50. Kuk F, Tyler R, Mims L: Subjective ratings of noise reduction hearing aids. *Scand Audiol* 1990; 19:237–244.
51. Kuk F, Tyler R: Relationship between consonant recognition and subjective ratings of hearing aids. *Br J Audiol* 1990; 24:171–177.
52. Byrne D: Evaluation measures of speech intelligibility and quality—Research and clinical application, in Studebaker GA, Bess F, Beck L (eds): *Vanderbilt Hearing-Aid Report II.* York Press, 1991, pp 195–200.
53. Studebaker G: Hearing aid selection: An overview, in Studebaker G, Bess F (eds): *The Vanderbilt Hearing-Aid Report: State of the Art Research Needs.* Upper Darby, PA: Monographs in Contemporary Audiology, 1982, pp 147–155.
54. Eisenberg L, Levitt H: Paired comparison judgments for hearing aid selection in children. *Ear Hear* 1991; 12:417–430.
55. Levitt H, Sullivan J, Neuman A, et al.: Experiments with a programmable master hearing aid. *J Rehab Res Dev* 1987; 24:29–54.
56. Cox R, Alexander G: Hearing aid benefit in everyday environments. *Ear Hear* 1991; 12;127–139.
57. Pearsons K, Bennett R, Fidell S: *Speech Levels in Various Noise Environments.* Bolt Beranek and Newman Report No. 32, Canoga Park, CA, 1977.
58. Hagerman B, Gabrielsson A: Questionnaires on desirable properties of hearing aids. *Scand Audiol* 1985; 14:109–111.

7

The Role of Subjective Measurement Techniques in Hearing Aid Fittings

DAVID A. FABRY, DONALD J. SCHUM

Introduction

As real-ear measurement continues to increase in popularity for hearing aid evaluation,[1] prescriptive formulae have become the method of choice for many audiologists to assess hearing aid success. Correspondingly, for the majority of these approaches, auditory threshold measures in quiet serve as the basis for defining "target" gain, and probe tube real-ear insertion gain (REIG) measures are used to verify the accuracy of the fit. When insertion gain matches prescriptive target gain within some criterion measure at a specified input level (usually 65 to 70 dB sound pressure level [SPL]), the procedure is considered a success (with the added hope that the patient does not return with problems). This strategy, however, neglects the fact that individual variations in preferred gain may occur for persons with similar hearing losses.[2]

Several other problems hamper this approach, including (1) there are nearly a dozen published prescriptive threshold formulae, and none has been demonstrated to be clearly superior to all others;[3] (2) it is difficult to quantify what is meant by an "adequate" match to target gain; (3) many prescriptive formulae do not include prescription of maximum hearing aid output levels; and (4) these methods do not suffice for many of the advanced circuits such as automatic signal processing (ASP) or programmable hearing aids that have low compression thresholds (i.e., 45–55 dB SPL) and variable compression ratios.

A primary issue becomes the accuracy of a hearing aid fitting model that uses only pure-tone thresholds and probe tube measurements for prescription and assessment of hearing aid performance, respectively. This strategy disregards the preferences of the person who ultimately provides the final determinant of hearing aid effectiveness: the patient. Structured speech-understanding tasks are available to assess differences between hearing aids or to assess long-term benefit. However, significant concerns have been raised as to the reliability, validity, and sensitivity of such techniques.[4] Furthermore,

136

in many cases, traditional speech understanding tasks apparently cannot differentiate between nonlinear circuit characteristics.[5] Subjective opinions may provide some indication of differences between hearing aids with similar electroacoustic response, when probe tube measures are of little use. Interestingly, subjective methods have long been used by engineering laboratories when attempting to differentiate sound transmission circuits.[6,7]

There are a variety of subjective rating measures that may be used by the audiologist for clinical evaluation and verification of hearing aid performance. These include ratings of aided speech intelligibility and speech quality, loudness judgments, and self-assessment of hearing handicap and hearing aid benefit. The focus of this chapter will be to contrast these measures with information obtained from "objective" measurements available to the audiologist. The principle question addressed in this chapter is whether subjective techniques can add useful information during hearing aid selection, setting, and verification.

The Value of Using Objective Measurement to Fit Hearing Aids

Objective measurements, for the purposes of the present chapter, are those that do not require a response from the patient. The most widely used objective techniques for hearing aid evaluations are real-ear probe tube measures. Additionally, some audiologists consider traditional word recognition testing to be another type of objective measure. It is not technically accurate to describe word recognition testing as an objective technique, since the listener provides a voluntary response. However, for the purposes of this chapter we will include this testing in a discussion of objective techniques for two reasons. First, the responses provided by the listener are generally automatic, requiring a minimal amount of cognitive evaluation. Typically, either the listener recognizes the word or does not recognize the word. The listener is not called on to provide a studied evaluation of the auditory signal. Second, this traditional evaluation technique provides a clear contrast with the sort of alternative measurement techniques to be discussed throughout the chapter.

Presently, prescriptive target formulae and real-ear measurements are used by over 65% of audiologists who dispense hearing aids.[1] Why has this approach become so popular? Most audiologists recognize that successful hearing aid fitting and evaluation involves more than simply matching insertion gain to some predetermined target based on audiometric thresholds. However, the use of insertion gain measurements has largely replaced Carhart's comparative approach[8] to hearing aid selection that was based primarily on speech threshold and recognition testing. Few audiologists use aided speech recognition testing to select between hearing aids for several reasons. For example, there is significant evidence that traditional word recognition testing does not reliably differentiate hearing aids.[4,9] Furthermore, most hearing aids dispensed today are custom in-the-ear (ITE) devices that are ordered directly from the manufacturer rather than selected from in-stock devices. As a result, hearing aids are often ordered by audiogram, matrix, or 2 cc full-on coupler gain, and then an appropriate fit is verified via real-ear assessment.

The advent of real-ear measurement test systems enables insertion gain measurements to be completed for the range from 200 to 8000 Hz significantly faster than functional gain. With careful insertion of the probe tube to within 1.0 cm from the tympanic membrane, accurate measurements within 3 dB of actual eardrum SPL can be achieved for frequencies below 5 kHz.[10] Furthermore, reported test–retest measurement error is less than 2.5 dB for the frequency range between 500 Hz and 4000 Hz.[11] Finally, real-ear measurements are possible on cooperative young children or difficult-to-test patients.[12]

Limitations of Objective Techniques

Prescriptive approaches to hearing aid selection have been available since at least the 1940s.[13] Most threshold-based approaches used today are modifications of the half-gain rule devised by Lybarger.[14] For sensorineural hearing losses, target gain at each frequency is simply the person's audiometric threshold multiplied by 0.5. Later approaches, including prescription of gain and output (POGO),[15] that of Berger et al.,[16] or that of National Acoustics Laboratories-Revised (NAL-R),[17] fine tune some of the computations in an attempt to ensure audible amplified speech.

The original developmental work on the NAL-R procedure[17] and subsequent evaluations[5,18] have demonstrated that auditory threshold, on average, serves as a reasonable foundation for selecting the appropriate gain and frequency response of a hearing aid. However, in most of these investigations, inter-subject differences were substantial. Apparently factors other than audiometric threshold contribute to overall hearing aid satisfaction.

Currently, the audiologist can chose from a variety of commercially available nonlinear hearing aid circuits. Most of these circuits can be adjusted to match a prescription (such as NAL-R) for lower input levels in quiet environments. In such listening conditions, most of these circuits are intended to be used as broadband linear amplifiers. It is only when the input level increases or when significant background noise is present that these circuits begin to behave differently. Prescriptive targets do not provide guidance in the selection or adjustment of nonlinear circuit characteristics. Specifically, two of the principal nonlinear circuits (ASP and K-Amp) which have been advanced for flat to gently sloping, mild to moderate sensorineural hearing loss are designed to behave in an opposite manner as the overall input level increases. There are no widely accepted fitting guidelines that provide direction when setting electroacoustic parameters such as compression threshold, compression ratio, attack time, and release time.

Most programmable hearing aids offer the option of the use of multiple memories. In most applications, each memory is established for a specific listening environment. Again, prescriptive targets are not specific for changes in listening environment. If one memory of a hearing aid is set to provide a NAL-R response for quiet environments, there are no specific, widely accepted rules for altering that response when the listener moves to a room with many other people speaking, is driving in heavy traffic, or when listening to music.

The Use of Subjective Techniques in Hearing Aid Research

The pioneering work of psychologists such as Thurstone, Weber, Fechner, and Stevens has demonstrated that human observers can provide valid and reliable subjective estimates of stimuli that vary along physical dimensions (see Purdy[19] and Watson,[20] for reviews). When properly prompted, an observer can provide either absolute or relative estimates along such dimensions as heaviness, length, brightness, pitch, and loudness. Given concerns over limitations with traditional measures of hearing aid performance, several research groups have looked to the field of experimental psychology for guidance in establishing and evaluating subjective techniques by which to assess amplification characteristics. Several techniques have been identified and investigated over the past few decades.

Magnitude Estimation

In magnitude estimation, the patient relates the signal presented at various intensities or signal-to-noise (S/N) ratios to its subjective magnitude. This may be accomplished in at least two ways. In the first, a standard speech stimulus is presented at some S/N ratio or overall intensity level, and the patient is instructed that it has a particular value, for example, 50%, that is called the *modulus*. Next, other speech passages are presented at other various signal-to-noise ratios or overall intensities, and the patient is instructed to assign different numbers to these that are ratios of the modulus.

An alternative approach is to omit the modulus. In this case, the patient is simply required to assign numbers to stimuli that reflect their subjective levels. Magnitude estimations have been used several times in the hearing aid literature. For example, when investigating the perceptual consequences of changes in the frequency response of a hearing aid, Lawson and Chial[21] had listeners provide magnitude estimations of speech quality. Follow-up developmental work has been reported by Studebaker and Sherbecoe.[22] The results of numerous studies have shown that magnitude estimations with and without a modulus result in similar findings.[23]

Magnitude Production

The reverse of magnitude estimation is magnitude production. In this approach, patients are presented with numbers and instructed to adjust speech intensity or to S/N ratio until it corresponds to the numbers.

Subject bias causes magnitude estimation and production to yield somewhat different results, especially at low and high stimulus levels. Specifically, patients tend to avoid extreme values in magnitude estimation, and they do not make extreme level adjustment in magnitude production. These bias effects are in opposite directions, so that the "real" function lies somewhere between the ones obtained from magnitude productions and estimations. Hellman and Zwislocki[24] discuss statistical techniques to compensate for this discrepancy. The interested reader is referred to their work.

Category Scaling

One method for achieving high face validity is via subjective ratings of speech intelligibility. In this method, the listener is presented with a bounded scale (0–10, 0–100, and so forth) and asked to judge a passage through a particular hearing aid or circuit configuration. The judgment can be along any one of several perceptual dimensions (e.g., speech intelligibility, speech clarity, speech quality, music quality, pleasantness, or harshness). Speaks et al.[23] found that estimates of speech intelligibility varied monotonically with more traditional measures of speech understanding. Gabrielsson et al.[25] describe the utility of having listeners rate both speech and music using a variety of different categories (e.g., spaciousness, clarity, brightness). Palmer et al.[26] found that listeners could even assign dollar values to the perceived quality of various hearing tasks.

The most extensive work in this area has been reported by Cox and McDaniel.[27–29] These investigators developed the Speech Intelligibility Rating (SIR) test in an attempt to provide a set of connected discourse passages that would optimize test reliability and face validity in one set of speech materials. The SIR is comprised of 20 passages of connected discourse that have been equated for intelligibility and duration; each passage is 48 seconds long and is paired with a segment of multitalker babble of equal duration. The listener's task is to rated the intelligibility of individual passages in quiet or in babble on a scale from zero to ten.

Cox and McDaniel[28] standardized the SIR for subjects with normal hearing and determined that the 90% confidence interval for two scores (based on three ratings each) was 1.8 scale units. That is, 90% of the time, two scores (averaged from three ratings each) that differ by a minimum of 1.8 will be truly different from each other. Cox and McDaniel,[29] using hearing impaired subjects, reported 90% confidence intervals of 1.75 scale units for the average of five ratings.

Surr and Fabry[30] compared SIR ratings from hearing impaired subjects who rated the intelligibility of three high frequency emphasis hearing aids that differed in mid-frequency amplification. Their data suggested that the SIR test was not sensitive to differences in frequency response slopes of 6–14 dB/octave between 1000 and 2000 Hz. Although rated intelligibility tests promise high face validity, the stimuli must be highly homogeneous for intelligibility and context to minimize inter and intrasubject variability. In addition, more time is required for completion of the SIR than for comparable, objectively scored test procedures, such as speech recognition threshold (SRT) in noise, because three or more passages must be presented to obtain a stable average rating.

Figure 7–1 provides three scales found helpful for research and clinical applications in the audiology clinic at the University of Iowa Hospital. Patients are presented with continuous discourse (e.g., Rainbow Passage) in quiet and various levels of cafeteria noise. The patient then provides a rating on one of the three indicated scales. We have found the "background noise" scale to be useful in providing a preliminary estimate of perceived differences between supposed "noise reduction" circuits. For some patients, the "clarity" and

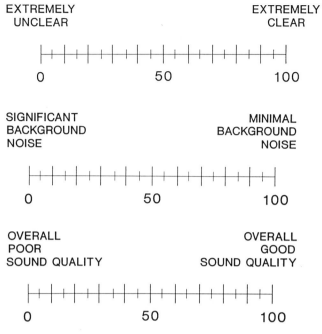

Figure 7–1. Three examples of category rating scales.

the "overall quality" scales yield different ratings. However, most of our experienced hearing aid users who have had a history of limited benefit from amplification will equate improved clarity with improved quality. This is not always the case with new hearing aid users. We are currently investigating the limits of sensitivity, reliability, and redundancy of these scales.

Paired Comparisons

When using the three techniques described above, the listener makes a judgment of the signal from a single hearing aid at any given time. Comparisons between hearing aids are performed later, "off-line." The relative performance of various aids is determined by comparing mean rated values. A more direct way to compare two different hearing aids is via direct paired comparisons. The listener listens to the signal through one device or combination of circuit settings and then through a second device or configuration. The listener then picks the member of the pair that is rated as superior along a given dimension. For some patients, this technique can lessen the "cognitive load" of the rating task. Some patients may be unable or unwilling to produce category ratings or magnitude estimates. However, they may be quite able to pick a member of a pair that is preferred on some dimension.

More than two hearing aids or circuit configurations can be evaluated by using one of a variety of tournament strategies. The principle tournament strategies used in hearing aid research include a complete round-robin (each hearing aid is compared with every other hearing aid), single-elimination tournament (a hearing aid is dropped from consideration once it loses to another in a head to head comparison), double-elimination tournament (a hearing aid is dropped after it loses two comparisons), and the modified simplex procedure (two or more electroacoustic dimensions are adaptively varied simultaneously). The most simple tournament to structure is the complete round-robin. However, since each hearing aid is compared with every other hearing aid, the round robin tournament takes the longest to complete. Elimination style tournaments appear to be sensitive to hearing aid "seeding."[31] The most efficient technique is probably the modified simplex,[32] as the superior hearing aid or circuit configuration is identified via an adaptive narrowing technique. However, this procedure is rather complicated to implement without computer control.

The tester has the choice as to whether the listener will hear each sample just once and then pick the winner or if repeated listening will take place. If repeated listening takes place, a structured ABA or ABAB presentation can be chosen, or the listener may be given the opportunity to switch back and forth between the samples as many times as is necessary before a decision is made. The tester will also need to make decisions as to what sort of signals will be used and which perceptual dimensions will be evaluated.

Paired comparison testing has been used in a number of instances over the past several years in an attempt to understand better patient responses to manipulation of various electroacoustic characteristics in hearing aids.[34-36] Byrne and Parkinson[37] reviewed several investigations that used the paired comparison technique and found the procedure to be reliable and generally sensitive. Furthermore, Eisenberg and Levitt[38] evaluated the utility of using the paired comparison technique with children of various ages. They report that the paired comparison technique is reliable and apparently valid for hearing impaired children as young as 6.5 years.

One important limitation of the paired comparison technique not encountered with category scaling or magnitude estimation should be pointed out. The paired comparison technique, in its classic form, only provides order information. If only two aids or circuits are being compared, the winner is obvious. However, if more than two items are in the tournament, the possibility of tied rankings occurs. For example, if three hearing aids (A, B, and C) are being compared and A beats B, B beats C, and C beats A, the audiologist still does not have information to help choose a superior hearing aid. When using category ratings or magnitude estimations, a specific score is assigned to each hearing aid. The likelihood of tied rankings occurring is less. To improve the sensitivity of the paired comparison technique, a strength of preference rating can be elicited from the subject.[39,40] Thus, not only does the listener pick the preferred member of the pair, but also rates the strength of preference (e.g., "A is slightly/moderately/significantly better than B"). The winner of the pair is assigned a numerical representation of the perceived difference compared with the loser. The inclusion of a strength of preference matrix potentially increases the sensitivity of such a procedure.

There are practical limitations to the use of the paired comparison technique when two or more actual hearing aids need to be compared.[41] However, when alternative circuit settings within one hearing aid need to be evaluated, the paired comparison technique would seem to be a reasonable option. With the advent of programmable hearing aids, the fitting hardware for most models has made the use of paired comparisons extremely accessible. In fact, in their fitting guides, several manufacturers of programmable hearing aids encourage the use of the paired comparison technique during circuit adjustments.

Measures Used for Self-Assessment of Hearing Handicap

The primary goal of hearing aid fitting procedures is to maximize word intelligibility. However, hearing aid satisfaction may be determined by a combination of word intelligibility, sound quality, and other factors. Furthermore, as was discussed previously, clinical speech measures may not be sensitive to subtle effects that distinguish one hearing aid from another. Also, the ultimate determination of hearing aid satisfaction—whether or not the person purchases the hearing aid—resides with the user's opinions about perceived benefit from amplification. All of the subjective techniques discussed thus far are intended to be used immediately after a listener hears an amplified sample. The listener is required to make a judgment concerning the perception of the material at that point in time under those specific listening conditions and along one specific perceptual dimension. This test environment allows for a high level of control. However, only limited generalizability to a broad range of listening environments is possible. It is not practical to test using a broad range of talkers, background noise types, background noise levels, and speech materials. Therefore, structured subjective judgments can be augmented quite effectively by using recollected judgments on the part of a listener.

Several questionnaires have been developed for self-assessment of hearing aid benefit.[42,43] Recently, the Profile of Hearing Aid Performance (PHAP), was developed by Cox and Gilmore[44] to supplement "objective" measures of speech recognition for several hearing aid clinical field trials. The PHAP consists of 66 statements that comprise communication in a variety of listening environments. Hearing impaired persons respond to each statement, based on their everyday experience, using a seven point scale, based on frequency of occurrence, ranging from "always" (99%) to "never" (1%). The 66 item test is divided into seven subscales combined into four scales. Cox and Gilmore[44] have standardized the test on a group of hearing impaired subjects, allowing both intra- and intersubject comparisons to be made for hearing aid conditions.

An example of such comparisons is indicated in Table 7–1, for a group of three (out of ten total) subjects who compared two hearing aids that were matched for gain and output at 50 and 90 dB SPL inputs but differed in compression threshold and compression ratio.[5] One device employed "full dynamic range" compression, and the other used input compression limitation. Subjects were fit with each hearing aid for a period of one month; subsequently, they were evaluated with the Speech Perception in Noise (SPIN) and PHAP tests and were ultimately forced to choose between the two hearing aids as the "preferred device if these were the only options for hearing aid use." SPIN results showed no significant differences between the two types of

Table 7–1.   Profile of Hearing Aid Performance (PHAP) Scores for Hearing Aids With Similar Frequency Responses but With Either "Full Dynamic Range" (FDR) or "Input Limiting" (IL) Compression*

| Subject | Condition | Scale (90% Critical Difference) | | | |
		SA (13.5)	SB (16.7)	SC (15.2)	ES (19.1)
T	FDR	16.0	50.4	50.6	56.2
	IL	15.0	47.6	40.5	30.2*
K	FDR	21.5	36.4	63.8	45.7
	IL	8.1	30.3	43.6*	29.6
C	FDR	32.1	49.8	59.9	47.5
	IL	30.1	40.8	75.5	71.0

*   Ninety percent critical differences from Cox and Gilmore[44] are indicated in parentheses; asterisks indicate that difference scores between two conditions exceed 90% values. See Cox and Gilmore[44] for a discussion of the scales SA, SB, SC, and ES.

Table 7–2.   Profile of Hearing Aid Performance (PHAP) Scores for Hearing Aids With the Same Frequency Responses, but With Either Fixed Release (FR) or Adaptive Release (AR) From Compression*

| Subject | Condition | Scale (90% Critical Difference) | | | |
		SA (13.5)	SB (16.7)	SC (15.2)	ES (19.1)
I	FR	27.6	50.7	42.9	27.7
	AR	23.1	50.6	42.9	23.6
O	FR	15	35.2	35.6	19.2
	AR	16.1	36.8	35.1	24.1
C	FR	21.2	32.1	34.7	25.0
	AR	22.1	35.2	32.1	25.5

*   Ninety percent critical differences from Cox and Gilmore[44] are indicated in parentheses; asterisks indicate that difference scores between two conditions exceed 90% values. See Cox and Gilmore[44] for a discussion of the scales SA, SB, SC, and ES.

compression devices, but the PHAP scores from scale environmental sounds (ES) indicated agreement with nine of ten subjects' overall preference.

Another evaluation in progress at the Mayo audiology clinic compares two hearing aids matched in frequency response that used either fixed- or adaptive-release time for compression. Preliminary results from this study reveal excellent test–retest PHAP scores (over one month's time) from several persons who reported no perceived differences between the two hearing aids (Table 7–2). Additional data are required to determine whether long-term changes in hearing aid satisfaction are reflected in PHAP scores and also to determine the efficacy of unaided, baseline, PHAP scores. Cox and Gilmore[44] also described another index derived from the PHAP, the Profile of Hearing Aid Benefit (PHAB), for use in making direct comparisons between unaided and aided conditions. The difference between aided and unaided responses is the measure of hearing aid benefit.

Advantages of Subjective Techniques

The work with subjective techniques as part of the hearing aid selection and verification process that has been reported thus far has revealed several distinct advantages for these nontraditional assessment techniques. Prescriptive fittings with follow-up real-ear verification has become ingrained as the preliminary step in the fitting of a hearing aid. However, for a variety of reasons, subjective assessment techniques should be investigated as a necessary part of the process.

Comparison to Word Recognition Testing

Traditional word recognition testing has been criticized as not being sensitive to differences between hearing aids.[4,9] The work of Studebaker and his colleagues (see Studebaker,[45] for a review) has suggested that the paired comparison technique may be more sensitive to differences between electroacoustically similar hearing aids than word recognition testing. Similar work by Leijon et al.[39] has suggested the same conclusion. In the work by Studebaker[45] and his colleagues and also in the work of Leijon et al.,[39] the test material typically consisted of an extended passage of continuous discourse. It should be noted, however, that Purdy and Pavlovic[46] found similar sensitivities between paired comparisons, magnitude scaling, category scaling, and word recognition testing when single sentences were used. Further work is needed to define fully the test conditions that maximize the sensitivity of the various subjective measures.

Dimensions Available for Evaluation

As illustrated by the work of Gabrielsson et al.[25] and Gabrielsson and Sjögren,[48] hearing aids can be differentiated on a variety of relatively independent dimensions. In a series of investigations into the adjectives most useful in providing differentiating information for sound reproduction systems in general and hearing aids in particular, Gabrielsson and colleagues found that dimensions such as "soft versus sharp", "full versus thin", and "bright versus dull" were useful in establishing differences between devices. Real-ear measures provide no information on the perceptual consequences of listening through a given amplifying system. Traditional word recognition testing will only provide information on overall speech understanding.

Although speech understanding is a primary concern when selecting and adjusting a hearing aid, there are other perceptual dimensions that can affect the patient's acceptance of the hearing aid.[49] In some but not all situations, a change on a given electroacoustic dimension may have opposite effects on rated speech clarity versus rated speech quality.[34,50,51] Just because speech is understood does not necessarily mean that it provides a pleasant listening experience. Therefore, speech understanding may at times have to be partially sacrificed for the sake of quality in order to guarantee patient acceptance. In other situations, speech understanding may remain unaltered for a variety of different circuit settings, although the patient may have a distinct preference for one particular configuration, based on judgments on some other dimension, such as "pleasantness," "sharpness," "hollowness," and so forth. For example, Kuk et al.[52] used adaptive paired comparisons to study the relationship between electroacoustic parameters and the perceived "hollowness" of the listener's own voice.

Evaluating Nonlinear Circuit Parameters

In recent years, hearing aid technology has progressed rapidly in an attempt to combat the deleterious effects of sensorineural hearing loss. Numerous circuits now on the market use a variety of adaptive and/or compression approaches to control background noise, maintain a comfortable and audible signal, and limit output without introducing certain forms of undesirable distortion. However, the market entry and exit of such advanced technology usually outpaces the corresponding controlled scientific evaluation of the performance of such circuits on hearing impaired patients. Since the clinician does not have the luxury of waiting for independent research to verify manufacturers' claims and since the performance of nonlinear circuits can vary widely from patient to patient,[53-55] it is important to be able to verify circuit effectiveness on each patient. Traditional word recognition testing often simply cannot tease out differences between nonlinear circuits or between settings on a given circuit.[5,56] Again, subjective testing techniques hold promise in improving test sensitivity on such dimensions. Furthermore, patients will vary as to how sensitive they are to changes along a given electroacoustic dimension. One patient may not notice any difference between a short versus a long compression release time. Another may have quite distinct preferences for one setting versus another. As more and more hearing aids incorporate nonlinear sound processing, the clinician needs to be aware that subjective judgments may need to be used in order to differentiate circuit differences fully.

User-Selected Frequency Responses

The advent of multiple-memory programmable hearing aids has created a dilemma for the dispensing audiologist: After the predetermined set of prescriptive "target" gain values has been programmed into one hearing aid memory, what should the other memories contain? To date, there are no published guidelines for empirically determining the optimal hearing aid electroacoustic parameters for any input signals besides speech in quiet.

Recently, Fabry and Stypulkowski[57] conducted a study that evaluated user-selected gain-by-frequency responses as a viable solution to the problem of programming multiple frequency responses for an individual hearing aid user. In that study, only two variables were manipulated: overall gain in the low and high frequency bands of a commercially available programmable hearing aid (Figs. 7–2, 7–3). Subjects manipulated gain to select the preferred frequency response for three different listening environments: speech in quiet, speech in noise, and recorded music.

Subsequently, the user-selected response for one of the three listening environments, for example, speech in noise, and the subject's NAL-R prescriptive target were programmed randomly into the hearing aid's memories;

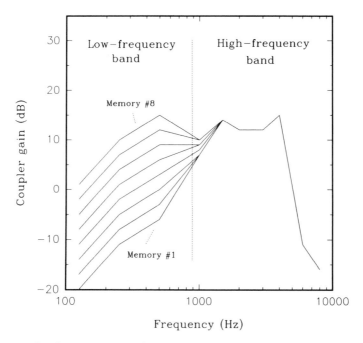

Figure 7–2. Configuration used for user-selected low frequency gain, with high frequency gain fixed at NAL target gain in all eight hearing aid memories of a programmable hearing instrument.

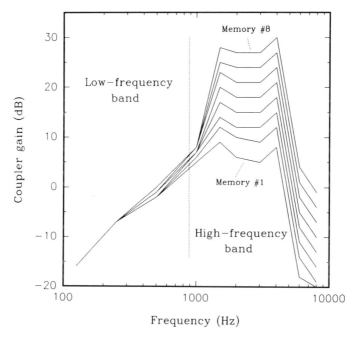

Figure 7–3. Configuration for user-selected high frequency gain, with low frequency gain fixed at NAL target gain in all eight hearing aid memories of a programmable hearing instrument.

subjects then wore the device for 2 weeks, but only for listening situations in which background noise was present. Subjects were instructed to alternate between memories to find the preferred frequency response for listening to speech in noise. This procedure was repeated for the other two listening environments (speech in quiet and recorded music). Fabry and Stypulkowski's conclusions[57] included the following: (1) In the laboratory, subjects selected frequency responses that differed in low and high frequency gain for listening to speech in quiet and when listening in background noise; (2) user-selected frequency responses differed from NAL-R target gain to varying degrees, with the greatest discrepancy for speech in noise; and (3) in real-world environments, seven of nine subjects used the gain-by-frequency response settings that they selected in the laboratory more than the NAL-R settings. This final result suggests that patients may provide relevant input for selecting optimal hearing aid electroacoustics for different listening situations.

Setting Maximum Output

Several investigators have reported that proper selection of hearing aid saturation sound pressure level (SSPL) below user discomfort is the single most important electroacoustic characteristic related to hearing aid acceptance.[58,59] Although most prescriptive formulae calculate target *gain* carefully, most do not use the same precision for determining maximum *output*. Some procedures predict loudness discomfort level (LDL) from a patient's quiet audiometric thresholds, which has been reported to be a highly inaccurate technique.[60] Other studies contend, however, that some procedures for measurement of LDLs are equally variable.[61] This issue is highly debatable, but some subjective measure of loudness can be used on an individual basis for determining target amplification levels and maximum hearing aid output. A magnitude estimation procedure similar to that used by Hawkins et al.[62] may be used to derive LDL. The patient's task is to judge the loudness of stimuli on a nine point scale from "Very Soft" to "Painfully Loud." Hawkins et al.[62] used an ascending approach for estimation of LDL and found it to be a stable measure over time (within 3 dB) when five judgments were made. An alternative method is to use the method of constant stimuli for noises bounded by threshold and 115 dB SPL (or the lowest level to which patients respond "Extremely Uncomfortable").

Another possible method that deserves further study is to use magnitude *production* for estimation of LDL. This would involve instructing the patient to adjust the audiometer attenuator dial to the level at which the stimulus is "Uncomfortably Loud." When patients are in direct control of stimulus intensity, they may be less conservative in their judgments than for either of the other two methods. Keep in mind that hearing aid users perform magnitude productions every day when they set the volume control of their hearing aid to "Most Comfortable."

When performing measures of loudness discomfort, a variety of specific decisions need to be made relative to stimuli and reference levels. A complete discussion of such issues is beyond the scope of this chapter, but the reader is referred to Stelmachowicz,[12] and Hawkins et al.[62]

Long-Term Verification

The use of some type of postfitting verification is likely to be essential, since overall satisfaction with a hearing aid is not reliably predicted based on audiometric or demographic variables known at the time of hearing aid selection.[64,65] Whereas traditional measures of sound field speech understanding are available, the use of questionnaire data collected from a patient after some significant period of new hearing aid use can provide information that may not be gleaned from sound field testing. For example, Cox and Alexander[66] followed new hearing aid users over a 10 week period, collecting both objective (Connected Speech Test) and subjective (Profile of Hearing Aid Benefit) information at selected postfitting times. These investigators found that the objective and subjective measures provided different pictures of the time course of obtained hearing aid benefit.

From a practical standpoint, questionnaire data can be collected from a patient via mail. This type of assessment may increase compliance with a follow-up program, as many patients may not be able to or are unwilling to keep scheduled follow-up appointments. The information gleaned from a mailed-in questionnaire can substitute for or augment information obtained live during a follow-up visit.

As part of the University of Iowa Hospital hearing aid program, all newly

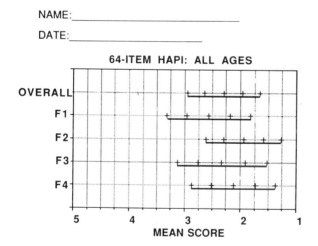

Results from the Hearing Aid Performance Invertory (Walden, Demorest, & Hepler, JSHR, 27, 49-56). Mean scores shown for overall 64-item test and for each of the following sub-factors: F1, speech in noise; F2, speech in quiet; F3, speech with reduced cues; and F4, non-speech signals. Responses were scored on the following 5-point scale: 1 = hearing aid(s) are "very helpful"; 2 = "helpful"; 3 = "very little help"; 4 = "no help"; and 5 = "hinders performance". For each scale, hatch marks from left to right indicate the 10th, 25th, 50th, 75th, and 90th percentiles, based on a sample of 128 hearing aid users from the age range of 19 to 87 years.

Figure 7–4.   Hearing Aid Performance Inventory summary sheet used for adults less than 65 years of age.

fitted adult patients are sent a copy of the Hearing Aid Performance Inventory[42] approximately 2 months after the fitting. Patients less than 65 years of age are sent the original version.[42] Patients over the age of 65 are sent a shortened version.[64] The patient responses are scored and the results are summarized using the forms shown in Figures 7–4 and 7–5. The summary sheets are then shared with other relevant professionals (e.g., the referring physician). The summary sheet presents the patient's self-perceived benefit from the new hearing aid to the 25th, 50th, and 75th percentiles of age-appropriate normative data. The information can be shared with the patient during subsequent follow-up contact.

In our experience, patients have found it useful to know how they perform with their new hearing aids compared with other users. We target patients who fall below the 25th percentile (report less benefit that 75% of other hearing aid users) for specific follow-up intervention (circuit modifications, communicative strategies, assistive devices, additional counseling on expectations, and so forth).

Again, even if follow-up objective measures could reliably demonstrate relative benefits from new hearing aid fittings, the patient still has the final word as to whether a fitting was successful. The audiologist who tries to convince the patient that the hearing aid should be providing benefit because a

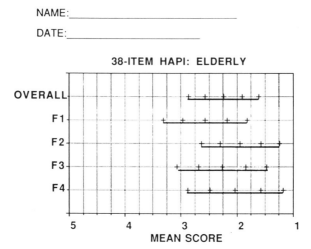

NAME:_____

DATE:_____

Results from the Hearing Aid Performance Invertory (Walden, Demorest, & Hepler, JSHR, 27, 49-56). Mean scores shown for overall 38-item test and for each of the following sub-factors: F1, speech in noise; F2, speech in quiet; F3, speech with reduced cues; and F4, non-speech signals. Responses were scored on the following 5-point scale: 1 = hearing aid(s) are "very helpful"; 2 = "helpful"; 3 = "very little help"; 4 = "no help"; and 5 = "hinders performance". For each scale, hatch marks from left to right indicate the 10th, 25th, 50th, 75th, and 90th percentiles, based on a sample of 75 elderly hearing aid users.

Figure 7–5. Hearing Aid Performance Inventory summary sheet used for adults 65 years of age or older.

prescriptive target was matched or because the sound field word recognition score increased by 18% may be projecting the image of being out of touch with the patient's needs. A structured approach to collecting the patient's perceived benefit in a variety of listening situations allows the audiologist to gain an appreciation of how well the new hearing aid meets the patient's needs and expectations.

Limitations of Subjective Measures

Whereas the procedural issues involved when performing word recognition and real-ear testing have received significant attention in the literature, the corresponding developmental literature for subjective testing is spotty. For example, a considerable literature has been developed on the assessment of LDL. However, little is know as to what measurement conditions may best differentiate various nonlinear circuits. There are a variety of unanswered questions as to the reliability, validity, and sensitivity of many of the recommended subjective measures.

The paired comparison technique would seem to hold promise in allowing listeners to make fine distinctions between hearing aid circuit settings. Studebaker et al.[36] reported that paired comparison measures of continuous discourse appeared to differentiate better between hearing aids than to word recognition testing. However, using different materials, Purdy and Pavlovic[46] found the sensitivity of these procedures to be similar. Schum and Collins[41] evaluated the reliability of the paired comparison technique in two timing modes: (1) when the listener could switch back and forth at will between two samples and (2) when the listener first listened to one sample and then, after a short time delay, to another sample (a replication of listening through one hearing aid, taking it off, and then listening through a second hearing aid). These investigators found the alternating listening procedure to be significantly more reliable than the sequential listening procedure. Thus, the exact conditions under which subjective measures can provide more reliable and valid assessment of hearing aid performance needs to be more clearly defined.

In terms of perceptual ratings of hearing aid performance, again there continue to be several unanswered questions. It is unclear how many different dimensions may need to be rated to best differentiate hearing aids. The work by Gabrielsson et al.[25] and Gabrielsson and Sjögren[47,48] was based on descriptors used by Swedish listeners. These adjectives were then translated into English. The appropriate follow-up verification study on the use of such descriptors by English speaking listeners has yet to be reported.

For any of the sound field subjective methods discussed, there is limited information available as to what speech and competition materials should be used. For example, the SIR[28] consists of 20 different passages to be used with ratings of intelligibility. It is obvious that the patient should not be familiar with the passage when attempting to rate how well it was understood (thus the need for unique passages for each rating). However, if the patient is rating along some other perceptual dimension such as "Clarity" or "Pleasantness," it is not known if unique passages are necessary for each rating. Furthermore, the shorter the passage and the fewer the number of required ratings, the quicker the evaluation process.

Unfortunately, the minimal passage length and the minimal number of required ratings for each type of subjective method have not been reported. However, it is quite certain that simply making an adjustment on a hearing aid and then stepping back and saying "Does that sound better?" is probably not sufficient to provide a valid and reliable subjective response from the patient.

It is also unclear whether subject experience affects the reliability or sensitivity of subjective judgments. Many clinicians would argue that an experienced hearing aid user will likely provide a more valid and reliable reaction to circuit modification than a first-time hearing aid user. The role of patient experience needs to be more fully explored. Finally, the specifics of the interaction between subjective responses and different types and levels of available competition are not known. In other words, are ratings of intelligibility most sensitive and reliable when done in quiet, in low levels of speech noise, at moderate levels of babble, and so forth?

Conclusion

The recent advances in hearing aid technology, including those devices that offer multiple frequency responses, multiband processing, and advanced compression circuits, require new techniques for hearing aid fitting and evaluation. So-called objective measures of hearing aid benefit, including real-ear measurement of eardrum SPL, have provided audiologists with a tool for making accurate, reliable, clinically feasible assessments of hearing aid function. These measures are based primarily on audiometric thresholds measured in quiet backgrounds. One detriment, however, of these new measures is that they remove the patient from active participation in the fitting process. This is a significant departure from the method used previously in fitting hearing aids, and it is not without limitations. Although prescriptive target formulae may be used to predict hearing aid satisfaction in general, personal preference differences remain across individuals with similar hearing losses.

The bottom line is that objective measurements, such as real-ear measurements and prescriptive formulae, may be used to set initial hearing aid characteristics with great accuracy, but subjective measures, such as rated intelligibility or self-assessment scales, may assist in fine tuning circuit settings and assessing long-term satisfaction with hearing aids. In addition, LDL measurements minimize rejection of hearing aids due to loudness discomfort, and may represent an improvement over predicting hearing aid maximum output from quiet auditory thresholds. Subjective techniques will allow for a greater utilization of the advanced programmable features of modern hearing aids.

References

1. Cranmer-Briskey KS: 1992 Hearing Instruments dispenser survey results. *Hear Instrum* 1992; June:8–15.
2. Bratt GW, Sammeth CA: Clinical implications of prescriptive formulas for hearing aid selection, in Studebaker GA, Bess FH, Beck LB (eds): *The Vanderbilt Hearing-Aid Report II*. Parkton, MD: York Press, 1991, pp 23–34.

3. Skinner MW: *Hearing Aid Evaluation*. Englewood Cliffs, NJ: Prentice-Hall, 1988, pp 149–190.
4. Walden BE, Schwartz DM, Williams DL, et al.: Test of the assumptions underlying comparative hearing aid evaluations. *J Speech Hear Dis* 1983; 48:264–273.
5. Fabry DA, Olsen WO: Targets, peaks, and use-gain settings. Paper presented at the annual meeting of the *American Speech-Language-Hearing Association*, 1991, Atlanta, GA.
6. McDermott BJ: Multidimensional analyses of circuit quality judgments. *J Acoust Soc Am* 1968; 45:774–781.
7. Munson WA, Karlin JE: Isopreference method of evaluating speech-transmission circuits. *J Acoust Soc Am* 1962; 34:762–774.
8. Carhart R: Tests for selection of hearing aids. *Laryngoscope* 1946; 56:780–794.
9. Shore I, Bilger RC, Hirsh IJ: Hearing aid evaluation: Reliability of repeated measurements. *J Speech Hear Dis* 1960; 25:152–170.
10. Gilman S, Dirks DD: Acoustics of ear canal measurement of eardrum SPL in simulators. *J Acoust Soc Am* 1986; 80:783–793.
11. Tecca J: Clinical application of real-ear probe tube measurement, in Sandlin R (ed): *Handbook of Hearing Aid Amplification, Volume II: Clinical Considerations and Fitting Practices*. Boston, MA: College-Hill, 1990, pp 225–256.
12. Stelmachowicz PG: Clinical issues related to hearing aid maximum output, in Studebaker GA, Bess FH, Beck LB (eds): *The Vanderbilt Hearing-Aid Report II*. Parkton, MD: York Press, 1991, pp 141–148.
13. Watson N, Knudson V: Selective amplification in hearing aids. *J Acoust Soc Am* 1940; 11:406–419.
14. Lybarger SF: U.S. Patent application SN 543, 278, 1944.
15. McCandless GA, Lyregaard PE: Prescription of gain/output (POGO) for hearing aids. *Hear Instrum* 1983; 34:16–21.
16. Berger KW, Hagberg EN, Rane RL: *Prescription of Hearing Aids: Rationale, Procedures, and Results*. Kent, OH: Herald Publishing, 1978.
17. Byrne D, Dillon H: The National Acoustic Laboratories' (NAL) new procedure for selecting the gain and frequency response of a hearing aid. *Ear Hear* 1986; 7:257–265.
18. Byrne D, Cotton S: Evaluation of the National Acoustic Laboratories' new hearing aid selection procedure. *J Speech Hear Res* 1988; 31:178–186.
19. Purdy SC: *Reliability, Sensitivity, and Validity of Magnitude Estimation, Paired Comparisons, and Category Scaling*, 1990. Unpublished doctoral dissertation, The University of Iowa, Iowa City.
20. Watson RI: *The Great Psychologists*, ed 4. Philadelphia: JB Lippincott Company, 1978.
21. Lawson GD, Chial MR: Magnitude estimation of degraded speech quality by normal- and impaired-hearing listeners. *J Acoust Soc Am* 1982; 72:1781–1787.
22. Studebaker GA, Sherbecoe RL: Magnitude estimations of the intelligibility and quality of speech in noise. *Ear Hear* 1988; 9:259–267.
23. Speaks C, Parker B, Harris C, et al.: Intelligibility of connected discourse. *J Speech Hear Res* 1972; 15:590–602.
24. Hellman RP, Zwislocki J: Loudness summation at low sound frequencies. *J Acoust Soc Am* 1968; 43:60–63.
25. Gabrielsson A, Schenkman BN, Hagerman B: The effects of different frequency responses on sound quality judgments and speech intelligibility. *J Speech Hear Res* 1988; 31:166–177.
26. Palmer CV, Killion MC, Wilber LA, et al.: Comparison of two hearing aid receiver-amplifier combinations using sound quality judgments. *Ear Hear* 1993 (in press).
27. Cox RM, McDaniel DM: Intelligibility ratings of continuous discourse: Application to hearing aid selection. *J Acoust Soc Am* 1984; 76:758–766.
28. Cox RM, McDaniel DM: Development of the speech intelligibility rating (SIR) test for hearing aid comparisons. *J Speech Hear Res* 1989; 32:347–352.
29. Cox RM, McDaniel DM: Evaluation of the speech intelligibility rating (SIR) test for hearing aid comparisons. *J Speech Hear Res* 1992; 35:686–693.
30. Surr RK, Fabry DA: Comparison of three hearing aid fittings using the Speech Intelligibility Rating (SIR) test. *Ear Hear* 1991; 12:32–38.
31. Montgomery AA, Schwarz DM, Punch JL: Tournament strategies in hearing aid selection. *J Speech Hear Dis* 1982; 47:363–372.
32. Neuman AC, Levitt H, Mills R, et al.: An evaluation of three adaptive hearing aid selection strategies. *J Acoust Soc Am* 1987; 82:1967–1976.
33. Punch JL: Quality judgments of hearing aid-processed speech and music by normal and otopathologic listeners. *J Am Audiol Soc* 1978; 3:179–187.
34. Punch JL, Parker CA: Pairwise listener preferences in hearing aid evaluation. *J Speech Hear Res* 1981; 24:366–374.
35. Zerlin S: A new approach to hearing-aid selection. *J Speech Hear Res* 1962; 5:370–376.

36. Studebaker GA, Bisset JD, Van Ort DM, et al.: Paired comparison judgments of relative intelligibility in noise. *J Acoust Soc Am* 1982; 72:80–92.
37. Bryne D, Parkinson A: Reliability and sensitivity of intelligibility and pleasantness judgments of amplified speech. *Aust J Audiol* 1987; 9:77–86.
38. Eisenberg LS, Levitt H: Paired comparison judgments of hearing aid selection in children. *Ear Hear* 1991; 12:417–430.
39. Leijon A, Lindkvist BA, Ringdahl A, et al.: Sound quality and speech reception for prescribed hearing aid frequency responses. *Ear Hear* 1991; 12:251–260.
40. McGee VE: Semantic components of the quality of processed speech. *J Speech Hear Res* 1964; 7:310–323.
41. Schum DJ, Collins MJ: Test–retest reliability of two paired-comparison hearing aid evaluation procedures. Paper presented at the annual meeting of the American Speech-Language-Hearing Association, 1985; Washington, DC.
42. Walden BE, Demorest ME, Hepler EL: Self report approach for assessing benefit derived from amplification. *J Speech Hear Res* 1984; 27:49–56.
43. Cox RM, Alexander GC, Gilmore C: Development of the Connected Speech Test (CST). *Ear Hear* 1987; 8:119S–126S.
44. Cox RM, Gilmore C: Development of the Profile of Hearing Aid Performance (PHAP). *J Speech Hear Res* 1990; 33:343–357.
45. Studebaker GA: Subjective judgments of hearing aid processed speech signals, in Collins MJ, Glattke TJ, Harker LA (eds): *Sensorineural Hearing Loss.* 1986, pp 291–303.
46. Purdy SC, Pavlovic CV: Reliability, sensitivity and validity of magnitude estimation, category scaling and paired-comparison judgments of speech intelligibility by older listeners. *Audiology* 1992; 31:254–271.
47. Gabrielsson A, Sjögren H: Perceived sound quality of sound-reproducing systems. *J Acoust Soc Am* 1979; 65:1019–1033.
48. Gabrielsson A, Sjögren H: Perceived sound quality of hearing aids. *Scand Audiol* 1979; 8:159–159.
49. Killion MC: Transducers, earmolds and sound quality considerations, in Studebaker GA, Bess FH (eds): *The Vanderbilt Hearing-Aid Report: State of the Art Research Needs.* Upper Darby, PA: Monographs in Contemporary Audiology, 1982, pp 104–111.
50. Tecca JE, Goldstein DP: Effect of low-frequency hearing aid response on four measures of speech perception. *Ear Hear* 1984; 5:22–29.
51. Punch JL, Beck LB: Relative effects of low-frequency amplification on syllable recognition and speech quality. *Ear Hear* 1986; 7:57–62.
52. Kuk FK, Plager A, Pape NML: Hollowness perception with noise-reduction hearing aids. *J Am Acad Audiol* 1992; 3:39–45.
53. Gordon-Salant S, Sherlock LP: Performance with an adaptive frequency response hearing aid in a sample of elderly hearing-impaired listeners. *Ear Hear* 1992; 13:255–262.
54. Kuk FK, Tyler RS, Mims L: Subjective ratings of noise-reduction hearing aids. *Scand Audiol* 1990; 19:237–244.
55. Schum DJ: Noise reduction strategies for elderly, hearing-impaired listeners. *J Am Acad Audiol* 1990; 1:31–36.
56. Kuk FK, Tyler RS, Stubbing PW, et al.: Noise reduction circuitry in ITE instruments. *Hear Instrum* 1989; 40(7):20–26, 58.
57. Fabry DA, Stypulkowski P: Evaluation of fitting procedures for multiple-memory programmable hearing aids. Paper presented at the annual meeting of the American Academy of Audiology, 1992, Nashville, TN.
58. Hawkins DB: Selection of a critical electroacoustic characteristic: SSPL90. *Hear Instrum* 1984; 28–32.
59. Walker G, Dillon H, Byrne S, et al.: The use of loudness discomfort levels for selecting the maximum output of hearing aids. *Austr J Audiol* 1984; 6:23–32.
60. Kamm C, Dirks D, Mickey R: Effect of sensorineural hearing loss on loudness discomfort level and most comfortable loudness judgments. *J Speech Hear Res* 1978; 21:668–681.
61. Cox R: Using ULCL measures to find frequency/gain and SSPL90. *Hear Instrum* 1983; 34(7): 17–21.
62. Hawkins DM, Walden BE, Montgomery AA, et al.: Description and validation of an LDL procedure designed to select SSPL90. *Ear Hear* 1987; 8:162–169.
63. Preves DA, Beck LB, Burnett ED, et al.: Input stimuli for obtaining frequency responses of automatic gain control hearing aids. *J Speech Hear Res* 1989; 32:189–194.
64. Schum DJ: Responses of elderly hearing aid users on the Hearing Aid Performance Inventory. *Am J Acad Audiol* 1992; 3:308–314.

65. Schum DJ, Nishiyama T: Success rates for new hearing aid users as a function of audiometric and demographic variables. Poster presented at the annual meeting of the American Academy of Audiology, 1993, Phoenix, AZ.
66. Cox RM, Alexander GC: Maturation of hearing aid benefit: Objective and subjective measurements. *Ear Hear* 1992; 13:131–141.

8

Fitting Strategies for Noise-Induced Hearing Loss

ROBERT W. SWEETOW

Introduction

At the Noise and Hearing Loss conference sponsored by the National Institutes of Health, it was estimated that of the approximately 28 million people in the United States with significant hearing loss, 10 million have losses attributable to high intensity noise.[1] Potentially hazardous sources of excessive exposure to noise include occupational noise, sociocusis, and music generated from personally worn headsets. Additionally, 50 million Americans use firearms, which expands the number of citizens exposed to high levels of noise.[2]

According to the Oticon Research Center,[3] a study performed by the Institute of Hearing Research in Nottingham, England, involving 25,000 randomly selected adults, revealed that approximately 1% of the population experiences bilateral high frequency hearing loss. If the statistics are recalculated to include unilateral loss, the prevalence increases to over 3%. Since noise-induced hearing loss (NIHL) is often insidious, it is impossible to determine how many citizens exposing themselves daily to harmful levels of noise may some day develop the symptoms that commonly accompany NIHL.

Despite these alarming prevalence rates, patients whose audiometric configurations suggest the cause of their hearing loss to be due to excessive noise exposure are currently woefully underserved by the use of amplification. This chapter (1) explores several reasons that may help to explain the lack of success in the past with conventional hearing aid fitting approaches for patients with NIHL; (2) examines fitting alternatives that have recently been introduced for this population; and (3) offers psychoacoustic considerations and practical fitting strategies for patients with NIHL.

Terminology and the Course of NIHL

A sudden loss of hearing from a single exposure of noise is called *acoustic trauma*. The gradual deterioration of hearing sensitivity occurring from several years of excessive noise exposure is referred to as *noise-induced hearing loss*. Understanding the nature of the hearing loss caused by exposure to intense noise can help to formulate methods of providing amplification. Mills,[4] for example, offers this explanation of the nature of hearing loss following exposure to impulse versus continuous noise:

> The nature of the hearing loss produced by acoustic impulses is probably different from the nature of the hearing loss caused by continuous exposures to steady state noise at moderate levels. That is, the excessive displacement of a basilar membrane by an intense acoustic impulse may produce mechanical ripping and tearing, whereas injuries produced by lower level acoustic signals may be caused by metabolic, biochemical or vascular effects, including the depletion of energy stores, mechanically induced changes in the shape of the tectorial membrane, and vasoconstriction within the cochlea. (p. 264)

The audiometric configuration resulting from noise exposure may be indistinguishable for either type.[5] Similarly, the audiometric configuration may mimic that produced by presbycusis. In each case, the resultant hearing loss can present the listener with significant communication difficulties. A typical progression of hearing loss as a function of exposure to industrial noise is shown in Figure 8–1.[6] Maximum damage seems to occur on the portion of the basal turn of the cochlea that tonotopically corresponds to 3000–6000 Hz. Originally, it was thought that the maximum hearing loss occurred in the 4000 Hz region, because the hair cells in this region were more susceptible to damage. Lehnhardt,[7] however, reported that auditory fatigue and recovery at 4000 Hz were no different than at other frequencies. Therefore, it is more likely that initial damage is greatest in the 4000–6000 Hz region because of the

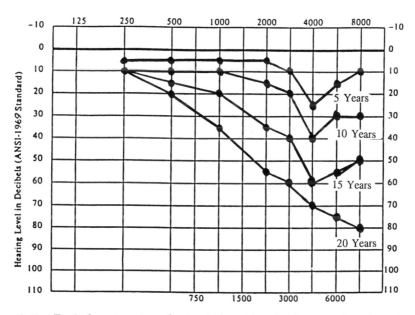

Figure 8–1. Typical progression of noise-induced hearing loss as a function of years of exposure. (Redrawn from Newby.[6])

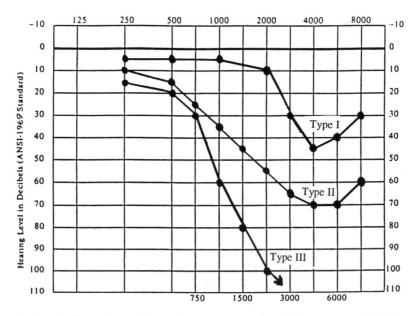

Figure 8–2. Audiometric configurations representative of three types of NIHL.

combination of the normal ear canal resonance, occurring at around 2700 Hz and because the frequency region most affected is usually one-half to one octave above the frequency of the offending noise. As the exposure continues, the "notch" typically seen at 3000–6000 tends to broaden to the frequency region below 3000 Hz, and the magnitude of hearing loss at 3000–6000 Hz increases.

The audiometric configurations of NIHL cover a wide range. However, for the purpose of clarity, only three representative audiometric configurations of NIHL are discussed in this chapter. Type I, which may be considered representative of an audiometric configuration typical of only several years of exposure to noise, is characterized by near-normal hearing through 2000 Hz. Type II, which may be considered representative of many years of excessive exposure to noise, is typically illustrated by audiograms revealing hearing loss extending into the lower frequencies (i.e., below 2000 Hz). Type III, which is less common, represents the more extreme case in which hearing is near normal for the low frequencies only, and the audiometric configuration has a precipitous slope into the high frequencies. These three audiometric configurations are illustrated in Figure 8–2.

NIHL Candidacy for Amplification

If one were to apply the conventional guidelines concerning candidacy for amplification developed approximately 20 years ago, it is obvious that only Type II and some Type III patients with NIHL would be considered prospective hearing aid users. A recent report by Griffing[8] suggests that, when hearing handicap scales are provided by patients who may not have met candidacy criteria by conventional guidelines, a pattern emerges suggesting that a large number of these individuals experience significant difficulties in communicating. In addition, the validity of these past guidelines concerning candidacy for amplification are being seriously questioned due to the recent introduction of advances in hearing aid technology as well as the findings from recent research describing the potential for mammalian hair cell regeneration.[9] Additional reports by Sweetow et al.[10] reflect benefit for Type I patients whose only complaint is the presence of tinnitus and who therefore might not be considered candidates for amplification strictly on the basis of degree of hearing loss. In reality, the only valid measure for determining candidacy for amplification is the extent of the communication problems experienced by the individual. Certain occupational demands (e.g., those experienced by judges or psychiatrists), further expand the need for amplification to an increasing number of Type I patients with NIHL.

Why Amplification Has Been Unsuccessful for Patients With NIHL

Historically, there have been a number of factors contributing to the lack of confidence shared by the public and hearing health care professionals regarding the benefit derived from hearing aids for this population. These include lack or misuse of appropriate handicap scales; misinterpretation of medicolegal formulas that underestimate the effect of hearing loss on word recognition because they are based only on the average hearing loss from 500 to 2000 Hz; and concentration on results based on mean group data rather than individual data. However, perhaps the most compelling reason for this bleak attitude is the history of poor results obtained by patients with NIHL wearing conventional amplification. Exploring these ideas further, six factors that may have contributed to the failure of amplification for NIHL patients emerge, and they are explored further in the following sections.

Lack of Motivation

Hearing aids are often dispensed to patients who lack motivation toward amplification. A poorly motivated patient is a poor candidate for amplification regardless of the degree of hearing loss.[11] Vanity, along with the unfortunate, but undeniable, social stigma often associated with hearing aids is combined with good word recognition scores in "quiet" produce hearing impaired listeners who are resistant to hearing aids. These potential candidates for amplification may have heard stories concerning hearing aids that make sounds uncomfortably loud, but not any clearer, and consequently reside in dresser drawers. Furthermore, one must consider the cost to benefit ratio (i.e., the expense associated with hearing aids may be unacceptable to a potential user who denies having anything more than a slight problem).

Primary Focus on Speech Recognition Measures

There are four primary reasons hearing impaired listeners have decreased word recognition skills: (1) reduced audibility of the speech cues that are important for correct recognition of speech; (2) cochlear distortions that are manifested as reductions in frequency selectivity, temporal resolution, gap detection, and frequency and/or intensity discrimination; (3) central auditory nervous system deficiencies; and (4) deficits in cognitive processing. It is extremely important to differentiate peripheral from central pathology as the cause for reduction of speech recognition ability, because only peripheral dysfunctions (reduced audibility and cochlear distortion) are subject to benefit from amplification. This distinction is particularly relevant for decision making for patients with NIHL who also have presbycusis compounded with central auditory involvement.

Regardless of the cause of diminished word recognition ability, speech recognition measures, particularly in quiet, are poor prognostic indicators of success with amplification for patients with NIHL. For many Type I patients, word recognition scores tend to be excellent when the words are presented in quiet. Thus, it is not possible to demonstrate improvement with amplification. Difficulty in word recognition arises, however, for these Type I patients in noisy environments. Crandell[12] found a low correlation between word recognition scores measured in quiet and those measured in noise. Furthermore, subjective ratings of aided intelligibility were similar despite differences in recognition scores. Smoorenberg[13] also reported a rather low correlation between identification of sentences presented in quiet versus those presented in noise.

It is highly likely, particularly with Type I and Type III patients with NIHL (as with presbycusis with central auditory problems), that comfortable listening in noise as well as a release from the stress and fatigue produced by straining to hear may be more important determinants of success with amplification than improved word recognition scores. Unwanted effects such as excessive loudness, the occlusion effect, or high internal noise levels generated by the hearing aid may lead to rejection of amplification even in the presence of better word recognition scores.

The Preponderance of Linear Amplification Fittings

The vast majority of hearing aid fittings in the United States utilize linear amplification. This was an understandable practice considering the technology available 20 years ago. Current theories concerning cochlear mechanics and recent technological advances providing enhanced signal processing, however, raise serious doubts about the applicability of linear amplification for patients with NIHL.

If the normal cochlea was, as once thought, linear, passive, and broadly tuned, then linear amplification would be appropriate for most hearing losses. However, recent findings indicate that this is certainly not an accurate description of the cochlea. The input–output function of the cochlea is nonlinear. At input sound levels less than 60 dB sound pressure level (SPL), a doubling of

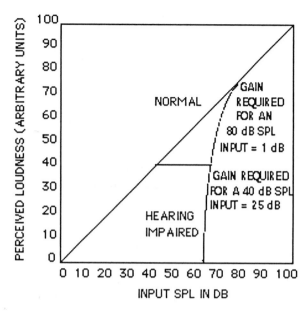

Figure 8–3. Loudness growth as a function of sound level for a normal and a sensorineural impaired NIHL Listener.

amplitude produces far less than a doubling of displacement of the basilar membrane. The active mechanical process of the outer hair cells "amplifies" these sounds while sharpening frequency selectivity. Recruitment results from damage to or loss of the active process in the cochlea, which enhances sensitivity for low input sound levels. Because this process is nonlinear, it results in an amplification of the basilar membrane response to low level sounds while leaving high level sounds relatively unamplified. If this active process is compromised, the response to low input sounds (below 60 dB) is unamplified and absolute threshold is elevated. However, the response to high level sounds remains nearly the same as in the normal ear.[14] An example of this concept is shown in Figure 8–3. In this example, the impaired listener would require gain of 25 dB for an incoming signal of 40 dB, but only 1 dB gain for an incoming signal of 80 dB in order to achieve "normal" loudness. Results such as these can be established using the Loudness Growth by Octave Band (LGOB) test,[15] which is part of the evaluation procedure for a currently available programmable hearing aid containing multichannel input compression.

The use of nonlinear amplification attempts to solve two important fitting problems. One, it minimizes the likelihood that amplified sound will reach the wearer's loudness discomfort level, which often forces the user to lower the volume control setting, resulting in components of the speech signal becoming inaudible. Two, it prevents moderate input levels from driving the aid into saturation. It is believed that the main cause of decreased word recognition of sensorineural impaired listeners in noisy situations is the presence of harmonic and intermodulation distortion produced by the hearing aid driven into saturation.[16]

Focus on Transparency in the Frequency Domain Rather Than in the Amplitude Domain

This factor is directly related to the preponderance of linear amplification just described. Dispensers of hearing aids have adhered to the principle of transparency in the frequency domain since the era of selective amplification. If an impaired listener has frequency regions of normal hearing, attempts are made to provide little or no amplification for those frequencies. This is, in fact, reflected in all of the prescriptive formulae currently in use. Only recently have we begun to appreciate the importance of transparency in the amplitude domain. As explained in the previous section, patients with NIHL, like other sensorineural impaired listeners, often have normal loudness and other psychoacoustic functions for stimuli presented at high intensity levels. It is therefore important to provide gain only for low and moderate intensity incoming stimuli and to provide little or no gain for high intensity incoming stimuli. Furthermore, it is incorrect to assume that there is a direct relationship between the degree of hearing loss at a specific frequency and the amount of gain required at that frequency for a given individual.

It is important to consider more than simply the presence of a hearing loss in determining the need for gain at that frequency. Masking experiments can be used to determine if a patient has a complete loss of functioning neurons over a certain range. This is particularly applicable for Type III patients with NIHL. Moore[17] documents an experimental procedure in which the threshold of a tone located between two bands of noise with a notch between them may increase as the notch increases instead of decreasing in the usual way. He theorizes that this will occur if the signal frequency falls in a range where there are no functioning neurons. This experimental procedure can be used to reveal a reduction or complete absence of high frequency neurons. When high frequency neurons are not functional, it makes little sense to provide high frequency amplification to restore audibility. Furthermore, subjects without functioning high frequency hair cells report that high frequency sounds such as pure tones are heard as "noise."[18] In such cases, it may be better either to filter out the high frequencies or to use a transposing filter.[19]

For the population with Type III NIHL and others with sloping high frequency hearing losses, questions have even been raised regarding the validity of the audiometric results. Terkildsen[20] reported that because of traveling wave principles (i.e., the slope of the envelope diminishing approximately 28 dB per octave), it is possible that for a sharply sloping precipitous hearing loss, certain audiometric thresholds may be determined by the configuration of the traveling wave and not by the actual perception at the tonotopical point on the basilar membrane. This could occur, for example, if the thresholds between adjacent octaves differ by more than 30 dB.

Excessive High Frequency Emphasis

A goal of all hearing aid fittings is to provide enough gain to render all speech sounds audible. This is often a difficult task when fitting patients with high frequency hearing loss. The spectrum of conversational speech indicates that

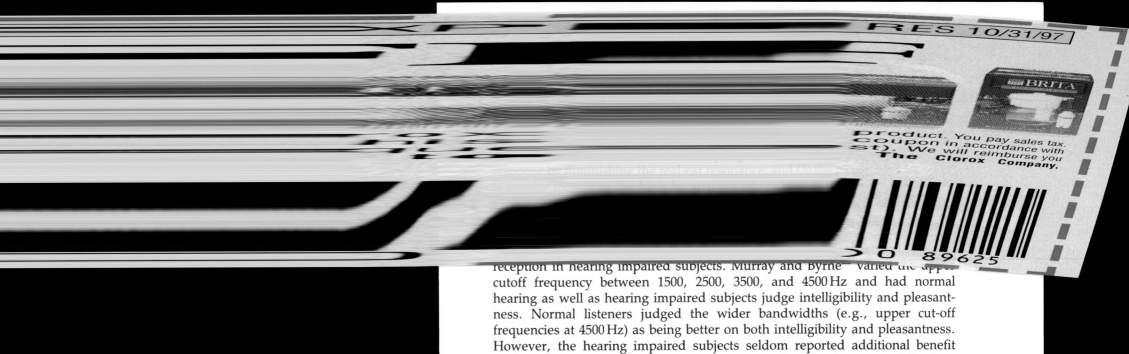

reception in hearing impaired subjects. Murray and Byrne varied the upper cutoff frequency between 1500, 2500, 3500, and 4500 Hz and had normal hearing as well as hearing impaired subjects judge intelligibility and pleasantness. Normal listeners judged the wider bandwidths (e.g., upper cut-off frequencies at 4500 Hz) as being better on both intelligibility and pleasantness. However, the hearing impaired subjects seldom reported additional benefit when bandwidth extended beyond 2500 Hz. Unfortunately, it was difficult to ascertain from this experiment whether the high frequency gain was sufficient above 2500 Hz to allow sounds to be audible for the impaired listeners. Sullivan et al.[23] indicated, on the other hand, that hearing impaired subjects experienced improved speech recognition with the addition of spectral information above 2000 Hz. They did not divide the spectral information above 2000 Hz into smaller bands, however, as did Murray and Byrne. Rankovic[24] stated that, for the majority of her subjects, speech recognition increased as the high frequency region was amplified; however, for subjects with sloping high frequency losses the conditions that produced the greatest high frequency gain resulted in decreased aided performance. Skinner[25] found that increasing high frequency gain by more than 20 dB above low frequency gain caused a decrement in performance for some, though not all, listeners. She speculated that spectral balance is needed to maintain optimal performance.

In another study, Sullivan et al.[26] found at least three factors affecting performance of listeners with steeply sloping losses: (1) the overall gain of the aid, (2) the presence of background noise, and (3) the type of performance measure. In quiet, amplification with the broadest response was reported to provide the best performance. This finding is similar to that reported by Punch and Beck,[27] who demonstrated that both normal and hearing impaired subjects associate better sound quality with speech containing low frequency energy.

Sullivan et al.[26] also indicated that they could obtain the same benefits by increasing the gain within a restricted bandwidth. They found that providing more high frequency energy resulted in improved scores for fricatives and affricatives. However, eliminating the high frequencies, while increasing the sensation level in the low and middle frequencies resulted in better recognition of plosives. They also reported that high frequency energy was more critical for syllable recognition in noise than in quiet. They concluded that, as audible bandwidth increases above 2000 Hz, speech recognition performance improves, but subjective judgments of speech intelligibility do not. This is in

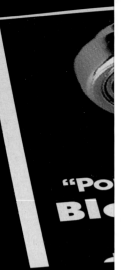

contrast with normal listeners, who report improvement in sound quality with increased bandwidth.

In an attempt to ascertain the minimum high frequency characteristics necessary to provide access to the important spectral cues for the sounds in English, Boothroyd and Medwetsky[28] analyzed the /s/ sound because of its high frequency content and importance to speech recognition. They found that the lowest prominent spectral peak for the /s/ sound was 4300 Hz for males and 7200 Hz for females. Furthermore, they found that the frequency of the lowest prominent spectral peak varied by as much as 1000 Hz, depending on coarticulation effects. For example, the /s/ sound in the /i/ context was 1000 Hz higher than it was in the /u/ context. Thus, if a hearing aid has an upper frequency limit that is lower than the lowest prominent spectral peak, (i.e., 4300 Hz for male speakers and 7200 Hz for female speakers), there may be occasions when the listener will fail to hear the /s/ sound or may confuse it with the /f/ or /th/ sounds. Some individuals could make these distinctions simply on the basis of the cues provided by formant transitions, but Zeng and Turner[29] found that hearing impaired subjects did not use these formant transition cues as efficiently as normal listeners and needed to hear the specific fricative spectra in order to provide correct identification.

Given these findings, combined with the difficulty generating audible high frequencies without creating feedback or distortion, it may be prudent to concentrate efforts on obtaining a better middle frequency response. This is particularly applicable to Stage III patients with NIHL who perceive high frequency sounds as "noise" or as being annoying. The importance of mid-frequency amplification (500–2000 Hz) was stressed by Staab.[30] He reviewed several studies that showed that lower frequencies contribute more to perception of continuous discourse than to identification of nonsense syllables. Rosenthal et al.[31] demonstrated that consonant reception improved when a low frequency band (220–440 Hz) was added to a high frequency band.

The articulation index[32] suggests that 70% of the cues for speech recognition are located between 500 and 2000 Hz. In fact, the frequency band of 500–1000 Hz contributes 35% to the power *and* 35% to the recognition of speech. Staab also emphasized the importance of formant transition perception in making consonant distinctions, and this information is centered in the mid-frequency regions. He concluded that too much emphasis is placed on trying to establish electronic high frequency emphasis and more should be placed on establishing a smooth response in the midfrequency region. Of course, this argument is not applicable to Type II and most Type I patients with NIHL whose unaided hearing is such that midfrequency amplification may be unwarranted and efforts at rendering high frequency consonants audible should be successful.

Inadequate Counseling

Since many patients with NIHL deny the presence of a hearing loss or lack sufficient motivation to treat it, they often demand to be convinced concerning the improvement that a hearing aid can provide. Since the main goal of

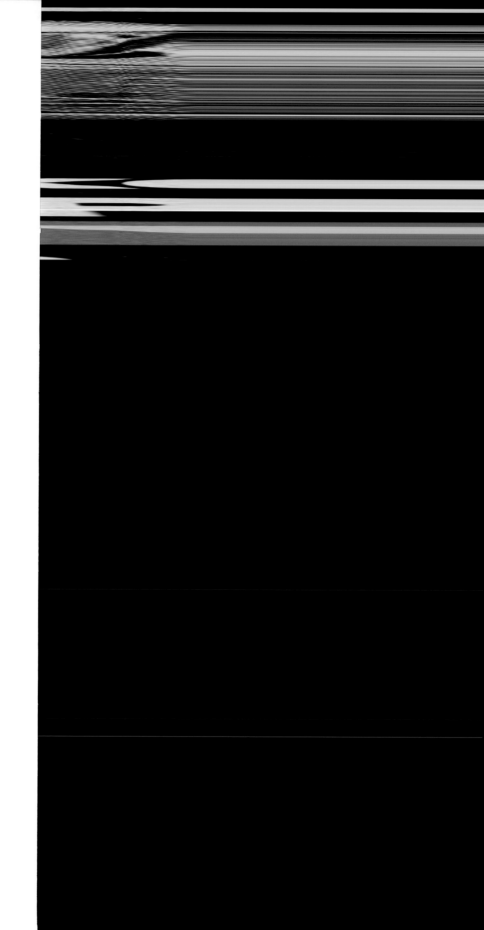

amplification is to facilitate the ease of communication, some Type I patients may be disappointed when they experience only minimal benefit during the initial evaluation of amplification. Proper counseling can alleviate this difficulty. Patients must be educated that prediction of long-term benefit from amplification is tenuous at best because of the initial adjustment and learning process that takes place. Most hearing aid wearers require several weeks before they adjust to the hearing aid.[33] Barfod[34] hypothesizes that a preliminary auditory analysis consisting of converting incoming acoustic signals into neural impulses is followed by a "recognition device" that matches these neural impulses to previously learned information to recognize phonemes properly. Frequency-dependent hearing aids modify the speech input and thus change the output of the preliminary auditory analysis by producing new patterns. Therefore, it takes considerable time for the user to adapt to the new pattern and to learn new "recognition" cues.

Patients also should be informed that there may be no measureable improvement in speech recognition performance, even if the hearing aid seems beneficial to the listener. An explanation for this apparent discrepancy is provided by Hafter and Schlauch.[35] They reason that this occurs because the hearing aid evaluation process may be reflected rather than the benefit from the hearing aid itself. Recognition scores may not be able to be improved for laboratory tasks void of extraneous demands on attention. Word recognition testing in quiet environments is an example a such a low demand task. Subjects in this situation might *prefer* amplified speech because it is easier to process; however, performance may not be improved because the hearing aid is not providing enough new information to the patient that could not be accessed simply by applying full attention. In other words, the hearing aid helps in quiet by allowing the subject to work less hard, but recognition scores, which were near the maximum (even unaided), are not significantly improved. The true test comes in noise or in "high demand environments" where attention is resource limited. In these conditions, the information provided by the hearing aid may no longer be redundant with processes the listener could have accessed on his own by paying full attention, so now the device may be shown to be of value. Thus, testing must be done in high demand conditions, such as created by sufficiently poor signal-to-noise ratios.

Fitting Strategies for Patients With NIHL

Signal processing strategies can be grouped into the following general categories: (1) frequency shaping, (2) adaptive amplification, and (3) compression.

Frequency Shaping

The use of potentiometers in combination with a variety of earmold configurations allows the fitter to achieve a fairly wide range of frequency responses that are appropriate for the Type II NIHL patient, but may not always be applicable for the Type I or Type III patient.

As suggested in the previous section, it is difficult not to provide any low or

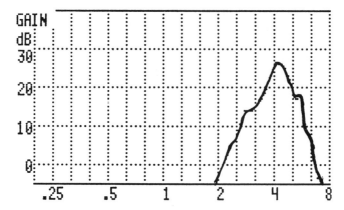

Figure 8–4. Frequency response of the Oticon E43 hearing aid measured in a 2 cc coupler.

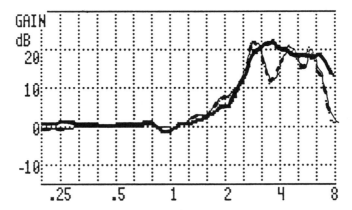

Figure 8–5. Real-ear unaided response (solid line) and real-ear occlusion response (dashed line) of a patient wearing an Oticon E43 hearing aid.

middle frequency real-ear gain with conventional hearing aids. Recognizing this fact, in 1990, one manufacturer (Oticon) introduced a postauricular hearing aid (E43) with a frequency-gain response that rises 24 dB/octave above 2000 Hz and provides essentially no gain below 2000 Hz (see Fig. 8–4). This hearing aid is coupled to a specially designed earmold that produces little, if any, alteration of the real-ear unaided response (REUR) (see Fig. 8–5). It is interesting to note that, during field testing of this hearing aid, Oticon found that 37% of the subjects with hearing loss confined to 3000–8000 Hz adjusted the volume control to avoid listening to the internal noise generated by the aid. The remaining 63% of the subjects adjusted the volume control to obtain satisfactory high frequency amplification. The manufacturer also reported that most of their test subjects preferred real-ear gain equivalent to 40% of their hearing loss at 4000 and 6000 Hz. This finding underscores the need for a different prescriptive formula for the Type I population.

Some conventional analog hearing aids also provide high frequency cut tone controls. Earlier, it was suggested that excessive high frequency amplification may be unnecessary and even detrimental to word recognition ability for certain listeners with Type III precipitously sloping NIHL. If this energy can be filtered out without adversely affecting audibility to the extent that speech becomes unclear, a more satisfactory fitting may result. In a later section, the role of digitally programmable hearing aids in identifying and fitting these patients is discussed.

The frequency-gain response selected by the fitter is often based on prescriptive formulae. Unfortunately, the use of these formulae is often inadequate for predicting the "desired" fitting parameters. A variety of reasons account for this shortcoming. First, subject preference and performance with hearing aids change as intensity levels are varied. Tecca and Goldstein[36] reported that subjects prefer more low frequency gain at a comfortable listening level, but less low frequency gain with higher input levels. Near threshold a patient might prefer a "four-fifths gain rule," but as loudness discomfort level is approached, the preferred gain might be one-fifth of threshold, or even 0.

Second, currently available prescriptive formulae are based on linear amplification. For hearing aids using compression, increasing input result in decreasing gain. Thus, the target is a function of intensity level, and the input levels that are most appropriate for defining target have not yet been established.

Third, the use gain preferred by some patients with NIHL may not be well predicted by any current prescriptive formula. Mueller et al.[37] suggest that NAL-R[38] and most other prescriptive formulae prescribe real-ear gain that is considerably greater than the use gain preferred by hearing impaired listeners exhibiting normal hearing through 2000 Hz. In fact, they found that the preferred use gain was only 20% of the hearing loss at 3000 Hz, far less than the use gain prescribed by NAL-R or the other formulae. However, in their experiment, Mueller et al. reported that most of their subjects' hearing aids produced excessive gain in the 2000 Hz region and that may have accounted for why the patients preferred a lower overall volume. Even so, one must recognize current technological limitations in providing adequate gain for the higher frequencies without providing *any* gain for the lower frequencies (e.g., below 2000 Hz). It is interesting to note that, although some listeners in the Mueller et al. study preferred as little as 5–8 dB of REIG, 10 of the 12 inexperienced hearing aid users preferred amplification and indicated improvement in communication.

Thus, when fitting the patient with NIHL, it is important to determine if exclusive amplification of the high frequencies is most useful for the listener or if amplification should also be provided in the mid-freqency region. In addition, one must take into consideration that requesting addtional high frequency gain, in instances when the REUR shows a particularly large resonant peak, may be fruitless since the manufacturer may have already incorporated the maximum gain possible into that circuit.

Adaptive Amplification

Crandell[12] indicated that for normal listeners, even a 1 dB enhancement in signal-to-noise (S/N) ratio can result in a 6%–8% improvement in speech recognition when evaluated with sentences from the SPIN test. Hawkins[39] reported an articulation function that rises at a rate of 7%/dB S/N. In other words, a 5 dB improvement in S/N theoretically could provide as much as a 35% increase in speech recognition for sensorineural hearing impaired listeners having good speech recognition abilities. One means of providing a perceptual, albeit not a physical, S/N improvement is to use a hearing aid that automatically reduces low frequency gain in response to the level of the input signal. That is, at low input levels the hearing aid provides a broad, flattened frequency response. However, as the input level increases, the signal processing provides progressively less low frequency gain without altering the high frequency gain. There are two major limitations to this approach. First, not all background noises have spectra limited to the low frequencies, and, second, these hearing aids would not be appropriate for Type I NIHL patients for whom virtually no low frequency gain would be desired, even when listening in quiet.

Research findings on hearing aids with automatic low frequency reduction have been mixed. The abundance of studies suggest that they do not usually result in significant improvement in speech recognition in comparison to a conventional linear hearing unless (1) the conventional aid provides an inappropriate frequency response or excessive maximum output for the subject's needs or (2) the background noise is limited to the low frequencies.[40,41] It is likely, therefore, that patients with Type II NIHL who indicate a preference for aids with automatic noise reduction circuitry are reacting in a positive manner to reduced listening efforts in noise and/or improved sound quality in comparison to listening through linear hearing aids.

Adaptive amplification also can be obtained using hearing aids containing K-Amp circuitry. For these aids, the high frequencies are emphasized for low input intensities, but, as input increases, the frequency response flattens, approximating the REUR.[42] This is another example of achieving transparency in the amplitude domain for signals that do not require any signal processing to make them audible to the hearing impaired listener.

Compression

It has been proposed in this chapter that the majority of patients with NIHL should be fit with hearing aids providing nonlinear amplification. Issues relating to the exact parameters defining the nonlinear parameters (i.e., optimal number of compression bands, compression kneepoint, compression ratio, time constants) remain to be resolved. Since aspects of compression are discussed elsewhere in this text, only a brief review of the relevance to fitting patients with NIHL is given here.

NUMBER OF COMPRESSION BANDS

Type I patients with NIHL generally will be fit with hearing aids having little or no low frequency gain. For these patients, single channel compression should be adequate. For Type II and Type III patients, however, *multichannel compression* may be beneficial since there may be a variation in the loudness growth patterns depending on frequency. Loudness growth cannot be predicted simply on the basis of the audiogram. Two patients with identical audiograms may present highly disparate loudness growth patterns. Similarly, an individual may present similar thresholds for two or more frequencies, yet highly different loudness growth slopes. In this case, there may be a need for compression (in varying degrees) for some frequencies but not for others. This can be determined by a procedure such as the Loudness Growth by Octave Band (LGOB) test mentioned earlier.

Multichannel compression systems offer flexibility to tailor compression parameters to the individual's needs. It should be noted that the number of compression channels should be limited to two or three. Leek et al.[43] indicated that reductions in spectral contrasts may add to the difficulty in detecting the spectral features in complex sounds. To avoid this problem, bandwidths of compression should be substantially greater than those of the auditory filters of the listener. Considering that sensorineural impaired listeners already have widened auditory bandwidths,[14] this means that no more than three channels of compression are viable. Moore[17] also confirmed that too many bands of compression can reduce spectral contrasts (between vowels and consonants and even within these two groups). He notes that a sensorineural impaired ear has about ten critical bands to process information (the normal ear has 35). He theorizes that unless the hearing aid has more than 10 bands, it will do little to reduce the masking effects of background noise. He asserts that adaptive filtering may be as effective in noise reduction as multichannel automatic gain control (AGC). Moore's theories notwithstanding, there continues to be a number of multichannel hearing aid users who report enhanced listening comfort in noise. Such improvement may not be achieved with single channel instruments.

Compression Threshold

Compression threshold (or kneepoint) can be defined as the lowest level at which compression becomes active. For hearing aids with input compression, the kneepoint is generally between 45 and 75 dB SPL. One advantage of lower compression thresholds is that the listener may not be aware of the system activating and deactivating (pumping and fluttering) since the hearing aid is in the compression mode most of the time. Kneepoints in the 70–75 dB range may result in frequent pumping and fluttering because of activation by normal conversational speech (particularly that generated by the user's own voice). Another advantage of the lower (45–55 dB) kneepoint is that compression is operating over a wider range (perhaps the full dynamic range of the listener). Since recruitment begins near threshold, it could be argued that the use of nonlinear amplification should operate over the entire dynamic range.

Compression Ratio

Compression ratio refers to the ratio of change in input level to the corresponding change in output level. Normal functioning outer hair cells act as a nonlinear "cochlear amplifier," providing up to 60 dB of gain for low input sounds (e.g., 0 dB) and no gain for high input sounds (e.g., 100 dB). The listener with impaired outer hair cell function has no "cochlear amplifier" for high input *or* low input sounds. Hypothetically, as a result, the normal listener may have a dynamic range on the order of 100 dB while the sensorineural impaired listener's dynamic range may be compressed to 40 dB. Thus, it can be argued that in order to restore "normal" nonlinearity to the sensorineural impaired ear, a compression ratio of no greater than 2.5:1 should suffice. High compression ratios (e.g., 8:1) with multichannel AGC having relatively low knee-points may degrade the relative intensity cues required to identify certain speech sounds.[44] However, Licklider and Pollack[45] demonstrated that with amplitude clipping so severe that no intensity contrasts existed among the speech sounds, speech was still intelligible to normal listeners. It should also be considered that even if spectral contrasts are reduced because of high frequency band compression (with linear low frequency processing), high frequency recruitment may compensate and reinstate the loudness differences.

Compression Time Constants

Several years ago, the concept of adaptive compression was introduced to minimize periods of inaudibility that occur as a result of listening in an acoustic environment characterized by loud transient sounds.[46] In this design, release time varies as a function of the duration of incoming noise. For example, a short burst of noise (such as a spoon dropping on a hard surface) produces a shorter release time than an ongoing noise, such as constant background chatter or machine noise). If the release time is too short, the S/N ratio is decreased. If the release time is too long, following transient noises, the aid remains in compression during a period of time in which the listener wants to listen to speech. Such compression activity may render speech components inaudible while the gain recovers to its desired level.

For hearing aids that do not have adaptive time constraints, it is best to have attack (and release) times that are longer for low frequency inputs than for high frequency inputs. This is because vowels have a longer duration than consonants, and most, though not all, noise is comprised mostly of low frequency energy. High frequency sounds fluctuate within a time frame of 40 ms and vowels may last for 500 ms. It is best to activate low frequency filtering for long duration sounds and not for fluctuating sounds of less than 40 or 50 ms. If different time constraints are not used for low versus high frequency inputs, normal conversational speech could activate an unnecessary adaptive filtered response. These considerations are incorporated into many of the digitally programmable hearing instruments.

Digitally Programmable Hearing Aids

As evidenced by the preceding discussion, knowledge correlating clinical data to the establishment of electroacoustic parameters for a given individual remains inadequate. Given the complexity and variety of needs exhibited by patients with NIHL, the flexibility provided by digitally programmable hearing aids is particularly advantageous to the fitter.

Programming the instrument and the patient's assessment of its performance must incorporate analysis of perceptual attributes. Emphasis must be placed on the individual's prioritized weighting of the importance of these attributes. These priorities should be established during the subjective (case history and interview) and objective (clinical testing) needs assessment. It is essential to prioritize issues, recognizing that certain compromises (e.g., noise reduction vs. speech intelligibility, intelligibility vs. tinny speech quality, gain vs. loudness comfort, feedback vs. high frequency gain) may be inevitable. Having established priorities, the dispenser can begin consideration of programming the various features available with digitally programmable systems. Listener preference (both to other voices and to their own) may represent the highest order of sensitivity. It certainly represents the most critical factor in getting a patient to use a hearing aid. The needs and preferences of the individual take precedence over any single assumption based on research data.

There are three primary advantages of programmable hearing aids. *Multi-channel compression* has already been discussed. The other primary advantages of these instruments are *flexibility in frequency shaping* and *user-controlled multiple memories*.

Flexibility in Frequency Shaping

It is difficult to obtain a target match in the 3000–4000 Hz region (using *any* of the prescriptive formulae) due to the loss of the natural resonance caused by complete or partial occlusion of the ear canal. Since audibility at this region is critical to speech recognition, it is advisable to begin programming the hearing aid so that target gain (or adequate consonant audibility and/or comfort) is achieved at 3000 and, hopefully, 4000 Hz. Then, the low frequency gain and slope can be set as desired. This can be accomplished either by changing the actual gain in the lower frequency band or by raising the transition or cross-over frequency in multi-channel hearing aids. Decisions involved in setting low frequency slope must incorporate both subjective (the patient's description of his acoustic environments) and objective (upward spread of masking and other masking functions) information. Priorities must be established regarding the need for low frequency reduction (perhaps to minimize certain background noises) versus the need for second formant and formant transition information.

In addition, one must be alert to problems that may occur due to high internal noise levels of hearing aids characterized by frequency responses yielding no low or mid-frequency real-ear gain. If these noise levels are audible to the Type I NIHL listener, the hearing aid may be rejected.

Conclusions regarding high frequency characteristics are equally significant. Earlier, it was stated that some patients with NIHL are better suited to a smooth frequency response in the mid-frequencies rather than a high frequency emphasis, due to nonfunctional high frequency neurons. A trade-off may exist between better audibility of the high frequency consonants versus comfort and quality. Once the desired parameters have been determined, amplification of the high frequencies can be systematically altered either by changing the high frequency channel gain or by altering the cross-over frequencies. For three channel systems, it is interesting to note that high frequency gain can be reduced by lowering the lower (F1) transition frequency.

Multi-channel programmable hearing instruments, particularly those with three bands, can be especially useful for Type III patients since gain can be minimized for the low frequencies, maximized for the middle frequencies, and then minimized for the high frequencies (if so desired). Also, for patients having unusual REURs, atypical frequency shaping can be fashioned to the individual's needs.

User-Controlled Multiple Memories

One of the more useful features available in some digitally programmable hearing aids is the capacity to utilize multiple memories. No single hearing aid is optimal for all listening environments.[47] Therefore, it seems logical to offer the patient choices of acoustic responses to best interface with the environment in which listening is taking place. This concept is not new. For years, some conventional analog hearing aids have offered user-manipulated tone control switches.

The optimal number of multiple memories to meet listening needs is unknown. The number of available program choices for listeners vary from two to as many as eight. There are no research data to support the concept that more memory choices are better. In fact, it is possible that too many choices might confuse the user and create difficulty in rapidly selecting the "correct" program choice. Even so, the psychological advantage of offering the patient some "control" over the listening environment is significant.

Some new users, particularly those with Type I NIHL, may find high frequency emphasis hearing aids objectionable and too "tinny." Sweetow and Mueller[48] reported a patient with normal hearing through 1500 Hz who effectively adjusted to a high frequency emphasis hearing aid by initially selecting a program containing a broader response and then progressively moving through to a higher emphasis response. The patient's primary hearing difficulty occurred during group meetings. At the time of the fitting, target gain was calculated and the instrument was programmed. This response is shown as response A in Figure 8–6. The patient objected to this response, saying that it sounded "tinny" and did not think the use of the hearing aid made a significant difference in his hearing ability. By manipulating the low cut and slope adjustment features, responses B, C, and D were set in the remaining three memory locations of the instrument. The patient now had the option of adding 15 dB of gain at 1000 Hz (response D), even though most prescriptive formulae would suggest that this response would overamplify the low frequencies. As the patient became accustomed to the programmable hearing aid, he gradually increased his use of response A by progressing through responses C and B. The flexibility of providing four different settings led to amplification acceptance that may not have occurred had he been offered only the amplification response shown in response A.

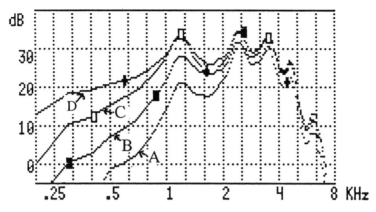

Figure 8-6. Full-on gain frequency response of widex Quattro Q8 in 2 cc coupler illustrating the use of multiple memories for adjusting to "new" sound processing.

It also may be practical to reserve one program for telephone use. Here too, it may be beneficial to frequency shape in order to limit amplification to below 3000 Hz, since most telephones do not transduce above this frequency, and so that feedback is limited.

One final issue related to digitally programmable hearing aids is their capacity to incorporate adaptive low frequency reduction (also termed *bass increase at low levels* [BILL]) and adaptive high frequency emphasis (also termed *treble increase at low levels* [TILL]). Programmable hearing aids can be adjusted to provide BILL merely by setting a low compression kneepoint in the low frequencies and a high compression threshold (or even a linear response) in the high frequencies. The opposite effect (TILL) can be achieved by setting a low compression threshold for the high frequencies and a linear or high compression threshold for the low frequencies. Both BILL and TILL programming (analogous to the K-Amp circuitry) would be more effective for the listener with Type II rather than Type I NIHL because of the regions of normal hearing present for Type I listeners. That is, both could generate too much audible low frequency noise in quiet environments. Furthermore, both strategies can be programmed into a single hearing aid using multiple memories. Then, the user can determine if one is more suitable than the other or perhaps if the need for both types of signal processing exists.

Other Considerations

Earmold Acoustics

The subject of earmold acoustics can easily occupy a chapter or even a textbook. For the purposes of this chapter, if a listener has normal or near-normal low frequency hearing (as do most patients with Type I NIHL) it is desirable, if not absolutely necessary, to minimize occlusion of the ear canal to the greatest extent possible. In a closed mold fitting, the loss of the REUR (often around 20 dB at 2500–3000 Hz) may be difficult for the hearing aid to overcome.

Equally as important is the unwanted enhancement of the low frequencies of the user's voice, as evidenced by the occlusion effect. It may be useful to have the patient vocalize words with both closed and open vowels (such as /i/ and /u/) to ascertain whether the occlusion effect is likely to be unacceptable to the user. Special earmolds, such as Continuous Flow Adaptors (CFA), Libby horns, open tube couplers, and deeply seated earmolds, can be of assistance in enhancing high frequency gain and minimizing occlusion. Within the limits imposed by feedback, patients with Type I or Type II NIHL seem best served by earmolds producing the least occlusion. Even some Type III patients can benefit from more open coupling if the desired frequency response is one that minimizes high frequency gain. If a significant amount (i.e., 30 dB or more) of high frequency real-ear gain is required, a more closed coupling system will be necessary.

Hearing Aid Style

As it is with earmold configuration, the REIG is greatly affected by the style of the aid. Specifically, it is difficult to achieve the type of frequency response (minimal low frequency with adequate high frequency gain) suitable for Type I or Type III patients using in-the-canal (ITC), or even certain IROS in-the-ear (ITE) hearing aids. Even so, Surr and Hawkins[49] report that 73% of new users select ITE hearing aids even when the advantages of behind-the-ear (BTE) hearing aids are explained. If the external auditory meatus is sufficiently large, use of an IROS configuration in an ITE may be helpful, but real-ear measures should be used to verify the amount of high frequency insertion gain. Similarly, these measures should be used to confirm the amount of low frequency insertion gain reduction, since this cannot be extrapolated simply on the basis of vent size.

Binaural Amplification

The superiority of binaural amplification will be expounded elsewhere in this text. For NIHL patients, as with other sensorineural hearing impaired listeners, speech recognition scores measured in quiet, sound treated rooms often are not sensitive enough to prove or disprove the notion of binaural superiority with regard to hearing aid use.[50] Even so, preference declarations and anecdotal reports of enhanced laterality and more comfortable listening through binaural systems abound.[51] A variety of factors may account for this subjective preference.

Elimination or minimization of head shadow is particularly important for listeners with high frequency hearing loss (i.e., the NIHL population). A central release from masking, termed *binaural squelch*,[52] may be operative. Absolute binaural thresholds are 2–3 dB better than monaural thresholds.[53] At suprathreshold levels, at which listeners receive amplified sound, summation increases by as much as 6–10 dB.[54] Thus, a hearing aid user can achieve the same loudness perception from binaural hearing aids set at a lower volume control setting than with a monaural aid. This may greatly reduce feedback problems. In addition, one might reason that if binaural stimulation sounds louder than monaural stimulation, it would be necessary to limit the maximum power of a hearing aid to keep it from exceeding the patient's loudness discomfort level. Hawkins[55] found that when subjects were asked to match the loudness of binaural and monaural stimuli, this summation effect occurred, but the subjects reported no reduction in binaural loudness discomfort levels versus monaural loudness discomfort levels. In fact, most indicated that the binaural stimuli could be more intense than the monaural stimuli before it produced discomfort. It follows that the dynamic range of listening is greater for binaural listening than for monaural listening. Thus, the general rule is that, unless a significant asymmetry exists between the ears in either sensitivity or word recognition ability, the standard should be trial with binaural amplification.

Verification Considerations

Verification of a successful hearing aid fitting for patients with NIHL should entail assessment of (1) speech recognition and judgments of sound quality, (2) real-ear insertion and saturation responses, and (3) subjective scaling.

Assessment of Speech Recognition and Judgments of Sound Quality

The primary goal of amplification is to enhance communication. For some hearing aid users, this corresponds to an improvement in speech recognition. For others, particularly those with Type I and some with Type III NIHL, the goal may be to ease listening effort. Both word recognition scores and judgments of sound quality should be obtained in quiet and in noisy environments. The ineffectiveness of speech recognition testing in quiet has previously been discussed. In addition, Beck[56] elucidated the inability of speech recognition tasks in noise to differentiate precisely among hearing aids. This is especially true when one utilizes monosyllabic word lists, which have questionable face validity.

A number of attractive alternative speech procedures have been proposed. The use of adaptive speech measures (i.e., maintaining a certain subjective intelligibility level, such as 50%) of connected discourse in various S/N ratios may be helpful in avoiding ceiling effects (e.g., word recognition scores that are too high to show improvement), as may be characteristic of Type I NIHL patients. The Speech Perception in Noise (SPIN) test[57] utilizes high predictability and low predictability items and can be effectively used. It has been shown, for example, that the need for extending the frequency response into the high frequencies becomes more apparent for low redundancy items. Cox and Alexander[58] propose use of the Connected Speech Test, but caution that a variety of input levels should be utilized in light of the fact that subjective preference of hearing aid processed sound may change as a function of intensity level.

Also, despite the apparent conclusion that speech recognition tests used for assessing patients with high frequency hearing losses should utilize speech materials designed specifically for this population (e.g., CUNY NST[59]), Lee et al.[60] demonstrated that these materials were no more sensitive than the conventional NU-6 word lists.[61]

Assessment of Real-Ear Insertion and Saturation Response

There is a disturbing trend recently for some manufacturers to claim that real-ear measurements are not valid for their particular hearing aids. This caution may be expressed in part because of the depth and nature of the coupling to the ear and in part because of concern that prescriptive targets cannot be adequately met by a particular product. Dirks and Kincaid[62] have indicated the difficulties encountered in accurately assessing the very high frequencies depending on probe microphone placement. Additionally, it is true that prescriptive formulae were developed for linear hearing aids and several unresolved questions remain concerning how target levels should vary as a function of input level. Moreover, it is likely that target gain is also a function of audiometric configuration and, perhaps, etiologic factors. Recall the earlier discussion that some patients with Type I NIHL prefer use gain equivalent to only 20% of the hearing loss.

Shortcomings of target insertion gains for patients with NIHL notwithstanding, it is this author's opinion that certain real-ear measures remain vital objectives of the hearing aid fitting verification procedure. Auditory mapping procedures such as proposed by Seewald[63] or Loven[64] utilize the Real Ear Aided Response (REAR) and the Real Ear Saturation Response (RESR) to ensure both audibility and that the individual's LDL is not exceeded. Similar to the rationale for using multiple input levels for speech recognition and quality assessment, the use of advanced compression techniques also requires that the REAR be measured using several different input levels.

Subjective Scaling

In view of the limitations of the validation procedures just discussed and of the fact that quality and comfort of listening, rather than improvements in word recognition performance, may be the most important factor determining success with amplification for NIHL patients, it is possible that one of the most valid ways of assessing aided benefit is with self-assessment scales. Several scales have been developed for this purpose.[65–68] Whether one chooses to utilize any of the published hearing aid benefit questionnaires or to devise an original one to meet the needs of a particular patient population, the use of subjective scaling is certainly useful. Audiologists must not forget that NIHL patients will not benefit from a hearing aid that is not worn, so the bottom line assessment measure is how an individual *feels* about the prescribed amplification, not how that individual scores on a battery of clinical measures in a controlled laboratory environment.

Conclusion

Significant technologic advances have been made for providing amplification to the hearing impaired population with NIHL. Further advances pertaining to digital feedback control, digital enhancement of speech components, and more effective noise reduction strategies are certain to follow. In the meantime, audiologists need to concentrate their efforts on developing concise and accurate clinical measures of the psychoacoustic skills and limitations of the individual patient. Among these could be measures of temporal masking, frequency resolving power, upward spread of masking, loudness growth, and speech detection in noise. It is anticipated that the use of otoacoustic emissions, particularly distortion products, in conjunction with noise notch masking tests may be of assistance in determining the functional status of outer hair cells so that the benefits of providing gain in certain frequency regions can be ascertained on an individual basis.

The use of programmable hearing aids having accessible "comparative" functions should continue to expand as audiologists utilize this flexibility in determining the electroacoustic parameters for each patient. The use of multi-channel compression, adjustable cross-over frequencies and the fine tuning of gain in narrow frequency regions will likely prove to be of great value as superior algorithms and fitting strategies are generated.

Technologic advances notwithstanding, counseling is critical. It should be explained that (1) amplification may not provide immediate or obvious benefit and (2) an *overall* improvement in speech recognition may not easily be realized. The improvement in speech recognition may be subtle and limited to fricatives and affricatives. Most important, it is vital that patients with NIHL be educated that ease of communication is a quality of life issue and that it may be the most important benefit to be derived from amplification.

References

1. Lankford JE: Noise pollution awareness needed by the 21st century. *Hear Instrum* 1990; 41(10): 6–13.
2. Kramer WL: Gunfire noise and its effect on hearing. *Hear Instrum* 1990; 41(10):26–28.
3. Oticon Research Center: *Testing and Evaluating a High Frequency Hearing Aid: E43.* Internal Field Test Publication. Copenhagen, Denmark: Oficon, 1989.
4. Mills JH: Relationship of noise to hearing loss. *Semin Hear* 1988; 9:255–266.
5. Ward WD, Frick JE: *Noise as a Public Health Hazard.* ASHA Report 4. Washington, DC: ASHA, 1969.
6. Newby HA: *Audiology,* ed 4. Englewood Cliffs, NJ: Prentice-Hall, 1979, pp 322–325.
7. Lehnhardt E: Die berufsschaden des ohres. *Arch Ohr Nas Kehlkopfheilkd* 1965; 85:11–14.
8. Griffing TS: A new approach to hearing instrument candidacy. *Hear Instrum* 1992; 43(3):23–35.
9. Corwin JT: Hair cell regeneration. *SHHH* 1992; 13:32–34.
10. Sweetow RW, Cato P, Levy MC: The tinnitus masking efficiency of high-frequency hearing aids. *Hear J* 1991; 44(4):24–34.
11. Alpiner JG: Aural rehabilitation and the aged client. *Maico Audiol Library Ser* 1987; 4:9–12.
12. Crandell C: Individual differences in speech recognition ability: Implications for hearing aid selection. *Ear Hear* 1991; 12(Suppl 6):100S–106S.
13. Smoorenberg GF: Hearing handicap assessment for speech perception using pure tone audiometry, in *Noise as a Public Health Problem; New Advances in Noise Research.* Part 1, vol 4. Stockholm: Swedish Council for Building Research, 1990, pp 245–246.
14. Kates J: Modeling normal and hearing impaired hearing: Implications for hearing aid design. *Ear Hear* 1991; 12(Suppl 6):162S–176S.
15. Pluvinage V: New dimensions in diagnostics and fitting. *Hear Instrum* 1988; 39(8):28–38.
16. Fabry DA: Programmable and automatic noise reduction in existing hearing aids, in Studebaker GA, Bess FH, Beck LB (eds): *The Vanderbilt Hearing-Aid Report II.* Parkton, MD: York Press, 1991, pp 65–78.

17. Moore BCJ: Characterization and simulation of impaired hearing: Implications for hearing aid design. *Ear Hear* 1991; 12(Suppl 6):154S–161S.
18. Moore BCJ, Glasberg BR, Hess RF, Birchall JP: Effects of flanking noise bands on the rate of the growth of loudness of tones in normal and recruiting ears. *J Acoust Soc Am* 1985; 77:1505–1513.
19. Velmans E, Marcuson M: The acceptability of spectrum-preserving and spectrum destroying transposition to severely hearing-impaired listeners. *Br J Audiol* 1983; 17:17–26.
20. Terkildsen K: Hearing impairment and audiograms. *Scand Audiol* 1980; 10(Suppl):27–31.
21. Pascoe D: Frequency responses of hearing aids and their effects on the speech perception of hearing impaired subjects. *Ann Otol Rhinol Laryngol* 1975; 84(Suppl 23):1–40.
22. Murray N, Byrne D: Performance of hearing impaired and normal hearing listeners with various high frequency cut-offs in hearing aids. *Aust J Audiol* 1986; 8:21–28.
23. Sullivan JA, Allsman CA, Nielsen LB: Hearing aid bandwidth for sloping, high frequency hearing losses, in Studebaker GA, Bess FH, Beck LB (eds): *The Vanderbilt Hearing-Aid Report II.* Parkton, MD: York Press, 1991, pp 287–294.
24. Rankovic CM: *An Application of the Articulation Index to Hearing Aid Fitting.* Ph.D. dissertation, University of Minnesota, Minneapolis, 1989.
25. Skinner MW: Speech intelligibility in noise-induced hearing loss: Effects of high-frequency compensation. *J Acoust Soc Am* 1980; 67:306–317.
26. Sullivan JA, Levitt H, Hwang J, Hennessey A: An experimental comparison of four hearing aid prescription methods. *Ear Hear* 1988; 9:22–32.
27. Punch J, Beck L: Relative effects of low frequency amplification on syllable recognition and speech quality. *Ear Hear* 1986; 7:57–62.
28. Boothroyd A, Medwetsky L: Spectral distribution of /s/ and the frequency response of hearing aids. *Ear Hear* 1992; 13:150–157.
29. Zeng F, Turner C: Recognition of fricatives by normal and hearing impaired subjects. *J Speech Hear Res* 1990; 33:440–449.
30. Staab WJ: Significance of mid-frequencies in hearing aid selection. *Hear J* 1988; 6:23–34.
31. Rosenthal RD, Lang JD, Levitt H: Speech reception with low frequency energy. *J Acoust Soc Am* 1975; 57:949–955.
32. French NR, Steinberg JC: Factors governing the intelligibility of speech sounds. *J Acoust Soc Am* 1947; 19:90–119.
33. Berger K, Hagberg E: Hearing aid users attitudes and hearing aid usage. *Mono Contemp Audiol* 1982; 3:24–27.
34. Barfod J: Speech perception processes and fitting of hearing aids. *Audiology* 1979; 18:430–441.
35. Hafter ER, Schlauch RS: Cognitive factors and selection of auditory listening bands, in Dancer AL, Henderson D, Salvi RJ, Hamernik RP (eds): *Noise Induced Hearing Loss.* St. Louis, MO: Mosby Year Book, 1992, pp 303–309.
36. Tecca J, Goldstein D: Effects of low frequency response on four measures of speech perception. *Ear Hear* 1984; 5:22–29.
37. Mueller HG, Bryant MP, Brown WD, Budinger AC: Hearing aid selection for high frequency hearing loss, in Studebaker GA, Bess FH, Beck LB (eds): *The Vanderbilt Hearing-Aid Report II.* Parkton, MD: York Press, 1991, pp 269–286.
38. Byrne D, Dillon H: The National Acoustic Laboratories' (NAL) new procedure for selecting the gain and frequency response of a hearing aid. *Ear Hear* 1986; 7:257–265.
39. Hawkins D: Methods of improving speech recognition in the presence of noise and reverberation. *Audiol Acoust* 1985; 9:10–12.
40. Stein L, Dempsey-Hart D: Listener assessed intelligibility of a hearing aid self adaptive noise filter. *Ear Hear* 1984; 5:199–204.
41. Van Tasell D, Larsen S, Fabry D: Effects of an adaptive filter hearing aid on speech reception in noise by hearing impaired subjects. *Ear Hear* 1988; 9:15–21.
42. Killion MC: A high fidelity hearing aid. *Hear Instrum* 1990; 41(8):38–39.
43. Leek MR, Dorman MF, Summerfield Q: Minimum spectral contrast for vowel identification by normal-hearing and hearing-impaired listeners. *J Acoust Soc Am* 1987; 81:148–154.
44. Plomp R: The negative effect of amplitude compression in multichannel hearing aids in the light of the modulation-transfer function. *J Acoust Soc Am* 1988; 83:2322–2327.
45. Licklider J, Pollack I: Effects of differentiation, integration, and infinite peak clipping upon the intelligibility of speech. *J Acoust Soc Am* 1948; 20:42–51.
46. Smriga D: Modern compression technology: Developments and applications, part 2. *Hear J* 1986; 39(7):13–16.
47. Libby ER, Sweetow RW: Fitting the environment—some evolutionary approaches. *Hear Instrum* 38(8):10–16.
48. Sweetow RW, Mueller HG: The interfacing of programmable hearing aids and probe microphone measures. Part 2. *Audecibel* 1991; 40(3):19–22.

49. Surr R, Hawkins DB: New hearing aid users' perception of the "hearing aid effect." *Ear Hear* 1988; 9:113–118.
50. Carhart RC: The usefulness of binaural hearing aids. *J Speech Hear Dis* 1958; 23:42–51.
51. Balfour PB, Hawkins DB: A comparison of sound quality judgments for monaural and binaural hearing aid processed stimuli. *Ear Hear* 1992; 13:331–339.
52. Koenig W: Subjective effects in binaural hearing. *J Acoust Soc Am* 1950; 22:61–62.
53. Haggard M, Hall J: Forms of binaural summation and the implications of individual variability for binaural hearing aids: *Scand Audiol* 1982; 15(Suppl):47–63.
54. Reynolds G, Stevens S: Binaural summation of loudness. *J Acoust Soc Am* 1951; 32:1337–1344.
55. Hawkins DB: Selection of SSPL90 for binaural hearing aid fittings. *Hear J* 1986; 39:23–24.
56. Beck L: Issues in the assessment and use of hearing aid technology. *Ear Hear* 1991; 12(Suppl 6):93S–99S.
57. Bilger R, Neutzel J, Rabinowitz J, Rzeczkowski C: Standardization of a test of speech perception in noise. *J Speech Hear Res* 1984; 27:32–48.
58. Cox R, Alexander G: Hearing aid benefit in everyday environments. *Ear Hear* 1991; 12:123–126.
59. Resnick S, Dubno J, Hoffnung S, Levitt H: Phoneme errors on a nonsense syllable test. *J Acoust Soc Am* 1975; 58:S114.
60. Lee LW, Humes LE, Wilde G: Evaluating performance with high frequency-emphasis amplification. *J Am Acad Audiol* 1993; 4:91–97.
61. Tillman T, Carhart R: *An Expanded Test for Speech Discrimination Utilizing CNC Monosyllabic Words.* Northwestern University Auditory Test No. 6 (Technical Report No. SAM-TR-66-55). Brooks Air Force Base, TX: USAF School of Aerospace Medicine, 1966.
62. Dirks DD, Kincaid GE: Basic acoustic considerations of ear canal probe measurements. *Ear Hear* 1987; 8:5S, 60S–67S.
63. Seewald R: The desired sensation level approach for children: Selection and verification. *Hear Instrum* 1988; 39(7):18–22.
64. Loven F: A real ear speech spectrum based approach to ITE preselection/fitting. *Hear Instrum* 1991; 42(3):6–13.
65. Cox RM, Gilmore C, Alexander GC: Comparison of two questionnaires for patient assessed hearing aid benefit. *J Am Acad Audiol* 1991; 2:134–145.
66. Cox RM, Alexander GC: Hearing aid benefit in everyday environments. *Ear Hear* 1991; 12:127–139.
67. Cox RC, Gilmore C: Development of the profile of hearing aid performance. *J Speech Hear Res* 1990; 33:343–357.
68. Walden BE, Demorest ME, Hepler EL: Self-report approach to assessing benefit derived from amplification. *J Speech Hear Res* 1984; 27:49–56.

9

Selecting and Verifying Hearing Aid Fittings for Symmetrical Hearing Loss

ROBERT DE JONGE

Introduction

The patient with a bilaterally symmetrical, typically sensorineural hearing loss is a common clinical occurrence. Traditionally, a person with this type of hearing loss has been considered the ideal candidate for binaural amplification. Yet many individuals who could benefit from a binaural fit are still being aided monaurally. The purpose of this chapter is to present information that should help the clinician to decide whether a binaural fit is justifiable. The basic research relating to binaural phenomena, and possible test protocols are reviewed. Additionally, patient and audiologist attitudes and beliefs concerning the use of two hearing aids are explored.

Binaural Hearing

The phenomenon of binaural hearing has been thoroughly investigated, and some excellent reviews of past research are available that deal with both normal and impaired listeners.[1-4] Binaural summation, localization, elimination of the head shadow effect, and binaural squelch are often cited as the major advantages of listening with two ears in the sound field. While hearing is not often thought of within the context of our balance system, it does provide significant information that helps us to orient ourselves in space. Loss of hearing in one ear, or using monaural amplification, limits this aspect of sensory experience.

Basic Variables Underlying Binaural Phenomena

Threshold for a binaural signal, presented diotically (i.e., identical signals at the two ears) via earphone, is better than that for a monaural signal by about

2–6 dB. At suprathreshold levels sounds presented binaurally are perceived as being louder than sounds of the same level presented to only one ear, the difference being about 9 dB for normal-hearing listeners.[5] For example, a 500 or 2000 Hz tone at 71 dB SPL delivered to both ears is judged as being equal in loudness to a monaural tone at 80 dB SPL. This difference, called *binaural summation*, could be viewed as a basic advantage of two-eared listening.

Most other binaural phenomena arise as a consequence of the two ears being located at either side of the head. A simple modeling of the situation considers the head to be a sphere with the ears positioned in the horizontal plane at opposite poles. Because of this arrangement sound coming from a source will be slightly different at the two ears both in spectrum and time. Since these differences are caused by the physical positioning of the ears, they are present for both children and adults, for individuals with unilateral and bilateral hearing losses, and for those with normal and compromised central auditory nervous systems (CANS). However, the ability to take advantage of these differences is dependent on the status of the periphery and CANS.

AZIMUTH AND ELEVATION: LOCATING A SOUND SOURCE

Figure 9–1 illustrates a point source located at a particular azimuth (angle). The listener is positioned so that the major axis is perpendicular to the ground. The sound source is located in the horizontal plane. The horizontal plane is parallel to the ground. Conventionally, 0° azimuth is located directly in front of the listener. Directly to the right is 90° azimuth. Directly to the left is 270° azimuth (or −90°). Elevations can also be specified as an angle if the source is located above or below the horizontal plane. The geometry of the situation can be quite complicated. But, under realistic situations the auditory system does quite well at locating sound sources at specific azimuths and elevations. For example, if

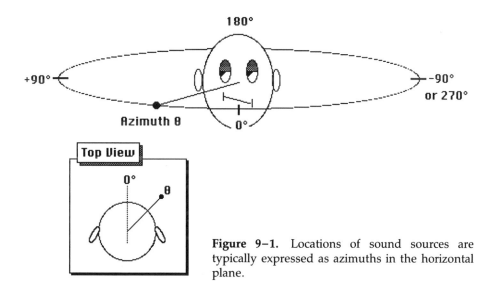

Figure 9–1. Locations of sound sources are typically expressed as azimuths in the horizontal plane.

the sound source is positioned in the horizontal plane (0° elevation), and moved slightly to the right and left, the listener can detect a change (minimum audible angle) of only 1 to 2° (see Mills[6] for a review of sound localization).

INTERAURAL TIME AND INTENSITY DIFFERENCES—THE HEAD
SHADOW EFFECT

The head serves as an obstacle in two ways. First, it simply separates the two ears by a certain distance. Sound travels a little more than 1 ft. each millisecond (msec). Depending on the azimuth of the source, the sound will reach one ear first (the near ear) and reach the second (the far ear) a short time later. The largest difference occurs when the azimuth is either +/− 90°. Although this varies with the exact diameter of the head and the speed of sound, the maximum time difference will be about 0.65 msec. The time difference becomes smaller as the azimuth decreases. At 0° azimuth, the time difference is zero.

The second way that the head serves as an obstacle is when it "shadows" one ear: the head shadow effect. The shadow is created when the sound wave reflects off the head. Intensity at the far ear is less than at the near ear. The

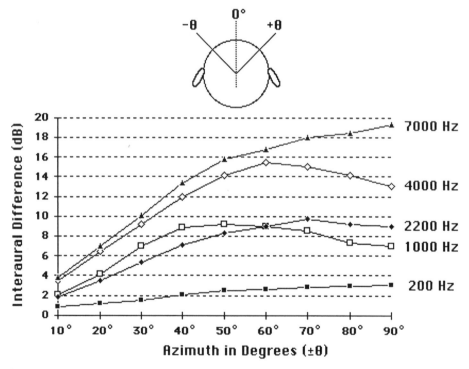

Figure 9–2. Interaural intensity differences, measured in db, as a function of azimuth. Differences in level are displayed for sound sources placed symmetrically about the midline. Results are shown for different frequencies. For example, at ±90° (a total angle of 180°) one source is placed directly in front of the right ear and the other in front of the left. At 200 Hz the ear difference would be about 3 dB. (Data are from Shaw.[8])

exact decibel difference between the two ears depends on the azimuth and the frequency (or wavelength) of the source[7,8] (see Fig. 9–2). These differences in SPL translate directly into differences in audibility.[9] For example, if the right ear is occluded, then threshold for a 4000 Hz tone will be determined by hearing in the left ear. If this tone is delivered through a loudspeaker positioned at a +90° azimuth, then the left ear is the shadowed, far ear. Compared with the tone's threshold at 0° azimuth, the +90° azimuth position will have a threshold about 13 dB poorer. In contrast, for the same azimuth, threshold for a 200 Hz tone would be only about 3 dB poorer.

When the sound wave encounters an obstacle, it has a tendency either to reflect off the object or to bend (diffract) around the object. If the dimensions of the object are large compared with the wavelength of the sound, the wave reflects off the object. High frequencies have short wavelengths and create the largest interaural differences. Conversely, low frequencies bend around the object, creating only small intensity differences.

When an individual is listening with only one ear, either because of unilateral hearing loss or being aided monaurally, situations will be present in which that ear will be the near ear. And, of course, the individual will naturally try to manipulate the listening environment so that the good ear is closest to the source. When this occurs, there is minimal disadvantage imposed by the hearing loss. In other circumstances, however, the good ear will be the far ear. When this occurs there will be a large disadvantage imposed.

Consider what happens in a typical situation. Speech, a complex signal containing a large range of frequencies, arrives at the listener from an azimuth associated with the speaker. The near ear will receive the full, unattenuated spectrum. The far ear, compared with the near ear, will receive a low-pass-filtered signal. The reduction in the higher frequencies will be more severe, and the reduction in intelligibility more pronounced, if the azimuth is closer to 90° than if it is at 0°.

The difference between the ears in time of arrival of the speech will create phase differences between the ears. How much of a phase difference will depend on the particular frequency. For example, a frequency of 1538 Hz has a period of 0.65 msec, the delay associated with a source presented at 90° azimuth. This frequency would be delayed precisely one cycle, so the far ear would be in phase with the near ear. However, a 769 Hz component of the speech signal would be delayed exactly one-half cycle and would be 180° out of phase at the two ears. Each frequency would have its own special relationship based on the azimuth of the sound source.

NOISE CANCELLATION BY THE CANS: BINAURAL SQUELCH

A realistic listening environment would also contain at least one noise source and often many more. In a reverberant sound field, echoes further complicate the situation by creating a diffuse field where noise appears to be omnidirectional. When the speaker is fairly close to the listener, within the critical distance,[10] incident sound is more intense than the reflections, and the signal is more "directional." Interaural phase and intensity relationships are likely to be different for the speech versus the noise. These differences are very important since the CANS can use them to improve speech intelligibility. Whenever the speech and noise are somewhat different at the two ears, the signal can be enhanced and the noise can be cancelled. When compared with a monaural condition (the ear is not in the head shadow), any improvement in intelligibility, related to interaural differences in time or intensity, is "binaural squelch." In terms of phase, it is believed that it is primarily interactions between the ears for the lower frequencies (roughly 1000 Hz and less) that are more important for creating the squelch effect. Cox and Bisset[11] measured binaural squelch by presenting NU-6 monsyllabic words to a loudspeaker located at 0° azimuth, and uncorrelated speech babble was presented from two horizontal arrays of loudspeakers located at ±90°. Binaural squelch was evaluated by comparing monaural performance to binaural. Their aided, hearing impaired listeners could tolerate 2–3 dB more unfavorable signal-to-noise (S/N) ratio when listening binaurally and still achieve the same intelligibility.

Improvements in Speech Perception for Normal-Hearing Listeners

When two ears are available to the listener, one is always "out of the shadow." For a monaural listener this is not true. Figure 9–3 was derived from data presented by Dirks and Wilson[9] and shows the large disadvantage that can be imposed by the head shadow. Thresholds for spondee words were obtained for normal-hearing individuals at different azimuths. Under the monaural conditions, one ear was occluded. The figure compares near ear and far ear listening with the binaural condition. At 0° azimuth, there really is no near or far ear, but both thresholds were about 3 dB poorer than for the binaural condition. This is what would be expected for binaural summation at threshold. When the "good" ear is in the shadow cast by the head (i.e., from +60° to +90°), thresholds were about 9–10 dB poorer than with binaural. Elimination of the head shadow is a very important aspect of binaural hearing. Reducing threshold by 10 dB is equivalent to increasing the sensation level of speech by 10 dB. Under the right circumstances this can result in a very large improvement in intelligibility. Assuming approximately 5% per dB slope to the intelligibility function, this could improve word recognition by 50%.[12]

An additional benefit derived from eliminating the head shadow occurs when speech is presented in noisy (competing message) situations, provided that the speech and noise emanate from different azimuths.[9] When speech (spondee words) and noise both come from 0° azimuth, intelligibility is virtually the same for the monaural near ear, monaural far ear, and binaural conditions. Binaural listening shows less than a 1 dB improvement in S/N ratio compared with the monaural conditions. However, under conditions in which the noise and speech are spatially separated (see Fig. 9–4) a binaural advantage of about 11.5 dB in S/N ratio can exist. Such an improvement in the S/N ratio reflects a combination of elimination of the head shadow effect and binaural squelch. For normal-hearing individuals this 11.5 dB improvement can mean a 70% increase in intelligibility (assuming approximately 6% per dB slope for spondee words).

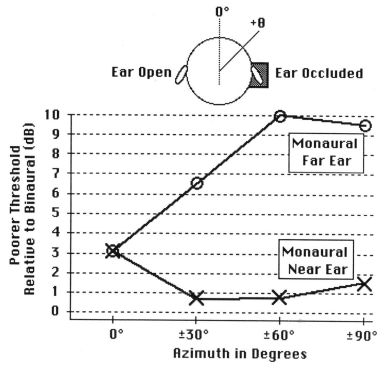

Figure 9–3. Spondee thresholds as a function of azimuth. Positive azimuths represent monaural listening with the open ear in the far ear condition. Negative azimuths are for the open ear when it is the near ear. Thresholds for both monaural conditions are compared with binaural thresholds (when both ears are open). Near ear and far ear thresholds were poorer than binaural thresholds. Compared with binaural performance, the head shadow was about 10 dB at +90°. (Data are from Dirks and Wilson.[9])

Objective Measures of Binaural Advantage: Hearing Impaired Listeners

There is no doubt that people with normal hearing experience substantial benefit from binaural hearing. Generally, people with impaired hearing perform similarly to normals on virtually any sort of auditory task involving speech perception. But, the impaired ears may not perform as well. The effects of any type of distortion that reduces intelligibility for normals may reduce intelligibility for the hearing impaired even more so. For example, the detrimental effects of noise and reverberation tend to increase with the magnitude of the hearing loss and are present for even mild losses with pure-tone averages of 30 dB HL.[13] The question of whether hearing impaired individuals will be able to benefit, as normals do, from binaural hearing is legitimate. Could the reduction in benefit usually seen with hearing impairment serve to make the binaural advantage negligible? Additionally, hearing aids add their own form of distortion and could produce time delays and phase changes that might negate any binaural benefit. However, even though aided listeners may

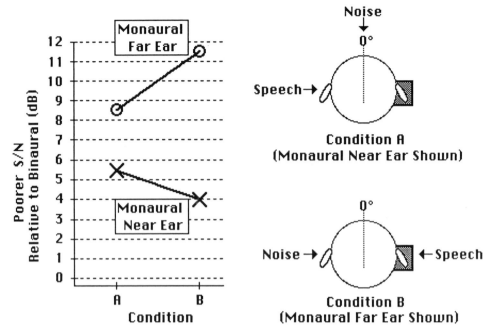

Figure 9–4. Poorer monaural spondee thresholds (compared with binaural) when listening in noise. For condition B, in which the unoccluded ear was "completely shadowed," the 50% recognition threshold was 11.5 dB poorer than the binaural condition. (Data are from Dirks and Wilson.[9])

not do as well as their normal-hearing peers, the binaural advantage appears to be present and worthwhile.

McCullough and Abbas[14] found that binaural advantages were present in the sound field for their five unaided, hearing impaired listeners. All listeners had falling, high frequency losses. Binaural squelch was typically 2–4 dB for all but one of the subjects. Some of the listeners, however, showed less binaural improvement from elimination of the head shadow than would be expected. Bronkhorst and Plomp[15] found that some hearing impaired listeners show minimal benefit from utilization of the head shadow effect, an effect that is present primarily for the higher frequencies. Almost all of these listeners had severely impaired high frequency hearing. This suggests that a hearing aid that restores the audibility of high frequency cues would have a beneficial effect on binaural gain. Markides[16] demonstrated that hearing impaired listeners (both conductives and sensorineurals), wearing ear level hearing aids do experience benefits very similar to normals. The reduction in head shadow effect was approximately 6–7 dB, and binaural squelch was 2–3 dB, as estimated at the 50% point on the intelligibility function for isolated monosyllabic words. The 10 dB combination (head shadow + squelch) increased intelligibility about 40% for monosyllables. Also, it is important to realize that these benefits accrued in both nonreverberant and reverberant environments. Most typical listening situations are reverberant. Hawkins and Yacullo[17] found 2–3 dB of binaural squelch for aided, hearing impaired listeners. The binaural advantage, obtained in realistic conditions (noisy and reverberant), was interpreted as being independent of reverberation time. When binaural hearing was used in conjunction with directional microphones, the improvement in S/N ratio was an additional 3–4 dB. Nabelek,[10] after reviewing previous research, also concluded that binaural benefit is present in noisy, reverberant environments, although use of amplification and excessive reverberation (reverberation times in excess of 2 seconds) can somewhat limit the benefit. Leeuw and Dreschler[18] found that directional hearing aids improve S/N ratio and benefit intelligibility and that the effect is even more pronounced for binaural fittings.

Cox et al.[19] evaluated binaural squelch in conditions in which the speech (NU-6 word lists) was delivered in uncorrelated speech babble to both normal and hearing impaired subjects. When the loudspeaker presenting the message was spatially separated from the loudspeaker presenting the babble, binaural squelch was about 4 dB for the normals. This resulted in a 26% improvement in word recognition for the binaural condition. Hearing impaired subjects, listening in the same environments with hearing aids, showed benefits amounting to an average of 19%. The 7% reduction relative to normal could be viewed as a degradation brought about by the hearing loss, hearing aids, or a combination of the two. This 19% improvement is similar to the 2–3 dB of binaural squelch found by Cox and Bisset[11] for aided hearing impaired listeners in a similar environment.

Markides[16] found errors in localization, when listening with only one hearing aid, to be greatest when the source was positioned on the off side. For example, if the hearing aid was worn on the left ear, errors in localization would be greatest at azimuths approaching 90°. The amount of error could be quite large: 60°–100°. In contrast, when binaural hearing aids were worn, errors were less than 20°. For monaural listeners, localization was only this good when the source was positioned directly at the near ear (−90° for aided left ear, +90° for aided right ear). Concerning ear asymmetry for localization cues, it was suggested that only 10 dB SL would be necessary. Thus, provided speech is properly amplified, unequal hearing loss should not be a contraindication to a binaural recommendation. A disadvantage to aided localization can be seen when the user would be capable of hearing the important spectral cues unaided, when the hearing loss is mild. Occluding the concha with the shell of an ITE, or the mold of a BTE, interferes with spectral cues normally offered by diffraction of sound by the pinna.[20]

Although "ease of listening" is usually considered a subjective benefit, it may be estimated from a subject's response time. The assumption is that, when little listening effort is required and the listener is more confident and certain as to what was said, the response will occur more quickly. When presented with monosyllabic words, hearing impaired listeners wearing binaural hearing aids do have shorter response times than when monaurally aided.[21] Feurstein,[22] in a study simulating conductive hearing loss, found that binaural listening was accomplished with less effort than monaural and that ease of listening correlated with word recognition ability. Binaural listening required less attentional effort than when listening monaurally with the far ear.

Central Auditory Effects, Amplification, and Sound Deprivation

As with peripheral hearing loss, any disturbance in central processing can compromise, but usually not eliminate, benefits from binaural processing.[23-25] For example, elderly individuals (63 to 74 years) can take advantage of binaural cues, but have smaller masking level differences[26] and can integrate binaural cues on a dichotic test in a normal fashion.[27] It has been suggested that, even for ears with symmetrical hearing loss, testing the ability to achieve a "fused binaural image" would help to establish candidacy for binaural amplification.[28]

In the case of lesions involving the primary auditory cortex, speech recognition is fairly normal for monaural signals, regardless of which ear the speech is delivered to. The deficit is most dramatically illustrated when a message is delivered to the ear contralateral to the lesion while a competing "noise" (which may be speech) is delivered to the other ear. This is an example of when binaural hearing could be poorer than monaural. However Kricos et al.[29] found there to be no relationship between perceived hearing aid benefit (as reported by subjects on a questionnaire) and central auditory function in a group of 24 elderly subjects. Central auditory function was assessed by subjects' performance on measures of word versus sentence recognition.

When the elderly exhibit central deficits it is assumed that relatively diffuse pathology exists randomly throughout the CANS, so they may be susceptible to a contralateral masking effect. This has been viewed as a contraindication for binaural amplification. Helfer[30] studied the performance of a group of nine older (>60 years) adults listening in a simulation of a realistic, noisy (+10 dB S/N), reverberant environment. She found that performance was similar to that of normals. Although the presence of reverberation lessened benefit somewhat, the older adults were able to take advantage of binaural cues to achieve improved intelligibility over the monaural condition. Also, from a purely acoustic standpoint, elimination of the head shadow effect serves to improve S/N ratio. Enhancing S/N ratio generally helps to improve understanding for those with an auditory processing deficit. While CANS pathology would not preclude benefit from binaural amplification, the clinician should be sensitive to this possibility,[31] especially since approximately three of every five hearing aid users are elderly.[32] Auditory processing disorders can degrade hearing aid performance, but there is little doubt that many such individuals can be successful hearing aid users.[33]

Related to auditory processing effects is the issue of whether "disuse atrophy" of the central auditory pathway can result from a combination of peripheral hearing loss and lack of acoustic stimulation. Hood[34] suggested that the fairly poor speech recognition ability seen in Meniere's patients may not be solely due to peripheral effects of the endolymphatic hydrops. The central auditory nervous system of these patients with unilateral hearing loss may be actively suppressing the distorted, conflicting input from the poorer ear resulting in a gradual deterioration in function. It has been demonstrated that sound deprivation can have adverse effects on development of the central auditory system. Webster and Webster[35] raised mice with simulated conductive hearing loss in one ear. When the rats were sacrificed, it was demonstrated that brainstem neurons serving the impaired ear were both smaller in diameter and fewer in number than those on the contralateral side receiving normal sound stimulation. Research of this sort indicates that the central auditory system does not develop independently of the environment. Rather, it suggests that neural systems develop in response to the demands placed on them by environmental factors.

Silman et al.[36] gave evidence to suggest that speech recognition ability may suffer in a sound deprived, unaided ear. They evaluated speech recognition ability in two groups of veterans. Although both groups had similar audiometric configurations, one group was fitted monaurally while the other received binaural amplification. When retested 4–5 years later, there were no differences between ears in either group for measures of sensitivity: pure-tone thresholds or speech recognition thresholds. However, the supra-threshold speech recognition ability of the unaided ears of the monaural group seemed to deteriorate. On the average, ears that went unaided had speech recognition scores 18% poorer than the ears that received greater acoustic stimulation (the aided ears of either the monaural or binaural group). Gatehouse[37] found evidence to suggest that ears with hearing loss became acclimated to listening at low levels. Relative to the aided ear (the ear not deprived of sound) speech recognition was poorer in the unaided ear for stimuli delivered at higher presentation levels.

It appears that the onset of the deterioration can be delayed by as much as 8–11.5 years[38] and that the deterioration is progressive. Stubblefield and Nye[39] found an average 10%–15% decrease in speech recognition over a 3–6 year period for the unaided ear of 60 patients with bilaterally symmetric hearing loss. Silverman and Silman[40] have further demonstrated that this deterioration may be reversible. They identified two subjects similar to those aided monaurally in the Silman et al.[36] study. With time, both of these subjects showed a progressive deterioration in speech recognition ability in the unaided ear. However, when fit binaurally, the decline ended and reversed itself to show an improvement. With time, the improvement in speech recognition amounted to about 25%–30%. Burkey and Arkis[41] also found that the effect was not permanent, but disappeared following a binaural fitting. However, they presented evidence to suggest that the deprivation effect is dependent on the magnitude of hearing loss. The loss in speech recognition ability was only present for those with poorer pure-tone averages (mean value of 48 vs. 34 dB HL).

While it is premature to warn patients about the risks of disuse atrophy and to use this rationale to encourage them to purchase a second hearing aid, certainly this phenomenon cannot be casually dismissed, especially in the case of children with developing nervous systems. Indeed, Fishbein[42] suggested that it would be prudent for dispensers to have binaural candidates who were to be fit monaurally sign a waiver. Perhaps future research will lend further support to the notion that binaural amplification will help to preserve speech perception skills.

Binaural Modifications to Fitting Strategies

It appears that the tacit assumption in the literature is that binaural hearing aids are typically fit in the same way as monaural aids. Libby[43] indicates that when the fitting is binaural, the selection procedure is performed with each ear separately. Byrne[44,45] states that the safest course is to fit binaural aids as two monaural fittings, as there is no research to suggest any alternative. Essentially, similar prescription, selection, and evaluation procedures would be followed for a binaural fit as would be performed for a monaural fit. Each ear would be dealt with separately. It was estimated that a binaural fit required 25% more time than a monaural one. Occasionally, minor modifications could be made. If one ear had difficulty with feedback or poor sound quality due to excessive high frequency emphasis, it might be possible to reduce high frequency gain in that ear, knowing that it would still be provided in the other.

Skinner[46] suggested that there are two approaches to fitting hearing aids binaurally. The first would be to fit one, allow the person to adjust, then fit the second. Alternatively, two aids could be fit initially. Cook[47] evaluated differences in adjustment to amplification using a questionnaire sent to 150 hearing impaired adults categorized into one of three groups. The first were monaural users, and the second group initially were monaural users, but had been fit with a second hearing aid. The third group was initially fit binaurally. Results indicated no statistically significant differences in adjustment difficulty between the three groups, except that the second group had more difficulty in adjusting to listening to music. This study did not support the belief that users have more difficulty adapting to two hearing aids.

To compensate for binaural summation, it has been suggested that slightly less gain be used for a binaural fitting. Reduced problems with feedback would be a benefit of this reduction in gain. Pollack[48] suggested that binaural users require 3–6 dB less gain than monaural users. This relatively small difference could be compensated for by volume control rotation, or the prescription could be modified. Skinner[46] indicated that SSPL90 should be reduced by 3 dB and gain be reduced by 5 dB to reflect increased binaural loudness. The reduction in gain and SSPL90 would be uniform across the spectrum.

In one study ten hearing impaired listeners with cochlear pathology showed loudness summation of 6–9 dB at frequencies of 500 and 2000 Hz.[5] Balfour and Hawkins[49] found 6.5 dB to be the average amount of binaural summation for speech and music stimuli. Hawkins et al.[50] found similar results (7.1 dB summation) with 20 hearing impaired listeners having bilaterally symmetrical, high frequency hearing losses. However, the binaural signals, while perceived as louder, were not judged as uncomfortable as monaural signals. In fact, the binaural signals were almost twice as loud before becoming uncomfortable. These listeners had identical loudness discomfort levels (LDLs) for binaural signals as for monaural, even though the binaural stimuli were louder. Since binaural summation improves threshold, this finding suggests that binaural users have a greater dynamic range. It also suggests that a binaural hearing aid fit, on the average, requires no special correction factor for SSPL90.

Loudness-Density Normalization

To explore further the issues relating to possible need for modification of the frequency response in binaural fittings, a model based upon Leijon's loudness-density normalization (LDN) procedure[51] was developed. The model was developed specifically to explore effects related to binaural summation and the changes in input spectrum to an ear produced by the head shadow effect. Leijon's method was appealing for several reasons. First, hearing aid prescriptive procedures, such as the revised NAL,[52] are typically intended to select gain based on a loudness criterion to amplify all speech bands to an equally comfortable loudness level. Second, recommendations for modifying the frequency response (i.e., 3–6 dB reductions) are based on listeners' perceptions of binaural loudness. Third, Leijon's calculations are based on an accepted model of loudness summation.[53,54] Fourth, Leijon's procedure has been validated upon a group of hearing impaired listeners.[55]

Leijon's calculations produce a real-ear insertion response (REIR) that purports to restore normal loudness contributions for amplified speech. The listener is assumed to have cochlear pathology with recruitment. Recruitment is either complete at 110 dB HL, or partial. The gain required to restore normal loudness for the speech peaks contained within each critical band is determined by an algorithm expressed by Leijon as a short computer program. His model was implemented here using a HyperCard stack developed by the author. The interested reader is directed to Leijon[51] for details of the calculations. The method was validated[55] with a group of 26 elderly hearing aid users with the mean audiogram shown in Figure 9–5. All users listened through their own

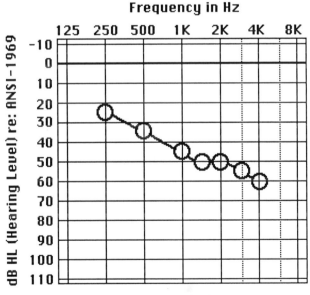

Figure 9–5. The audiogram used to determine the frequency responses in Figures 9–6 through 9–11. This is the mean audiogram of subjects used in a validation study of intelligibility and quality judgments of the LDN procedures.[55]

hearing aids to speech presented in a noise background via loudspeaker. The input spectrum was shaped to give an effective frequency response corresponding to the revised NAL procedure or to Leijon's LDN procedure (other frequency responses were also simulated, but are not presented here). Recordings from an FM radio transmission were used for subjective quality ratings, and sentence material was used for intelligibility testing. Results indicated that intelligibility was similar for the two frequency responses, and both were acceptable. However, the quality judgments for the LDN response were slightly superior to the NAL-R response (statistically significant at the 0.2% level).

Predicted Changes in Frequency Response (REIR)

A comparison between the NAL-R response and two LDN responses is given in Figure 9–6. LDN-C calculates REIR based on the assumption that loudness recruitment is complete at 110 dB HL. Generally, it shows a response flatter than the NAL-R curve, requiring slightly greater low frequency emphasis with less high frequency gain. The LDN-P curve (partial recruitment) recommends a response with essentially the same high frequency gain as NAL-R. LDN-P assumes that loudness is not complete at 110 dB HL. Since the LDN-C curve

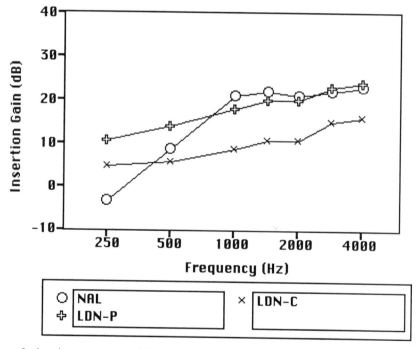

Figure 9–6.   A comparison of the gain recommended by the NAL procedure versus the loudness-density normalization procedure for the audiogram in Figure 9–5. LDN-C assumes recruitment is complete at 110 dB HL, whereas LDN-P assumes partial recruitment. The input spectrum is average conversational level speech at an overall level of 65 dB SPL.

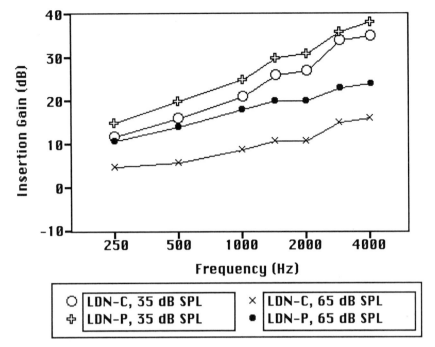

Figure 9–7.   REIR varies depending on the input level to the hearing aid and upon the assumptions concerning how the ear recruits, either complete (LDN-C) or partial (LDN-P) recruitment. Gain is greatest for low input signals (speech at an overall level of 35 dB SPL) versus average conversation level speech (65 dB SPL).

was judged to be more pleasant sounding, but equal in intelligibility to NAL-R, it was concluded that the goals of processing speech so that it is both intelligible and of good quality are not incompatible.[55]

Figures 9–7 and 9–8 illustrate how the LDN procedures indicate that real ear insertion gain (REIG) should vary with input level. Generally, less gain is needed as the input level increases. Fairly soft sound requires a greater amount of gain to normalize loudness. As input level increases for a recruiting ear, less gain is needed to create a normal loudness perception. If the ear has a sloping high frequency loss (Fig. 9–5), then a more pronounced high frequency emphasis is required for softer sounds. Qualitatively, these results are consistent with the manner in which the K-Amp circuitry processes sound.[56,57] Kruger and Kruger[58] found that, of 45 patients fit with hearing aids using a K-Amp circuit, 44 were considered successful users and 25 of those were binaural fittings.

The information presented previously at ±60° for the head shadow effect was used to generate Figure 9–9. For the far ear, the effect of the head shadow is similar to low-pass filtering of the speech. Relative to the near ear, the far ear would require an REIR with a greater high frequency emphasis. This effect is more pronounced for speech input at a softer level. This finding suggests that a frequency response that might be appropriate with one speaker on the near ear side of the monaurally aided listener may not have enough high frequency

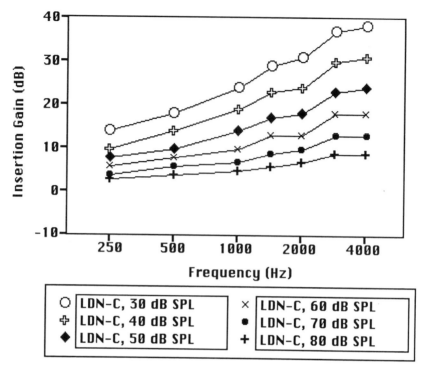

Figure 9-8. Differences in REIR (LDN-C) based on the SPL of speech input to the hearing aid. At low levels, more gain with a pronounced high frequency emphasis is required to normalize loudness. At higher levels, less gain and a flatter response is needed.

gain when a second speaker is on the unaided side (i.e., when the person is communicating with two people, one slightly to the right and the other to the left). This disadvantage would not be present for a binaural user when communicating with more than one person.

How binaural hearing aids might function differently for children is a topic of considerable importance, especially as it might affect their ability to monitor their own speech. Cornelisse et al.[59] made sound field measurements of average conversational speech levels (ACL) at a distance of 30 cm in front of the speaker and at an ear-level position similar to the location of a hearing aid. Measurements were made for children, adult males, and adult females. Results indicated that the overall level of the children's own speech was approximately 5 dB greater at the ear-level position (results for the adults were similar). The spectrum at ear level had a more pronounced low frequency emphasis (about 5 dB greater at 500 Hz) and less high frequency energy beyond 2000 Hz (the 4000 Hz region was about 5 dB less). However, from Figure 9-10 in can be seen that the differences in REIR required to normalize the loudness of speech at these two locations are minimal.

In the last example, another question might relate to what differences would be required for the case of a binaural fitting with loudness summation. Also, in

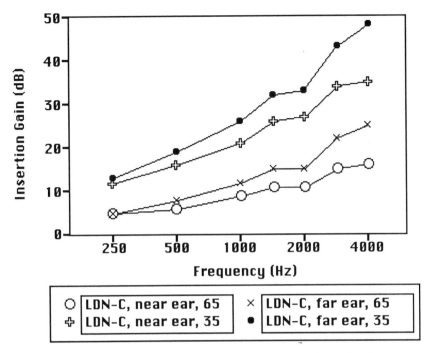

Figure 9–9. Differences in REIR required to normalize loudness for the near ear and far ear for a sound source located at ±60°. The speech spectrum (input levels of 35 and 65 dB SPL) has been modified to reflect the attenuations produced by the head shadow effect shown in Figure 9–2.

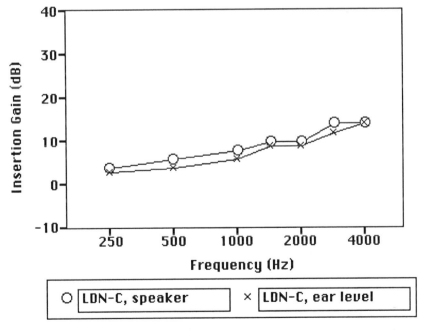

Figure 9–10. Differences in the REIR predicted by the LDN procedure for a child listening to a speaker located at a 0° azimuth (68 dB SPL input) versus monitoring his or her own speech at ear level (73 dB SPL input). The speech spectrum was modified to include spectral changes according to measurements made by Cornelisse et al.[59]

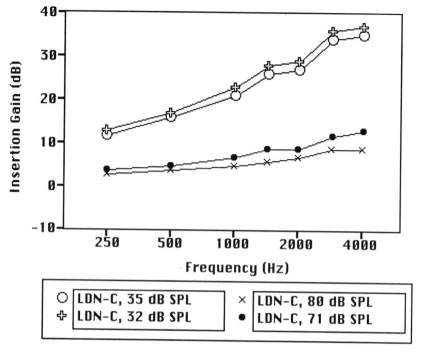

Figure 9–11.   Small differences in the REIR needed to normalize loudness for monaural versus binaural fittings. The assumption is that the binaural fitting increases loudness (relative to monaural) equivalent to a 3–9 dB change in input level. The 3 dB change was for a softer speech input level of 35 dB, and the 9 dB change was for an input of 80 dB SPL.

general, how different must an REIR be to compensate for binaural summation of approximately 3 dB at threshold and 9 dB at suprathreshold levels?[50] The REIRs presented in Figure 9–11 were created based on the assumption that binaural loudness summation could be viewed as an equivalent change in the input level. Granted this assumption, it would appear that binaural fitting would require less gain than monaural, but the difference is fairly small, approximately equal for all frequencies, and roughly the same for softer and louder speech. This also suggests that probably little change in REIR would be needed for a child monitoring his or her own speech when listening binaurally.

Binaural Considerations for Children

In Australia, the National Acoustic Laboratories' policy is to fit binaurally unless there is a specific contraindication.[45] During the period from 1977 to 1985, 80%–90% of children under the age of 4 years were fit binaurally. Ross et al.[60] believe that binaural amplification is the method of choice for most hearing impaired children. For the vast majority of children binaural hearing improves the ability to comprehend speech, both in quiet and noise. This improvement in speech comprehension is assumed to result in better speech and language development. Children would be better able to hear the productions of the speech–language models around them, and they would be better able to monitor their own productions. Binaural amplification is thought to make difficult listening less fatiguing and would provide for better localization in the classroom. Matkin[61] suggests that this improvement in localization would benefit speechreading. A quicker localization would allow the child to attend to the speaker more rapidly, allowing the association of facial and acoustic cues. Binaural summation would permit a reduction in overall gain, reducing problems with feedback and the risk of the child acquiring noise-induced hearing loss.

Franklin[62] suggested modifying the frequency response of a binaural fitting for profoundly impaired children so that one ear would receive a low frequency emphasis and the other ear a high frequency emphasis. The high frequency aid would provide most of the segmental features in speech and would usually be placed on the right ear since the left hemisphere is dominant for consonant perception. Removing the low frequencies from this aid would reduce problems with unwanted background noise and upward spread of masking by the low frequencies. Pitch, rhythm, and intonational cues (suprasegmental features) would be conveyed to the right hemisphere by the low frequency emphasis aid on the left ear. She noted improvements of 12–18 dB in thresholds with this type of fitting.

Maxson[63] reviewed some of the factors that have caused skepticism toward the idea of binaural amplification being the fitting of choice: risk of developing noise-induced hearing loss in both ears instead of just one, extrapolating the results of research from adults to children, difficulty in obtaining ear-specific information from children, body aids not providing true binaural hearing, and cosmetic complaints from parents. She addressed these concerns and concluded that binaural amplification is beneficial, appropriate, and the most advantageous fitting for practically every hearing impaired child. Hearing aid selection and evaluation were carried out in an ongoing clinical, aural rehabilitation context. She indicates that, although clinicians tend to make binaural recommendations, even without definitive and documented support, there is a need to document binaural advantages. This has not been readily accomplished.

Hearing impaired children 6.5 years of age, and occasionally younger, have been found able to participate in a hearing aid evaluation procedure requiring paired comparison judgments of the clarity of amplified speech.[64] Grimes et al.[65] evaluated 24 aided, hearing impaired children 9–17 years of age. The sound field arrangement was such that head shadow effect was not assessed; only binaural squelch was measured using sentence material in multitalker babble. Results showed no statistically significant differences between the monaural and binaural scores. A similar result (lack of statistical significance) was found by Hawkins[66] when using spondee words and the Phonetically Balanced Kindergarten (PB-K) word lists. This illustrates the difficulty in using speech audiometry for the clinical assessment of individual patient differences, especially when the differences may be quite small. They concluded that it was not possible to demonstrate binaural superiority, but that this cannot be considered sufficient reason to dismiss binaural amplification as the fitting of choice.

Binaural Considerations in Verification Strategies

If the primary goal of the fitting is to provide a hearing aid that produces pleasant sounding, intelligible speech, then the two primary issues would appear to be the head shadow effect and binaural squelch. Byrne[44] indicated that it is probably unnecessary to document the advantage arising from the head shadow effect. The improvements in S/N ratio that give rise to enhanced intelligibility are readily predictable from the physical arrangements of the ears on the head. The head shadow is primarily present for the higher frequencies, and the listener requires audibility of the high frequency portions of the spectrum to realize its benefit. Real-ear probe microphone measurements, performed in the same manner as for a monaural fitting, could be used to effectively document whether appropriate REIG is being achieved for the higher frequencies in each ear.

Traditionally, speech audiometry has been used to evaluate whether a hearing aid is superior to the unaided condition and which of several hearing aids might be the best.[67] Improvement in speech recognition could be used to evaluate the benefit of binaural versus monaural. Limitations in the reliability and precision of speech recognition testing severely limit its usefulness for measuring small differences between conditions.[68] For example, to be certain that results were statistically significant (0.05 level), at an intelligibility level of 68% correct for a monaural score the binaural score would have to be greater than 88% for a 25 item word list, 84% for a 50 item word list, and 80% for a 100 item, word list.[69] About one-half of a group of normal-hearing subjects had test–retest differences exceeding 10% for a 50 item word list presented in noise.[70] For evaluating binaural squelch, values of 2–3 dB would not be uncommon, and the improvement in intelligibility could only be 10–15%. Many listeners with a binaural advantage might not be measured as such simply due to limitations in the precision of the test.

Mueller et al.[71] found that a 20 item synthetic sentence test was not effective in determining binaural advantage in a group of 24 adults. Using the nonsense syllable test and W-22 monosyllables delivered at 0° azimuth in quiet, Danhauer et al.[72] found no statistically significant binaural advantage. Their 15 patients expressed definite preferences for binaural amplification in typical listening situations, but it was not possible to document these preferences using speech audiometry. They stated that the traditional practice of searching for binaural benefit in the sound booth seems fruitless. Cox et al.[19] found that only 8 of 15 aided hearing impaired subjects demonstrated a significant binaural advantage when using a 50 item NU-6 word list. Using a 200 item test, ten of the subjects showed significant binaural improvement. This suggests that in some cases binaural benefit may be present, but the precision of the test may not be sufficient to uncover it. This study also indicated that it is difficult to construct a valid demonstration of binaural advantage, especially in a typical audiometric test room. Small changes in azimuth brought about by variation in loudspeaker position or subject position could have substantial influence on the results.

Cox et al.[73] investigated the possibility of using subjective estimates of intelligibility. Subjects indicated what percentage of words they believed they understood. High positive correlations (0.82–0.92) were found between listeners' subjective estimates and the percentage of words they actually understood. This suggests that listeners probably have valid perceptions of how intelligible speech sounds through a hearing aid. Unfortunately, the subjective estimates were more imprecise than the objective measurements.

Balfour and Hawkins[49] were successful in using a paired-comparison format to evaluate sound quality judgments for a group of 15 adults with mild, bilaterally symmetrical sensorineural hearing loss. The subjects listened via insert earphones to speech and music mixed with noise. The stimuli were recorded in the sound field through two hearing aids that were worn on a Knowles Electronics Manikin for Acoustic Research (KEMAR). Subjects preferred the binaural aids for all eight listening dimensions (brightness, clarity, fullness, loudness, nearness, overall impression, smoothness, and spaciousness). Binaural preferences were strongest for overall impression, fullness, and spaciousness. The authors were optimistic about the use of a paired comparison format for demonstrating to potential users the benefits of binaural amplification. Sullivan and Agnew[74] described a tool, the binaural equalizer, to be used in binaural fittings and evaluations. It is a hand-held, battery-operated sound source producing a high frequency noise spectrum, the greatest energy being present in the 2000–6000 Hz region. They felt it was useful for demonstrating binaural advantage to prospective users and reported that 73% of 92 patients who were fit binaurally on an experimental basis retained both instruments.

Recordings presented via KEMAR can be useful for rapidly comparing stimuli. However, to ensure that recordings are valid, meticulous care must be given to all aspects of the recording process.[75] Problems with individual variation in earmold configurations, ear canal and middle ear impedance, open molds with sound entering the ear directly, and controlling for the canal resonance are some of the potential problems. Care must be taken to ensure that time and intensity differences between ears are preserved and that the sound spectrum at the eardrum during earphone playback would be the same as if the listener were actually in the sound field. Variation in low frequency response could affect quality judgments and binaural squelch. Preparation of such recordings by the individual clinician would be problematic.

Cox and Rivera[76] used a 66 item self-report inventory (Profile of Hearing Aid Benefit-[PHAB]) for assessing hearing aid benefit. The PHAB has questions that evaluate performance in a variety of communication situations (e.g., noise, reverberation, use of visual cues). While they did not specifically utilize this to evaluate binaural performance, it could be used within the context of a 30 day trial period. Unfortunately, the reliability of the PHAB was such that the authors concluded that it would be best used for research purposes on groups of subjects rather than for individuals in a clinical situation.

Monaural and binaural hearing aids have been compared during a 30 day trial period.[77] Twenty-six potential hearing aid users with moderate, bilaterally symmetrical audiograms used binaural or monaural hearing aids on an alternate week basis for 4 weeks. They were evaluated using a questionnaire. The subjects were neither encouraged nor discouraged from binaural use. The advantage to this type of evaluation is its face validity. Subjects were allowed to use hearing aids for an extended period in situations that were typical for them. A disadvantage is that it was not possible to control the equivalency of the monaural and binaural listening conditions. Subjects reported that localization was better with binaural. They generally felt that binaural hearing aids were better in quiet than in noisy situations. They preferred monaural aids in noisy environments. This was an unexpected finding, since binaural hearing is supposed to improve listening in noisy situations. However, it was unclear whether the subjects preferred monaural listening because of one aid or if they preferred listening with one unamplified ear.

The loudness–density normalization procedure predicts that in high level input situations much less real-ear gain would be needed. Hypothetically, since the average subject had only moderate hearing loss, perhaps they preferred to have at least one ear listen without the distortion that can occur in linear aids driven to saturation. A detailed description of the hearing aids used was not reported. Monaural user preference in noise, or difficulty in using binaural in noisy situations has been found in other surveys of hearing aid users.[78–80] Erdman and Sedge[80] reported better speech clarity in noise as an advantage and increased ambient noise as a disadvantage of binaural hearing aid use.

Of the 26 potential hearing aid users, Schreurs and Olsen[77] found at 6 months follow-up that 17 had purchased monaural aids and only eight had purchased binaural aids. Of the hearing aid users, 32% chose binaural. This is in contrast to the 73%[74] and 83%[80] binaural user rates reported by others. Erdman and Sedge[80] found that at 3 months follow-up 25 of 30 first-time hearing aid users used binaural aids full-time, part-time, or occasionally (17 of the 30, 57% used binaural on a full-time basis). Byrne[45] reported that, after 3 months, 10 of 43 patients issued binaural aids were using monaural ones. Binaural use rate was 77%. Of 150 initial binaural fittings, Chung and Stephens[78] reported 74% were still binaural users after at least 6 months. Harford,[81] apparently using a similar binaural trial, stated that of over 1,000 patients during a 6 year period, only 5% returned the second aid and became monaural users. Erdman and Sedge[82] asked 30 monaural hearing aid users, who would not have to pay for a second aid, to evaluate binaural hearing aids on a 30 day trial basis. Of the 30, 27 (90%) indicated a preference for binaural. Interestingly, a number of the monaural users from the first group were so pleased with the second aid that they were openly annoyed at not being given the option of using binaural initially. In a similar situation Lowe[83] reported a possible malpractice case. A monaural user, who later became a binaural user, felt that she should have been informed of the binaural option at the first fitting.

In an effort to determine if cost was a factor in accepting or rejecting a second aid, Erdman and Sedge[82] identified a second group of 30 subjects who were not eligible for free hearing aids. After evaluating first monaural and then binaural on a trial basis, all 30 decided to purchase a second hearing aid (100% binaural use rate). The cost was $210 per aid. Of 25 patients initially fit binaurally with K-Amp hearing aids, 24 (96%) remained binaural.[58] With the exception of the initially negative report,[77] it appears that, when the hearing impaired are given a chance to make an informal comparison of binaural to monaural, a significant number will decide to become binaural users.

Concerning hearing aid evaluation strategies, one commonly held belief seems to be that acceptable patient performance on an appropriate clinical test procedure is necessary before the audiologist can legitimately recommend a hearing aid. For example, Bronkhorst and Plomp[15] indicate that a prerequisite for properly advising a patient, or for selecting a hearing aid, would be a reliable clinical test for assessing speech perception in noise. They go on to state that development of such a test is complicated by the large number of variables involved with patient hearing loss, type of test material, presentation method, and acoustics of the listening environment. Comparing binaural to monaural would be an additional complication. Cox et al.[19] state that a need "continues to exist for a procedure which can be used with some confidence in a clinical setting to test whether a binaural hearing aid fitting is more advantageous than a monaural fitting for a particular individual."

Another belief, expressed by Libby,[84] suggests that too much emphasis has been placed on clinical test procedures to demonstrate an elusive binaural advantage. He indicated that these test procedures are more appropriate for designing research studies to show average or group trends than for individual patients in a clinical setting. Patients should not be denied binaural amplification just because it cannot be demonstrated clinically. Harford[81] suggests that, considering the wealth of information available concerning binaural benefit, perhaps the emphasis should be on justifying the use of only one hearing aid. He felt that there were no dependable clinical tests that would tell him who would and who would not benefit from binaural amplification. Pollack[85] expresses the attitude that for the vast majority of users the binaural advantage is so obvious that the recommendation should be made even if it cannot be supported empirically. Concerning the issue of whether a clinical demonstration of binaural advantage is necessary, Byrne[44] indicates that, considering the few cases in which a binaural fitting may be disadvantageous it may be preferable to fit all binaurally unless there is a specific audiologic or medical contraindication. Economically, it may be more expedient to waste a few aids than to incur the expense of the additional testing.

Attitudes and Opinions Toward Binaural Amplification

For the year 1990, it was estimated that 50.6% of the hearing aids sold were binaural,[86] and 49.4% were monaural. Hearing instrument specialist sales of binaural aids were slightly higher than audiologist sales (56.2% vs. 47.3% for private practice audiologists, and 48.9% for audiologists in a clinical setting). Another survey estimated total binaural sales during 1991 at 60.6% for all users and 53.1% for new users.[87] This represents a steady increase in binaural sales since 1984 when only 24.5% were binaural. Overall, 55.8% of the monaural users expressed their satisfaction with their hearing aid, and 60.2% of the binaural users were satisfied. This difference is not statistically significant.

Surveys have polled user preferences regarding binaural and monaural amplification. Brooks and Bulmer[79] found generally favorable attitudes toward binaural amplification in a study of 204 patients. There were 605 positive comments, such as binaural aids were helpful, superior to one aid, beneficial in company, easy to use, provided better sound localization, boosted confidence, were invaluable, and were relaxing. There were only 63 negative comments, such as the aids were difficult to balance, embarrassing, noisy, clumsy, uncomfortable, tiresome, difficult to manipulate, inconvenient, useless, and not worth the effort. Similar results were reported in another survey of 200 patients fit with binaural aids.[78] Chung and Stephens[78] found that males were more likely to continue using binaural aids than females, people with more severe hearing losses were more likely to be frequent binaural users, and asymmetric hearing loss was not a contraindication to binaural use (88% of those with asymmetrical hearing losses continued to be binaural users as opposed to 70% of those with symmetric losses). It has been suggested that the more socially active, outgoing personality type is a more promising binaural hearing aid candidate.[72] In a study with 30 subjects, Erdman and Sedge[80] found the following advantages of binaural amplification: improved speech clarity, stereo effect, balanced hearing, relaxed listening, better speech clarity in noise, natural quality, tinnitus relief, lower volume setting, and enhanced localization ability. Disadvantages were difficulty balancing volume, increased ambient noise, cosmetic concerns, noise when driving an automobile, and awkward when using the telephone.

Mueller[88] evaluated factors influencing prospective users' attitudes toward amplification. The 282 patients were retired military personnel, adult males, mostly ranging in age from 60 to 70 years. Even though two hearing aids would be dispensed at no charge, only 120 patients (43%) indicated a preference for binaural. Of those preferring binaural, some of the main reasons were that two aids would produce better hearing, would be more natural and balanced, the loss was severe enough to warrant two, and advice was received from a professional. Of those preferring monaural, reasons were that hearing loss was not severe enough, no improvement was expected from a hearing aid, advice from other users, and advice from a medical professional. It was concluded that, when a professional made a binaural recommendation, the patient was strongly influenced by it. This is consistent with another study that indicated that 26.6% of first-time owners were influenced by an audiologist in their purchase decision.[87] This was the third most important factor, ranking behind poorer hearing and suggestions by family members. The audiologist was more influential than either the family doctor, otologist, or hearing aid specialist.

The "hearing aid effect" is the negative attitude the hearing aid wearer perceives to be elicited in others by the presence of the hearing aid. Surr and Hawkins[89] reviewed the responses concerning the hearing aid effect from 86 patients who completed a pre- and post-fitting questionnaire. Of these subjects, 73% chose ITE aids and 27% BTE aids. The ITE users chose binaural fittings 54% of the time, and 41% of the BTE users chose binaural. The authors were favorably surprised that only about 10% of these subjects sensed negative attitudes from others. The most common negative belief was that 26% of the subjects anticipated that they would be viewed as being older. After using the hearing aids only 11% felt that they actually were viewed as being older. Generally, pre-fit negative expectations did not seem to come true. In terms of binaural advantages, 69% of the binaural users reported that others noticed improvement in their hearing, whereas only 46% of the monaural group noticed this. The binaural group felt they were more alert (55%) than did the monaural group (31%). On the negative side, 37% of the binaural users felt that people noticed their aids, but only 20% of the monaural users felt that the aid was noticed. However, people did report that their hearing loss prior to the fit was more noticeable than their hearing aid. In general, 94% of the patients believed they heard better with the hearing aid(s).

Summary

A considerable body of literature exists that demonstrates the benefits of binaural listening for people with normal hearing. The person with symmetrical sensorineural hearing loss also experiences similar benefit. Hearing impaired listeners, wearing two hearing aids in noisy, reverberant, realistic environments experience the benefits of binaural hearing. The major benefits accrue from binaural summation, binaural squelch, and elimination of the head shadow effect. Binaural summation allows the user wearing two aids to experience the same loudness, but with less gain than the monaural user. This reduces the chance of feedback occurring before a comfortable listening level is achieved. Binaural signals, while louder, may not be judged as uncomfortable, thus allowing the binaural listener a greater dynamic range than the monaural listener. Binaural squelch permits listeners with two hearing aids to achieve better intelligibility in noisy situations. Provided sufficient high frequency gain, the binaural listener will perform better than the monaural listener due to elimination of the head shadow.

The improvement related to the head shadow effect is relatively large and primarily caused by the acoustics of the head and position of the ears. Real-ear probe microphone measurements are useful for documenting the presence of an appropriate REIR in the higher frequencies. The average improvement expected due to binaural squelch is fairly small and difficult to document clinically. Some clinicians assume that it is necessary to document this improvement; others do not. In general, binaural hearing aids are selected and evaluated in the same manner as monaural aids. Theoretical predictions indicate only small changes to the REIR.

People who are fit with binaural hearing aids are generally satisfied. They report improvements in speech intelligibility, sound quality, spatial balance, and localization ability. Patients are influenced by the recommendations audiologists make. If allowed to make an informal comparison of monaural to binaural hearing aids, most patients will prefer binaural. Given an opportunity to use binaural hearing aids in their typical listening environments, over a period of 30 days, most hearing impaired individuals will purchase two aids. If the hearing aids are purchased, the majority will continue to be used over at least a 3 to 6 month period.

References

1. Durlach NI, Colburn HS: Binaural phenomena, in Carterette EC, Friedman MP (eds): *Handbook of Perception*, vol IV. New York: Academic Press, 1978, pp 365–466.
2. Durlach NI, Thompson CL, Colburn, HS: Binaural interaction in impaired listeners: A review of past research. *Audiology* 1981; 20:181–211.
3. Hausler R, Colburn S, Marr E: Sound localization in subjects with impaired hearing. *Acta Otolaryngol* (Suppl) 1983; 400:1–62.
4. Valente M: Binaural amplification. *Audiology* 1982; 7:79–93.
5. Hall JW, Harvey ADG: Diotic loudness summation in normal and impaired hearing. *J Speech Hear Res* 1985; 28:445–448.
6. Mills AW: Auditory localization, in Tobias JV (ed): *Foundations of Modern Auditory Theory*, vol 2. New York: Academic Press, 1972, pp 301–348.
7. Shaw EAG: Earcanal pressure generated by a free sound field. *J Acoust Soc Am* 1966; 39:465–470.
8. Shaw EAG: Transformation of sound pressure level from the free field to the eardrum in the horizontal plane. *J Acoust Soc Am* 1974; 56:1848–1861.
9. Dirks D, Wilson R: Binaural hearing in sound field, in Libby ER (ed): *Binaural Hearing and Amplification*, vol I. Chicago: Zenetron, 1980, pp 105–122.
10. Nabelek AK: The effects of room acoustics on speech perception through hearing aids by normal-hearing and hearing-impaired listeners, in Studebaker GA, Hochberg I (eds): *Acoustical Factors Affecting Hearing Aid Performance*. Baltimore: University Park Press, 1980, pp 25–46.
11. Cox R, Bisset JD: Relationship between two measures of aided binaural advantage. *J Speech Hear Res* 1984; 49:399–408.
12. Olsen W, Matkin N: Speech audiometry, in Rintelmann WF (ed): *Hearing Assessment*. Baltimore: University Park Press, 1979, pp 133–206.
13. Harris RW, Swenson DW: Effects of reverberation and noise on speech recogntion by adults with various amounts of sensorineural hearing impairment. *Audiology* 1990; 29:314–321.
14. McCullough JA, Abbas PJ: Effects of interaural speech-recognition differences on binaural advantage for speech in noise. *J Am Acad Audiology* 1992; 3:255–261.
15. Bronkhorst AW, Plomp R: A clinical test for the assessment of binaural speech perception in noise. *Audiology* 1990; 29:275–285.
16. Markides A: *Binaural Hearing Aids*. London: Academic Press, 1977.
17. Hawkins DB, Yacullo W: Signal-to-noise ratio advantage of binaural hearing aids and directional microphones under different levels of reverberation. *J Speech Hear Dis* 1984; 49:278–286.
18. Leeuw AR, Dreschler WA: Advantages of directional hearing aid microphones related to room acoustics. *Audiology* 1991; 30:330–344.
19. Cox R, DeChicchis AR, Wark DJ: Demonstration of binaural advantage in audiometric test rooms. *Ear Hear* 1981; 2:194–201.
20. Preves DA, Orton JF: Localization ability as a function of hearing aid microphone placement, in Libby ER (ed): *Binaural Hearing and Amplification*, vol II. Chicago: Zenetron, 1980, pp 293–303.
21. Causey GD, Bender DR: Clinical studies in binaural amplification, in Libby ER (ed): *Binaural Hearing and Amplification*, vol II. Chicago: Zenetron, 1980, pp 75–96.
22. Feurstein JF: Monaural versus binaural hearing: Ease of listening, word recogntion and attentional effort. *Ear Hear* 1992; 13:80–86.
23. Antonelli AR: Auditory processing disorders and problems with hearing aid fitting in old age. *Audiology* 1978; 17:27–31.
24. Olsen W, Noffsinger D, Carhart R: Masking level differences encountered in clinical populations. *Audiology* 1976; 15:287–301.
25. Roush J: Aging and binaural auditory processing. *Semin Hear* 1985; 6:135–146.
26. Pichora-Fuller MK, Schneider BA: Masking level differences in the elderly: A comparison of antiphasic and time-delay dichotic conditions. *J Speech Hear Res* 1991; 34:1410–1422.
27. Kaplan H, Pickett JM: Effects of dichotic/diotic versus monotic presentation on speech understanding in noise in elderly hearing-impaired listeners. *Ear Hear* 1981; 2:202–207.
28. Mercola P, Wenke-Mercola C: A new test procedure for determining binaural candidacy. *Hear J* 1985; 37(3):19–31.
29. Kricos PB, Lesner SA, Sandridge SA, Yanke RB: Perceived benefits of amplification as a function of central auditory status in the elderly. *Ear Hear* 1987; 8:337–207.
30. Helfer KS: Aging and the binaural advantage in reverberation and noise. *J Speech Hear Res* 1992; 35:1394–1401.

31. Hayes D, Jerger J: Aging and the use of hearing aids. *Scand Audiol* 1979; 8:33–40.
32. Cranmer K: Hearing instrument dispensing. *Hear Instrum* 1989; 40(6):6–15.
33. Stach B, Louiselle L, Jerger J: Special hearing aid consideration in elderly patients with auditory processing disorders. *Ear Hear* 1991; 12(Suppl):131S–137S.
34. Hood JD: Problems in central binaural integration in hearing loss cases. *Hear Instrum* 1990; 41(4):6, 8–9, 56.
35. Webster DB, Webster M: Neonatal sound deprivation affect brainstem auditory nuclei. *Arch Otolaryngol* 1977; 103:392–396.
36. Silman S, Gelfand SA, Silverman CA: Late-onset auditory deprivation: Effects of monaural versus binaural hearing aids. *J Acoust Soc Am* 1984; 76:1357–1362.
37. Gatehouse S: Apparent auditory deprivation effects: The role of presentation level. *J Acoust Soc Am* 1989; 86:2103–2106.
38. Silverman CA: Auditory deprivation. *Hear Instrum* 1989; 40(9):26–32.
39. Stubblefield J, Nye C: Aided and unaided time-related differences in word discrimination. *Hear Instrum* 1989; 40(9):38–39, 42–43, 78.
40. Silverman CA, Silman S: Apparent auditory deprivation from monaural amplification and recovery with binaural amplification: Two case studies. *J Am Acad Audiol* 1990; 1:175–180.
41. Burkey JM, Arkis PN: Word recognition changes after monaural, binaural amplification. *Hear Instrum* 1993; 44(1):8–9.
42. Fishbein H: Binaural amplification vs. auditory deprivation. *Hear Instrum* 1991; 42(10):58.
43. Libby ER: Measures to verify achievement of desired real-ear gain in adults. *Semin Hear* 1991; 12:42–52.
44. Byrne D: Clinical issues and options in binaural hearing aid fitting. *Ear Hear* 1981; 2:187–193.
45. Byrne D: Binaural fitting practices in the national acoustic laboratories. *Hear J* 1986; 38(11): 41–44.
46. Skinner MW: *Hearing Aid Evaluation.* Englewood Cliffs, NJ: Prentice-Hall, 1988, p 241.
47. Cook AL: *A Survey of Adjustment between Three Groups of Amplification Users.* MS thesis. Central Missouri State University, Warrensburg, MO, 1983.
48. Pollack MC: Special applications of amplification, in Pollack MC (ed): *Amplification for the Hearing Impaired,* ed 3. New York: Grune Stratton, 1988, pp 295–328.
49. Balfour PB, Hawkins DB: A comparison of sound quality judgments for monaural and binaural hearing aid processed stimuli. *Ear Hear* 1992; 13:331–339.
50. Hawkins DB, Prosek RA, Walden BE, Montgomery AA: Binaural loudness summation in the hearing impaired. *J Speech Hear Res* 1987; 30:37–43.
51. Leijon A: Hearing aid gain for loudness-density normalization in cochlear hearing losses with impaired frequency resolution. *Ear Hear* 1991; 12:242–250.
52. Byrne D, Dillon H: The national acoustic laboratories' (NAL) new procedure for selecting the gain and frequency response of a hearing aid. *Ear Hear* 1986; 7:257–265.
53. ISO 532. *Acoustics—Methods for Calculating Loudness Level.* Geneva: International Organization for Standardization, 1975.
54. Zwicker E: Scaling: Loudness and its calculation, in Keidel WD, Neff WD (eds): *Handbook of Sensory Physiology,* vol V/4. Berlin: Springer Verlag, 1975, pp 401–448.
55. Leijon A, Lindkvist A, Ringdahl A, Israelsson B: Sound quality and speech reception for prescribed hearing aid frequency responses. *Ear Hear* 1991; 12:251–260.
56. Killion MC: A high fidelity hearing aid. *Hear Instrum* 1990; 41(8):38–39.
57. Killion MC, Staab WJ, Preves DA: Classifying automatic signal processors. *Hear Instrum* 1990; 41(8):24–26.
58. Kruger B, Kruger FM: The K-AMP hearing aid: Clinical impressions with fittings. *Hear Instrum* 1993; 44(2):30–31, 35.
59. Cornelisse LE, Gagné JP, Seewald RC: Ear level recordings of the long-term average spectrum of speech. *Ear Hear* 1991; 12:47–54.
60. Ross M, Brackett D, Maxson AB: *Assessment and Management of Mainstreamed Hearing-Impaired Children: Principles and Practices.* Austin, TX: Pro-Ed, 1991, pp 205–206.
61. Matkin ND: Wearable amplification: A litany of persisting problems, in Jerger J (ed): *Pediatric Audiology: Current Trends.* San Diego: College Hill Press, 1984, pp 125–145.
62. Franklin B: Split-band amplification: a HI/LO hearing aid fitting. *Ear Hear* 1981; 2:230–233.
63. Maxon AB: Binaural amplification of young children: A clinical application of Ross' theory. *Ear Hear* 1981; 2:215–219.
64. Eisenberg LS, Levitt H: Paired comparison judgments for hearing aid selection in children. *Ear Hear* 1991; 12:417–430.
65. Grimes AM, Mueller HG, Malley JD: Examination of binaural amplification in children. *Ear Hear* 1981; 2:208–210.
66. Hawkins DB: Comparisons of speech recognition in noise by mildly-to-moderately hearing-impaired children using hearing aids and FM systems. *J Speech Hear Dis* 1984; 49:409–418.

67. Carhart R: Tests for selection of hearing aids. *Laryngoscope* 1946; 56:780–94.
68. Shore I, Bilger RC, Hirsh IJ: Hearing aid evaluation: reliability of repeated measures. *J Speech Hear Res* 1960; 25:152–170.
69. Thornton AR, Raffin MJ: Speech-discrimination scores modeled as a binomial variable. *J Speech Hear Res* 1978; 21:507–518.
70. Gengel RW, Miller L, Rosenthal E: Between and within listener variability in response of CID W-22 presented in noise. *Ear Hear* 1981; 2:78–81.
71. Mueller HG, Grimes AM, Jerome JJ: Performance-intensity functions as a predictor for binaural amplification. *Ear Hear* 1981; 2:211–214.
72. Danhauer JL, Mitsunaga FF, Danhauer KJ: Wearer's personality may enhance benefit of binaural amplification. *Hear J* 1991; 44(8):22–31.
73. Cox R, Alexander GC, Rivera IM: Comparison of objective and subjective measures of speech intelligibility in elderly hearing-impaired listeners. *J Speech Hear Res* 1991; 34:904–915.
74. Sullivan RF, Agnew J: A useful tool for binaural fittings. *Hear Instrum* 1991; 42(3):32–33.
75. Cox R, Studebaker GA: Problems in the recording and reproduction of hearing aid-processed signals, in Studebaker GA, Hochberg I (eds): *Acoustical Factors Affecting Hearing Aid Performance.* Baltimore: University Park Press, 1980, pp 169–195.
76. Cox R, Rivera IM: Predictability and reliability of hearing aid benefit measured using the PHAB. *J Am Acad Audiol* 1992; 3:242–254.
77. Schreurs KK, Olsen WO: Comparison of monaural and binaural hearing aid use on a trial period basis. *Ear Hear* 1985; 6:198–202.
78. Chung SM, Stephens SDG: Factors influencing binaural hearing aid use. *Br J Audiol* 1986; 20:129–140.
79. Brooks DN, Bulmer D: Survey of binaural hearing aid users. *Ear Hear* 1981; 2:220–224.
80. Erdman SA, Sedge RK: Subjective comparisons of binaural versus monaural amplification. *Ear Hear* 1981; 2:225–229.
81. Harford ER: Hearing aid selection for adults, in Pollack MC (ed): *Amplification for the Hearing Impaired,* ed 3. New York: Grune & Stratton, 1988, pp 175–212.
82. Erdman SA, Sedge RK: Preferences for binaural amplification. *Hear J* 1986; 38(11):33–36.
83. Lowe RG: Are audiologists guilty of malpractice if they do not recommend binaural amplification? *ASHA* 1988; 30(11):39–40.
84. Libby ER: Editorial: Binaural amplification—State of the art. *Ear Hear* 1981; 2:183–185.
85. Pollack MC: To binaural or not to binaural: That is the question! *Elect Com* 1988; 8–9.
86. Cranmer K: Hearing instrument dispensing—1991. *Hear Instrum* 1991; 42(6):6–13.
87. Kochkin S: MarkeTrak III: Higher hearing aid sales don't signal better market penetration. *Hear J* 1992; 45(7):47–54.
88. Mueller HG: Binaural amplification: Attitudinal factors. *Hear J* 1986; 38(11):7–10.
89. Surr RK, Hawkins DB: New hearing aid users' perception of the "hearing aid effect." *Ear Hear* 1988; 9:113–118.

10

Fitting Binaural Amplification to Asymmetrical Hearing Loss

ROBERT E. SANDLIN

Introduction

Forty-two years ago, Carhart[1] observed that *The problem of hearing aid selection is currently the most controversial aspect of clinical audiology.* Unfortunately, even today one of the major problems facing the clinical audiologist is determining the criteria by which hearing aids are selected and fitted to those with hearing impairment. Although advances in electroacoustic performance permit audiologists to employ various forms of signal processing, there still exists no general consensus for supporting any one fitting protocol. That is, in the more than 50 year history of electronic hearing aid use, audiologists have failed to reach a consensus on a number of important issues relating to the fitting of hearing aids. For example, no consensus is present as to what specific aspects of auditory function need be measured. Even if such a consensus could be reached, there is no agreement on how such measurements should be used to determine the electroacoustic properties of the recommended hearing aid(s). In addition, consensus is lacking on the type of electroacoustic performance the hearing aid should have to best interface with the acoustic requirements of an impaired auditory system. It is little wonder that current audiologists often reflect indecision when selecting and fitting hearing aids.

The fitting of a hearing aid device is a very subjective procedure. One is involved not only with the magnitude of the hearing impairment, but also must be concerned with the social and psychological consequences of hearing aid use. The wide variety of asymmetrical hearing losses and the subsequent problems associated with fitting this type of hearing loss would seem to demand that audiologists adopt an attitude embracing experimentation in the assessment of need and benefit.

Purpose and Definitions

The purpose of this chapter is to review current thought regarding the selection and verification strategies for fitting asymmetrical sensorineural hearing loss. It is important to remember that no clear-cut consensus is currently available to guide the audiologist when fitting this population. The range of opinions, attitudes, and strategies regarding asymmetrical hearing loss, and the subsequent fitting of hearing aids to this type of loss, is very broad.

First, it is important to propose a reasonable definition of asymmetrical hearing impairment. In its broadest sense, asymmetrical hearing impairment can be defined as interaural differences in threshold sensitivity. However, this is not a very functional definition when making decisions concerning hearing aid use for this very broad hearing impaired group. For example, in one individual one ear could be within normal limits while the opposite ear has a profound hearing loss in which the ear is "unaidable." In another individual, both ears could be equally impaired in audiometric configuration, but one ear may be significantly different than the other ear relative to speech recognition scores. In still another individual, the audiometric configuration could be significantly different, requiring special consideration in determining the electroacoustic properties of the recommendrd hearing aids. Speech recognition scores may differ considerably between ears, creating additional concerns in the decision-making process. In other cases, the loudness growth function may differ significantly from one ear to another. Regardless of what conditions contribute to asymmetrical impairment, the amplfication needs may vary greatly from one ear to another.

Perhaps a working definition of *asymmetrical hearing loss*, relative to the application of hearing aids, would be the following: *Given that an asymmetrical hearing loss implies a significant difference between ears regardless of magnitude, the use of amplification must improve hearing performance so that it can be verified by objective and subjective evaluations. Such differences can be expressed in terms of pure-tone threshold improvement, most comfortable listening levels, word recognition scores, loudness growth compensation, and positive subjective response to amplified sound in everyday listening environments.*

In this definition, subjective evaluation is a major consideration. Depending on the severity of the hearing loss, patients perceive benefit when benefit, as measured by traditional fitting procedures, cannot be measured. This may be especially true if one is using speech recognition scores as the major criterion for determining improved aided hearing.

The majority of patients with bilateral hearing impairment have asymmetrical hearing losses. That is, the threshold sensitivity for those discrete frequencies assessed in the evaluation process is not identical for each ear. The clinical issue is whether the magnitude of difference between the two ears can determine whether to fit the better ear, poorer ear, or both ears. If the audiologist cannot demonstrate the benefit of two hearing aids when fitting asymmetrical losses, should any effort be made to fit a hearing aid to each ear?

Briskey[2] suggests the following criteria when considering binaural fitting of those with asymmetrical loss:

1. The average hearing loss at 500, 1000, and 2000 Hz should be within 15 dB HL or less between ears.
2. Two of these three frequencies must be 15 dB HL or less between ears.

3. The speech recognition scores between ear should be within 8% of each other.
4. The decibel values of the uncomfortable loudness level (ULL) in each ear should be within 6 dB of each other.
5. The most comfortable loudness level (MCL) in each ear should be within 6 dB of each other.
6. There should be a high activity index. (The activity index is based on the lifestyle of the individual. For example, if the lifestyle is rather sedentary, perhaps binaural amplification should not be considered. On the other hand, if the other criteria are met and the patient has a very active lifestyle, then binaural hearing aid amplification may be the better choice.)

Briskey[2] reminds us that not all the criteria need to be met for a successful binaural fitting; for example, *binaural fitting can be achieved by considering either 1 or 2; any two of 3, 4, and 5; and always have 6. (p. 505)*

The recommendations given by Briskey[2] may be straightforward in suggesting the possibility for achieving maximum benefit from binaural amplification. However, these recommendations tend to underestimate the advantages gained by those with asymmetrical loss who do not meet all the suggested criteria. One may embrace the need to adhere to strict criteria when justifying a binaural fitting, to document sound source localization, binaural summation, and speech recognition in environmental noise. Nonetheless, there are advantages for fitting binaural hearing aids to patients whose hearing loss is significantly different between ears to the point where they may not fully enjoy the binaural advantage of improved speech in noise. However, current clinical practices indicate that many asymmetrical losses can benefit from applying amplification to both ears, even though they may not be able to enjoy completely the binaural advantages, which are easier to demonstrate when interaural differences are not present. Courtois et al.[3] maintain that *It is amazing that such a small asymmetry as 15 dB between the two ears, such a small difference as 8% in speech discrimination is, by some audiologists, considered a contraindication of binaural treatment. (p. 243)*

It is a matter of deciding how to demonstrate benefit from providing amplification to both ears that is of clinical importance. Skinner[4] describes two approaches to fitting bilateral asymmetrical hearing loss. The first approach is to fit one ear and have the patient determine benefit over a defined period of time. The other approach is to fit the individual initially with binaural amplification; then, during the trial period the patient is asked to listen to binaural amplification for some of the time and utilize monaural amplification for the remaining portion of the time. By so doing, an informed decision can be reached as to the value received for monaural versus binaural amplification. This view implies, and rightly so, that one's subjective analysis of perceived benefit is tantamount to assessing value received from amplification. To assume there is a magnitude of interaural differences that precludes the use of binaural hearing aids appears to be less than clinically astute. Skinner does not tell us, however, what kind of assessment should be made during the experimental period to determine whether the binaural or monaural system provided greater benefit.

Hawkins[5] discusses several approaches that have been used in the decision-making process regarding monaural versus binaural hearing aid amplification. The first approach seems to be "prove binaural is better, then I'll recommend it." Proponents of this approach tend to utilize speech recognition scores to demonstrate superiority of monaural versus binaural performance. However, the reliability and/or validity of this method of evaluating binaural advantages has been questioned repeatedly[6,7] in that the variability of speech recognition scores may exceed the difference between any two hearing aid conditions. A second approach is to "recommend binaural amplification unless there is a clear reason not to." This approach tends to rely more on patient subjective preferences during a specified trial period when determining the binaural or monaural advantage. The philosophy for not fitting two hearing aids to a patient with asymmetrical hearing impairment because of the presence of interaural differences in word recognition scores or pure-tone threshold differences has been pointed out by Hawkins[5] as having "little evidence in the research literature to support this position" (p. 147).

Opinions regarding the efficacy of fitting binaural amplification to asymmetrical loss vary greatly. There is no compelling research data that suggest that the presence of asymmetrical hearing loss should, a priori, result in rejecting a recommendation to dispense binaural amplification. Binaural advantages for asymmetrical losses have been demonstrated by a number of investigators.[8–14] However, Davis and Haggard[15] reported decreased speech recognition in the presence of noise for those having asymmetrical hearing loss when fit with binaural amplification. They suggested that when interaural threshold difference is 15 dB or greater, there may be a contradiction for binaural amplification. The conclusions of Davis and Haggard[15] may serve only to cloud the issue of fitting asymmetrical loss with two hearing aids. Staab[16] advises that:

> Potentially, every individual with a hearing impairment may be a candidate for hearing aid use. Concepts that dictate hearing aid candidacy on the basis of specific levels or types of losses should be discarded. Generalizations might still be used, but should be just that—generalizations. The emphasis should be on the handicap and the problems a particular hearing loss presents. (p. 368)

Although Staab did not directly address asymmetrical hearing impairment, it is clearly implied in his statement that the decisions audiologists make must not be governed solely by generalized fitting concepts, and from them overgeneralize what is and is not appropriate for an individual hearing impaired person. Similar concerns were expressed by Walden and colleagues[17] pertaining to the assumptions underlying hearing aid evaluation processes.

Clearly, there needs to be some general consensus for a recommended guideline concerning the clinical practices to be followed when fitting asymmetrical hearing loss. In view of the existing controversy, consider the following as a workable definition of asymmetrical loss and the subsequent selection and fitting of hearing aids: *Regardless of the interaural differences, amplification*

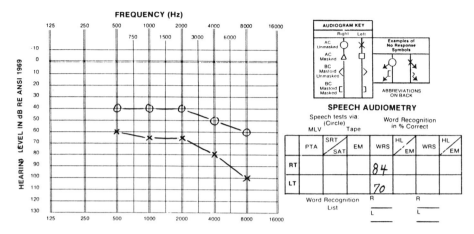

Figure 10-1. Pure-tone audiogram indicating a mild to moderate hearing loss in the right ear and a moderate-severe to profound hearing loss in the left ear.

should be evaluated to determine the efficacy of hearing aid use, if the amplified sound can be made audible. Such evaluation should include a trial period during which time the patient is exposed to listening environments experienced in the conduct of day to day activities.

Granted, this is a loose definition, but it is one that embraces the importance of empirically determining the advantage or disadvantage of hearing aid use in the presence of asymmetrical hearing loss. In view of the divergence of opinion regarding hearing aid use by those with asymmetrical loss, various asymmetrical losses (Figs. 10-1 through 10-3) may present a dilemma to some audiologists.

In Figure 10-1, the right ear has a pure-tone average (PTA) of 40 dB HL. A word recognition score of 84% was obtained when speech stimuli were presented at a comfortable level. For the left ear, the PTA is 63 dB HL and the word recognition score was 70%. Is this individual a reasonable candidate for binaural amplification, or does one fit only the better ear?

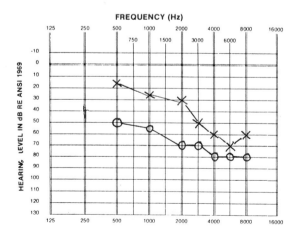

Figure 10-2. Audiogram indicating a moderate to severe hearing loss with a gradually sloping configuration for the right ear. Results for the left ear reveal a slight to moderate hearing loss with a steeply falling configuration between 2000–3000 Hz.

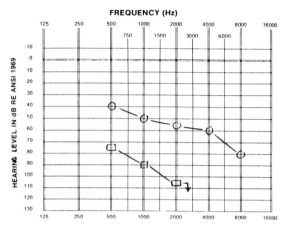

Figure 10–3. Audiogram indicating a mild to severe hearing loss for the right ear with a gradually sloping configuration. Results for the left ear reveal a severe to profound hearing loss at 500–2000 Hz with no measurable hearing beyond 2000 Hz.

The asymmetrical loss illustrated in Figure 10–2 reveals a PTA of 23 dB HL in the left ear and a PTA of 58 dB HL in the right ear. Note that the better ear has an average loss of approximately 25 dB. In asymmetrical losses of this type, the question is whether one should fit the better ear in addition to the poorer ear.

Figure 10–3 presents an even greater challenge. In this case, the PTA in the right ear is 48 dB HL. The PTA for the left ear is 90 dB HL, with no measureable hearing beyond 2000 Hz. Few would question a recommendation for fitting the right ear. The question is whether one should recommend a second hearing aid for the poorer ear, in view of the magnitude of hearing loss. If one were to fit the left ear, what clinical rationale would be used to justify the decision for doing so? The audiometric types presented (Figs. 10–1 through 10–3) will be discussed in greater detail in this chapter.

Recommended fitting strategies presented in this chapter are those that have been developed by the author over the last 20 to 25 years, as well as the reasoned and welcomed contributions of colleagues and patients during that time. To state with absolute impunity that such fitting strategies are those to be employed by all who select and fit hearing aids would be a gross breech of logic. Nonetheless, it is fair to state that the fitting strategies described in this chapter have been very useful in meeting the amplification needs of patients with asymmetrical hearing loss. The reader must remember that the fitting strategies discussed have been modified over the years as additional information and experiences were gained regarding the complex behavior of the impaired auditory system. Additionally, one must take into account the significant, recent advances in hearing aid design and function, which permit a much more efficient interface with the existing hearing loss.

Objective Versus Subjective Responses

Since the introduction of hearing aids, there has been controversy involving the appropriate approaches for selecting and fitting hearing aids. Currently, there is no indicator that the controversy will be resolved in the near future.

Objective Methods

By an *objective measure*, one means that some electroacoustic or psychoacoustic performance goals have been set that should be met by the amplification system. For example, of the many prescriptive formulas in use today,[18–22] the primary objective of the fitting strategy is that the measured real-ear gain match the prescribed real-ear gain. That is, once PTAs have been measured (250–6000 Hz) the fitting formula prescibes an amount of gain at each test frequency that will amplify average conversational level to the MCL of the patient. In addition to providing target gain requirements, some formulas include the computation of the prescribed saturation sound pressure level SSPL90 in their assessment protocol.

Objective methods assume that the optimal amplification needs of the individual have been met if target gains are achieved. In practice, however, this assumption may be invalid in that the patient's qualitative reaction to the prescribed amplified signal may be less than positive. That is, even if target gain has been achieved, the patient may not like the sound quality and may simply reject amplification. In support of this scenario, Humes and Houghton[23] reported that matching obtained gain to the prescribed gain of the hearing aid does not always guarantee that the user is receiving optimal benefit from amplification. That is, *matching obtained gain to prescribed gain does not ensure that the hearing instrument wearer is receiving significant benefit from amplification. Benefit must be verified directly with each wearer* (p. 43). Such observations regarding instrument performance and patient acceptance would seem to support the necessity of monitoring the subjective responses of those utilizing hearing aids. Additionally, relative to the numerous fitting methods, no general agreement is present among the authors of each method as to which formula provides the "ideal" required real-ear gain. Most current fitting methods were established on patients with sensorineural loss, using linear amplification coupled to an occluding earmold.

Subjective Responses

Understanding the importance of patient (i.e., subjective) reactions to amplified sound is critical in selecting and fitting hearing aids to those with confirmed asymmetrical hearing loss. The audiologist should be aware that there are several possible behaviors found among inexperienced users of amplification having asymmetrical loss. One behavior is that of an immediate acceptance of amplification with little or no negative reactions or extended period of adjustment. A second possibility includes those patients who adjust fairly well to amplification but the trial period may need to be extended. Finally, there is the third possibility, wherein the patient reports considerable difficulty in adjusting to amplification and never completely accepts the hearing aid regardless of its electroacoustic performance.

It is not only the attitude of the patient that is of considerable importance in the successful selection, fitting, and utilization of hearing aids, but that of the audiologist as well. If audiologists fail to appreciate the value of empirical evidence (trial and evaluation) regarding asymmetrical hearing loss and hearing aid benefit, they may deny the hearing impaired person advantages arising from binaural amplification. If there is rigid adherence to general rules concerning candidacy for binaural hearing aid use, much may be lost to the hearing impaired patient who fails to meet whatever restrictive standards are employed.

One is not suggesting that all persons having asymmetrical loss can benefit from binaural amplification. There are those who may gain greater benefit from contralateral routing of the signal (CROS), BICROS, or power CROS amplification than can be realized with binaural amplification. The point here is the need to *consider* evaluating binaural amplification when measurable hearing is present in the poorer ear, which may possibly be made audible through the use of amplification and is satisfactory to the patient. That is, binaural amplification provided superior peformance than when amplification was coupled to either ear monaurally.

Technologic Advances and Fitting Asymmetrical Hearing Losses

With the recent introduction of sophisticated signal processing in current hearing aids, the clinician now has a greater opportunity to provide hearing aid amplification yielding greater user satisfaction than was possible in the past. For example, most patients with asymmetrical hearing losses have significant interaural differences in dynamic range. In general, the narrower the dynamic range, the more difficult it will be to provide the appropriate amplified signal when using linear amplification because of the disproportionate growth in loudness. Certainly, hearing aids with compression cricuitry have contributed to the greater success with which asymmetrical losses can be fit. The benefit of input and output compression circuitry as a means of interfacing with the amplification needs is well established. More importantly, hearing aids are now available in which the frequency response can be divided into two or three separate "bands" that are adjusted by selecting one or two cross-over frequencies. In addition, the gain, compression ratio, kneepoint of the compression, and attack or release time can be controlled independent of the other band(s). This type of control in shaping the frequency-gain and output response has lead to greater satisfaction for patients with reduced dynamic range, but have marked interaural differences in threshold sensitivity and dynamic range (Fig. 10–4). The audiometric data illustrated in Figure 10–4 indicate that patients with this configuration may be poor candidates for binaural amplification if one were to use strictly the criteria described earlier.

Prior to recent technologic developments in nonlinear hearing aid devices, it was difficult to meet amplification needs of those with a narrow dynamic range. Several hearing aid systems are now available that permit the audiologist to provide improved amplification to better "match" the existing hearing loss with the amplified signal. It is commonly agreed that when hair cell loss is present in the cochlea due to drugs, aging, or disease processes, there is a change in the rate of loudness growth. Furthermore, the greater the damage to the hair cell population, the more restricted is the dynamic range. The more restricted the dynamic range, the greater the rate of loudness growth. It is

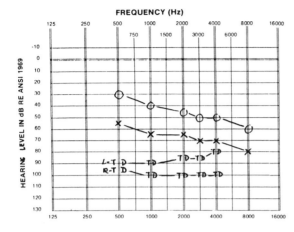

Figure 10–4. Audiogram showing symmetry in audiometric configuration, but asymmetry in the dynamic range.

possible that the patient may have one ear in which loudness growth is significantly different than the other (see Fig. 10–4). Obviously, the same hearing aid response cannot equally meet the demands for each ear. Fortunately, hearing aids are now available in which the compression ratio can be controlled within specified frequency bands, and thereby better meet the acoustical needs of the patient

Ménière's Disease and Asymmetrical Loss

One example of a disease process resulting in asymmetrical hearing loss is Ménière's disease. This disease process usually results in unilateral hearing loss, vertigo, tinnitus, and a sense of fullness. In addition, the affected ear usually reveals a sensorineural hearing loss that is rising in configuration and has reduced word recognition scores and an intolerance to loud sounds (i.e., recruitment). In this case, the audiologist must decide whether to fit CROS amplification to the nonaffected normal ear or to fit a hearing aid directly to the poorer ear. Whenever there is a narrowing of the dynamic range, interaural differences become more apparent.

Whenever these differences exist, the fitting of hearing aids presents a challenge to the audiologist. It is the firm conviction of this author in these cases that the poorer ear should be fit with an appropriate hearing aid. The use of the words *appropriate hearing aid* suggests that, for the most part, linear amplification will not optimally resolve the amplification needs of these patients because of the presence of reduced dynamic range. Earlier, it was briefly mentioned that abnormal growth of loudness was present as a result of specific disease precesses affecting normal cochlear behavior. Ménière's disease is one of those disease processes. Care must be exercised by the audiologist in not overamplifying the affected ear exhibiting reduced dynamic range. Assessment of the patient's ULL for the amplified frequency range will assist in avoiding over amplification at any single frequency.

For many, the problems associated with Ménière's disease will resolve over time. If the clinician decides to fit a CROS hearing aid without assessing the value and contribution of amplifying the pathologic ear, it may very well constitute an error in judgment—not only a clinical error but one that may compromise the patient for whom benefit was intended.

Assuming that the nonaffected ear is within normal limits, it is difficult to fit a CROS hearing aid properly. Ideally, one would not want a CROS system to supply any amplification to an ear in which hearing is within normal limits at 250–6000 Hz.

One of the major advantages of CROS amplification is that of providing awareness and discrimination of sounds arising from the side of the poorer ear. The greatest benefit derived from such fittings occurs in a quiet listening environment. For those environments in which background noise is appreciable, the value received from CROS amplification becomes negligible.

On the opposite side of this coin is the careful selection of the frequency-gain response to best correspond with the Ménière's ear's capacity to handle acoustic information. Is it a better resolution than the restricted performance of one ear only? There is no doubt that threshold sensitivity can be significantly enhanced by hearing aid use for the poorer ear. With attention given to the utilization of the existing technology, which has better control of the output limiting of a hearing aid, it is quite possible to achieve equal, or nearly equal, sensitivity of the good ear.

These statements are not intended as a condemnation of CROS amplification. However, these suggestions are intended to indicate the value of empirically evaluating the extent to which amplification can be employed when asymmetrical hearing loss exists.

As mentioned earlier, Ménière's disease usually results in sudden onset of unilateral hearing loss, nausea, dizziness, and vertigo. Each of these concomitant symptoms may be resolved over time. Hearing may return to normal, or nearly so. During the process of recovery, amplification requirements will change. If the patient has been fitted with a hearing aid to the affected ear, the clinician may be best advised to consider selecting a programmable hearing aid to adapt to the fluctuations in hearing. As the electroacoustic needs of the patient change, adjustable parameters could be changed to meet the patient's amplification needs. Rather than having to return the hearing aid to the manufacturer for modification, it would be a simple matter to reprogram the frequency-gain response and output characteristics to match better the changing auditory sensitivity.

Case Studies Involving Asymmetrical Hearing Loss

Patients have been selected to illustrate a wide variety of asymmetrical hearing losses. Additionally, only those patients benefitting from hearing aid amplification will be presented. The patient selection is not intended to overstate the value of clinical judgment in fitting asymmetrical hearing loss. Selections were made, rather, to underscore the importance of assisting individuals in gaining better appreciation of their acoustic world through the judicious use of binaural amplification, when such is possible.

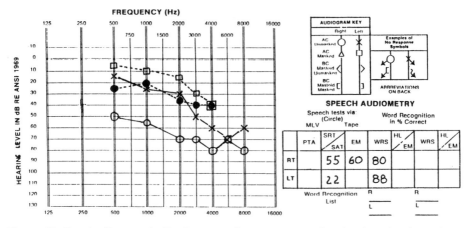

Figure 10–5. Audiogram indicating a moderate to severe hearing loss for the right ear with a gradual slope. Results for the left ear reveal a slight to moderate-severe hearing loss from 500–4000 Hz with slight recovery at 8000 Hz. Open squares represent aided left ear response and filled circles represent aided right ear responses.

Case One

Figure 10–5 represents an audiogram from a 62-year-old male with bilateral hearing loss of long duration. Through the urging of his son, an otolaryngologist, he was referred to a dispensing audiologist. There is a significant disparity in threshold sensitivity between the right and left ears, with the left reporting better hearing. The left ear has a slight to moderate–severe loss at 500–4000 Hz, with slight improvement at 8000 Hz. The right ear has a moderate to severe hearing loss gradually sloping in configuration. If conventional fitting criteria were applied to this case, the patient could be fit with monaural amplification to either ear or perhaps be fit with a left BICROS hearing aid. However, when CID W-22 words were presented to the right ear, a word recognition score of 80% was obtained at MCL. For the left ear, the speech recognition score at MCL was 88%. This patient had no prior experience with amplification and indicated a desire to be fit with amplification to only the left ear. Nonetheless, the patient was counseled to evaluate binaural amplification to determine if improved word recognition in noise could be realized when hearing aids were coupled to both ears in comparison to when a hearing aid was coupled only to the left ear.

Binaural in-the-ear (ITE) hearing aids were recommended. Each aid had signal processing functions specifically prescribed to provide maximum benefit for the patient's bilateral, asymmetrical hearing loss. The ULL for each ear was markedly different. For the right ear, his ULL was greater than 100 dB HL, whereas for the left ear, the ULL was 95 dB HL. With current technology, the need to provide amplification with different output limits can be accomplished without difficulty. In the aided condition, little change is obtained in speech recognition scores for the right ear when speech was delivered at MCL. The

MCL is now 50 dB HL. For the left ear, the aided MCL is 50 dB HL, and the speech recognition score is 96%.

In addition, aided threshold values for the left ear are better than those for the right. Even though the conventional audiometric criteria are not met for recommended binaural hearing aid amplification,[2] the patient performs better with binaural amplification than with monaural amplification to either ear alone. To emphasize this point, observe that the differences between threshold sensitivity for 250 through 4000 Hz are markedly less in the aided mode.

Following a trial evaluation in a number of everyday listening situations, the patient soon appreciated the value of binaural amplification. When the patient had the opportunity to compare binaural amplification to monaural amplification, the advantages of binaural hearing were clearly evident in almost all listening situations.

Had this patient been fitted with monaural amplification to the left ear, it would have been very difficult for him to process acoustic information arriving from the unaided side. Coupled with the magnitude of hearing loss, along with the head shadow effect, the patient's acoustic world existed only on his left side. This is true not only for speech signals, but for other information bearing signals as well.

It cannot be stressed too strongly that patients with asymmetrical hearing loss should be evaluated with binaural amplification, if acoustic benefit can be derived by directly aiding the poorer ear as well. There may be medical conditions dictating against binaural amplification. Clearly, if contraindications are not present then clinical trial of binaural amplification should be initiated.

Case Two

Figure 10–6 reveals the audiologic data for a 74-year-old female with a long-standing bilateral, asymmetrical hearing impairment. She presented with a mild to moderate-severe sensorineural hearing loss for the left ear. There was a moderate to severe loss for the right ear. Speech recognition scores were 88% in the left ear and 32% for the right ear when CID W22 word lists were presented at MCL. ULLs were 85 dB HL for the right and 95 dB HL for the left ear.

The patient was aware of the marked disparity in speech recognition ability between ears. However, she strongly favored binaural amplification, for it created a "balanced hearing environment" that could not be achieved with monaural amplification. She did not feel that the interaural differences in speech recognition presented any obstacle sufficient enough to deter her from trying binaural amplification.

Interestingly enough, at a later date she indicated a desire to be evaluated again, with specific reference to her left ear. Subjectively, she felt that the acoustic level of speech signals to that ear should be greater than was provided with her current hearing aid. Note that she did not question the value of the additional amplification to the right ear, but wished to improve the efficiency with which the better ear performed. At the time of this writing, she was using binaural ITE hearing aids.

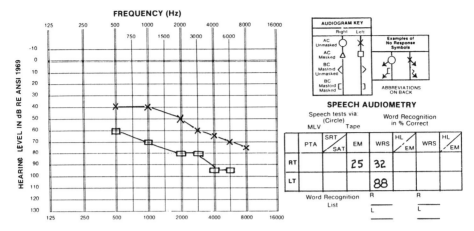

Figure 10–6. Audiogram indicating a moderate to severe hearing loss for the right ear with a gradual slope. Results for the left ear reveal a mild to moderate-severe hearing loss at 500–8000 Hz with a gradual sloping configuration between 1000–8000 Hz.

Again, had the audiologist followed traditional fitting guidelines, the patient may not have been considered a candidate for binaural amplification because of the large interaural difference in word recognition scores. One may argue that the differences in recognition scores was large. As such, the right ear could not really contribute a great deal to understanding the intended message. Nonetheless, the patient functioned better because she felt the binaural amplification system provided a more natural sound and she was better able to recognize speech in her everyday listening environments.

Case Three

Figure 10–7 reports the audiometric results of a 68-year-old male. The hearing loss is asymmetrical, with hearing in the left ear being significantly better. The patient had been using a left BICROS since 1986. Note that the word recognition score for the *right ear* was 76%, when presented at MCL. There was no significant tolerance problem. Even in view of these audiologic findings, the patient was not considered a candidate for binaural amplification by the audiologist who fit the patient with a left BICROS hearing aid.

The patient was dissatisfied with the performance of the left BICROS hearing aid and seldom wore it. Furthermore, he reported that sound localization was not improved with the BICROS fitting and there was no significant improvement in word recognition.

Following a hearing aid evaluation in early 1992, the patient was fitted with binaural ITE hearing aids with automatic low frequency reduction. When assessing "real-life" differences between monaural and binaural amplification, the latter yielded superior performance in essentially all listening environments. He reported improved sound localization in those environments where noise was present.

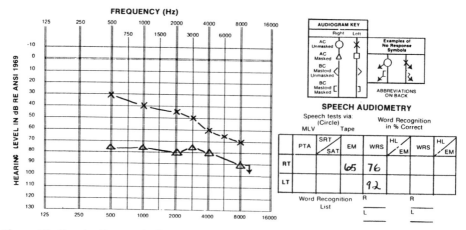

Figure 10–7. Audiogram indicating a severe to profound hearing loss for the right ear that is flat in configuration. Results for the left ear reveal a mild to moderate-severe hearing loss that is sharply sloping in configuration.

It is reasonable to assume that this patient could have realized the benefit of binaural amplification 6 years earlier if binaural amplification were recommended instead of the BICROS instrument. One can only assume that the clinician fitting the initial BICROS system was convinced that the presence of asymmetry argued against using binaural amplification.

Case Four

Figure 10–8 illustrates a fairly common asymmetrical hearing loss. Examination of the audiometric data suggests an asymmetrical hearing loss in which the left ear reveals hearing within normal limits through 1000 Hz, followed by a severe to profound hearing loss at 2000–8000 Hz, which is precipitously falling in configuration. Word recognition at MCL is 76%. The right ear reveals a mild to moderate-severe hearing loss gradually sloping in configuration. The word recognition score is 82% at MCL. The question is whether the left ear should be fitted with a hearing aid. There is no question that the right ear is a candidate for amplification.

In this case, little can be gained by aiding the left ear, in view of the magnitude of loss. This patient would probably perform best with a hearing aid fitted to the right ear alone. If possible, the gain of the hearing aid should be adjusted so that the threshold sensitivity at 500 and 1000 Hz approaches the threshold sensitivity of the left ear at the same frequencies. In this manner, binaural function is greatly enhanced, permitting the patient to achieve better sound localization and improved word recognition in noise. Now, one may question whether this is a contradiction to one's philosophy of fitting asymmetrical losses. I do not think so, in that the loss of hearing above 1000 Hz is so precipitous that current hearing aid devices cannot make that impaired range audible without risking over amplification of the frequency range falling within normal limits.

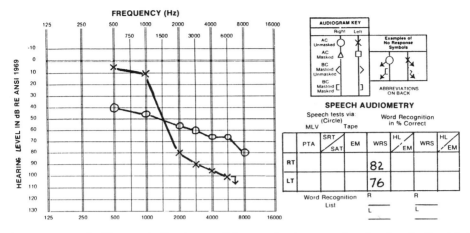

Figure 10–8. Audiogram indicating a mild to moderate-severe hearing loss in the right ear that is gradually sloping in configuration. Results for the left ear indicate hearing to be within normal limits at 500–1000 Hz, followed by a severe to profound hearing loss at 2000–8000 Hz that is precipitously falling in configuration.

Contraindications for Fitting Binaural Amplification

As indicated in Figure 10–8, and stated earlier in this chapter, it would be foolish to suggest that every asymmetrical hearing loss, regardless of magnitude, lends itself to hearing aid use. There have been efforts in the past to define an unaidable ear. However, in the opinion of this author, there are only three conditions for which asymmetrical loss would not benefit from consideration for recommending binaural amplification:

1. In those instances in which, when performing functional gain measures, there is no measurable hearing in the unaided and aided condition at the limits of the audiometer. For these patients, a CROS or BICROS arrangement with the amplified signal forwarded to the better ear would be more appropriate.

2. In those instances in which there is medical evidence contraindicating the use of amplification coupled to the poorer ear. However, such cases should be reconsidered for binaural amplification when the medical condition is resolved and the physician approves the evaluation of hearing aids.

3. In those instances in which the patient has an asymmetrical hearing loss and has tried binaural amplification and experienced little or no benefit from the addition of the second hearing aid to the poorer ear.

Ultimately, the patient makes the decision regarding the benefit or lack of benefit from binaural amplification. While this suggestion may offend some audiologists, it is a rational suggestion. Far too frequently, the clinician assumes that the electroacoustic characteristics present in the recommended aid are those acceptable to the user. This statement is not to indict, necessarily, the fitting rationale employed in the selection process, but rather it is intended to remind the audiologist that patients react subjectively to amplification. If this reaction is negative, it can be sufficient cause to reject whatever benefit may have been realized. This is also true for those with asymmetrical loss. If the clinician is willing to recommend binaural amplification when this recommendation is appropriate and support the patient's response of perceived benefit, there may be some pleasant clinical rewards.

Verification of Hearing Aid Fitting and Performance

In truth, there are only three ways in which hearing aid performance can be verified: (1) real-ear performance based on some pre-selected criteria; (2) patient evaluation of perceived benefit and acceptance after a period of use in everyday listening environments; and (3) psychoacoustic assessment of patient performance in unaided and aided conditions.

Electroacoustic Assessment

Electroacoustic assessment is an objective method of verification that implies that the frequency-gain response of the hearing aid meets the prescribed gain or other criteria offered as guidelines by a fitting formula. Based on earphone thresholds for discrete frequencies, the frequency-gain response of a hearing aid should provide sufficient gain so that the measured real-ear gain approximates the prescribed real-ear gain established by adhering to some fitting formula. Real-ear probe tube measurements is the preferred objective method for validating the amount of real-ear gain provided by the hearing aid. The assumption is, assuming prescribed gain is achieved, that the patient has been provided satisfactory amplification. In reality, however, achieving prescribed gain may provide only a first approximation (Libby, personal communication). As mentioned earlier, there is often the need, regardless of the fitting formula utilized, for adjusting the frequency-gain response to achieve patient acceptance and optimal electroacoustic performance.

When fitting asymmetrical hearing loss, a given fitting method is of limited value. For example, if the patient has a severe to profound hearing impairment in one ear, recommended prescribed gain may not be reached, regardless of the hearing aid selected. In these instances, the verification task is that of determining whether the dynamic range of conversational speech is as audible as possible. With recent changes, however, in some fitting formulae, namely, the NAL and POGO II, closer approximation of electroacoustic needs can be achieved for those with severe to profound hearing impairment.

With the advent of programmable hearing aids, the task of determining the appropriate electroacoustic response of a hearing aid for a specific listening environment is a rather formidable one. That is, existing fitting formulae provide only a single recommended gain response. The assumption is that, when prescribed gains are achieved, the hearing aid is thought to be satisfactory in most, if not all, listening environments. With the introduction of programmable hearing aids with multiple memories, however, the audiologist is faced with the task of specifying different electroacoustic responses to meet the demands of the different listening situations. To provide some objectivity to the decision-making process, some hearing aid manufacturers provide a fitting formula recommended for specific listening conditions. Obviously, such fitting methods can be verified by real-ear measurement.

Patient Evaluation of Perceived Benefit

In this chapter I have supported the notion of using patient responses to modify the initial frequency-gain response, which may have been selected using one or more prescriptive formulae. The premise on which such assumptions are made is simply that the patient will make the final decision concerning acceptance or rejection of amplification. For some patients with asymmetrical hearing loss, the only way in which one can assess the benefit gained from amplification is by having the patient try amplification to determine if the amplified signals provide satisfactory listening. For example, if the patient has a severe to profound hearing loss in one ear and a moderate hearing loss in the other, what value is gained by fitting a hearing aid to the poorer ear? There are no universally accepted guidelines on which to base the possible contributions of the poorer ear. Only two avenues are open for evaluation. One is whether sounds are audible when amplification is provided to the poorer ear. The other is whether the audibility of sounds, regardless of how restricted the frequency range is, provides some useful information about the acoustic environment in which the person functions. To determine the latter, some form of a self-assessment scale or inventory may be succesfully employed.

Psychoacoustic Assessment of Hearing Aid Utility

Prior to the development of real-ear measurement equipment and the subsequent advantages offered to the audiologist, psychoacoustic assessment was the only quasi-objective method of assessing hearing aid performance on the patient. Aided and unaided acoustic measurements in calibrated sound field provides useful information about the contributions of the hearing aid(s). Improvement in threshold sensitivity, word recognition scores, and assessment of unaided and aided MCL and UCL thresholds are all useful indicators of aided benefit.

Psychoacoustic assessment (i.e., functional gain measures) is still of value today and a very useful tool in deciding whether patients are benefitting from amplification. This is especially true for some asymmetrical hearing losses wherein real-ear assessment is limited in the kinds of information that can be provided in making decisions about benefit. Assessing the patient's responses to speech and pure tones presented in a sound field yields information as to aided audibility and speech recognition. Such information is most useful in counseling the patient as to the benefit and limitation of the dispensed hearing aid(s). However, complete reliance on speech recognition performance as a means of determing the efficiency of a given hearing aid is suspect at best.[24]

Jerger (personal communication, 1987) states:

Although systems for the measurement of real ear gain of hearing aids represent a significant technologic advance over analogous closed coupler measurements in quantifying the frequency response of a hearing aid system, it is important to remember that successful fitting of a hearing aid involves much more than the determination of the optimal frequency response. The audiologist must answer the following questions.

1. Is the use of any hearing aid appropriate?
2. What is the best arrangement and configuration of the hearing aid system (e.g., BTE, ITE, canal aid; monaural vs. binaural: CROS, BICROS, etc.)?
3. Does the patient perform adequately with the recommended aid in the sense of understanding speech in realistic environments?
4. Is there a better solution than a hearing aid (i.e., assistive listening device)?

To answer these questions, a thoughtful and responsible audiologist must necessarily incorporate into the evaluative system measures that go far beyond the real ear frequency response. They will typically involve some measure of the patient's ability to understand real speech in a realistic environment. They may involve quality judgments, paired comparisons, adaptive measures of signal-to-noise ratio, or more traditional speech audiometric measures. Whatever their nature, however, they will broaden the evaluative spectrum beyond the narrow confines of frequency responses.

Recommended Guidelines in Determining Hearing Aid Candidacy

Probably no text dealing with hearing aid fitting strategies would be complete without some suggested guidelines to determine when patients are candidates for binaural, monaural, or a CROS fitting. The reader should keep in mind, however, that the primary intent of this chapter has been justification for binaural amplification for asymmetrical hearing loss. Therefore, comments about binaural application shall be restricted to those hearing losses evidencing significant interaural differences in auditory behavior to acoustic stimuli, either speech or pure tone. The working assumption presented here is that the better ear is either normal or has a degree of hearing loss in which amplification would be beneficial is unquestionable.

-   **Rule One:** Do not determine, a priori, that the utilization of binaural amplification is not appropriate simply because interaural differences are present that may fall within untested criteria recommending that binaural amplification may not be appropriate.
-   **Rule Two:** Always be aware of technologic advances that may significantly alter what can be provided electroacoustically for making the amplified signal one that provides information to those with asymmetrical hearing impairments.
-   **Rule Three:** Never underestimate the value of the patient's subjective response to amplified sound.
-   **Rule Four:** In those cases in which the patient or the audiologist are unsure of the value received from amplification applied to the poorer ear, never hestiate to carry out a carefully constructed trial period to determine benefit.

The purpose of the trial period is to permit the patient to determine the degree to which contributions from the poorer ear may add to signal detection and information processing.

- **Rule Five:** Given an asymmetrical hearing loss, if the poorer ear cannot respond to an acoustic signal at the output limitations of the audiometer, then CROS or BICROS systems may be most appropriate, depending on the magnitude of hearing loss in the better ear. That is, if the input signal is not audible, little can be gained in fitting the poorer ear, although some tactile sensation may be present.

- **Rule Six:** Given an asymmetrical hearing loss, if the poorer ear greatly degrades the recognition of information-bearing signals when such signals are presented binaurally, a CROS, BICROS, or power CROS configured instrument is recommened, depending on the magnitude of hearing impairment in the better ear.

  It is important for the augiologist to remember that the recognition of monosyllabic words in an acoustically controlled test environment does not correlate highly with understanding connected discourse in changing ambient backgrounds. The patient should be permitted to assess "running speech" during the fitting process to determine how it is perceived by the poorer ear.

- **Rule Seven:** Given an asymmetrical hearing loss, if the poorer ear presents with an active disease process, it is best to withhold amplification until appropriate treatment is provided. If both ears have active disease processes, any effort to fit hearing aids is ill advised, regardless of the magnitude of hearing loss.

- **Rule Eight:** Given an asymmetrical, bilateral hearing loss, fit only the better ear if audible sounds for the poorer ear are within normal limits. Although infrequent, it is possible for the poorer ear to have hearing thresholds well within normal limits for a restricted frequency band. All other sounds are not audible even with amplification.

- **Rule Nine:** In the final analysis, the fitting of asymmetrical hearing losses often represents clinical judgment rather than adherence to hard and fast fitting rules based on hearing level. Always discuss, openly and completely, with the patient the advantages and limitations of amplification applied to the poorer ear. The patient needs to be an integral part of the evaluation process.

Summary and Conclusions

Fitting hearing aids to asymmetrical hearing loss presents clinical challenges to audiologists. There is no general consensus as to what can and should be accomplished in prescribing amplification for these patients. For some audiologists, if performance criteria are not met in the presence of asymmetrical loss, then binaural amplification is not recommended. For example, if the interaural threshold difference is greater than 15 dB HL at 500, 1000, and 2000 Hz, or if there is an interaural difference in word recognition score greater than 8%, then binaural amplification may not be recommended. Such rigid criteria are no longer appropriate in view of the technologic advances made in hearing aid design and performance. As illustrated by the several cases referred to in this chapter, these restrictive criteria are to be questioned, since many patients with asymmetrical hearing loss benefit from binaural amplification, even though "traditional" criteria for binaural candidacy were not met.

The purpose of this chapter was to offer a reasonable suggestion for the fitting of binaural amplification to asymmetrical losses. It was not the intent to suggest that all asymmetrical hearing losses are amenable to binaural amplification. Rather, most asymmetrical losses should be evaluated and the determination of benefit should be made following a trial period of hearing aid use. Nor was it the intent of this chapter to indict or to question the use of CROS or BICROS hearing aids. There is no doubt that the use of such hearing aid configurations has been of significant benefit to those who could not demonstrate value from binaural fitting.

In the final analysis, the intent of this chapter was to encourage clinical curiosity and experimentation. One should question established criteria that dictate the use of hearing instruments. While most accepted criteria for assessment and fitting of hearing aids will meet the challenge, consider the valuable knowledge gained when some do not. Not only has the audiologist gained additional clinical insight in meeting amplification needs, but the hearing impaired patient may be better served.

Audiologists should be quick to accept change or modification in fitting protocols if sufficient data are presented questioning that which is traditionally followed in making decisions about hearing aid use and its subsequent benefit. The willingness to question and the desire to change in light of new and compelling clinical evidence is a virtue to be embraced by us all.

References

1. Carhart R: Hearing aid selection by university clinics. *J Speech Hear Disord* 1950; 15:105–113.
2. Briskey RJ: Binaural hearing aids and new innovations, in Katz J (ed): *Handbook of Clinical Audiology*, ed 2. Baltimore: Williams & Wilkins 1978, pp 501–507.
3. Courtois J, Johansen PA, Larsen BV, et al: Hearing aid fitting in asymmetrical hearing loss, in Jensen JH (ed): *Hearing Aid Fitting: Theoretical and Practical Views*. 13th Danavox Symposium, Copenhagen: Stougaard Jenson, 1988, pp 243–255.
4. Skinner M: *Hearing Aid Evaluation*. Englewood Cliffs, NJ: Prentice Hall, 1988.
5. Hawkins DB: Selection of hearing aid characteristics, in Hodgson W (ed): *Hearing Aid Assessment and Use in Audiologic Habilitation*, ed 3. Baltimore: William and Wilkins, 1986, pp 128–151.
6. Byrne D: Clinical issues and options in binaural hearing aid fitting. *Ear Hear* 1981; 2:187–193.
7. Studebaker G, Cox R, Formby C: The effect of environment on the directional performance of headworn hearing aids, in Studebaker G, Hochberg I (eds): *Acoustical Factors Affecting Hearing Aid Performance*. Baltimore: University Park Press, 1980, pp 81–105.
8. MacKeith A, Coles R: Binaural advantages in hearing of speech. *J Laryngol* 1971; 75:213–232.
9. Markides A: *Binaural Hearing Aids*, London: Academic Press, 1977.
10. Causey D, Bender D: Clinical studies in binaural amplification, in Libby E (ed): *Binaural Hearing and Amplification vol 2*. Chicago: Zenetron, Inc., 1980, pp 75–96.
11. Nabalek A, Mason D: Effect of noise and reverberation on binaural and monaural word identification by subjects with various audiograms. *J Speech Hear Res* 1981; 24:375–383.
12. Byrne D, Dermody P: Localisation of sound with binaural body-worn hearing aids. *Br J Audiol* 1975; 9:107–115.

13. Dermody P, Byrne D: Auditory localisation by hearing-impaired persons using binaural in-the-ear hearing aids. *Br J Audiol* 1975a; 9:93–101.
14. Dermody P, Byrne D: Loudness summation and binaural hearing aids. *Scand Audiol* 1975b; 4:123–28.
15. Davis A, Haggard M: Some implications of audiological measures in the population for binaural aiding strategies. *Scand Audiol* 1982; 15(Suppl):167–179.
16. Staab W: Selecting amplification systems, in Sandlin R (ed): *Hearing Instruments Sciences and Fitting Practices*. Livonia, MI: National Institute for Hearing Instruments Studies. 1985, pp 387–437.
17. Walden B, Schwartz D, Williams D, et al.: Test of the assumptions underlying comparative hearing aid evaluations. *J Speech Hear Dis* 1983; 48:255–263.
18. McCandless G, Lyregaard P: Prescription of gain/output (POGO) for hearing aids. *Hear Instrum* 1983; 34(1):16–21.
19. Berger K, Hagberg N, Rane R: A method of hearing aid prescription. *Hear Instrum* 1978; 29(7):1, 12–13.
20. Byrne D, Dillon H: The National Acoustics Laboratories (NAL). New procedures for selecting the gain and frequency response of a hearing aid. *Ear Hear* 1987; 7:257–265.
21. Libby R: The 1/3–2/3 insertion gain hearing aid selection guide. *Hear Instrum* 1986; 3:27–28.
22. Cox RM: A structured approach to hearing aid selection. *Ear Hear* 1985; 6:226–239.
23. Humes LE, Houghton R: Beyond insertion gain. *Hear Instrum* 1992; 43(3):32–35.
24. Thornton A, Raffin M: Speech discrimination scores modeled as a binomial variable. *J Speech Hear Res* 1978; 21:507–518.

11

Selecting and Verifying Hearing Aid Fittings for Unilateral Hearing Loss

Michael Valente, Maureen Valente, Martha Meister, Kelly Macauley, William Vass

Introduction

Patients with unilateral hearing loss can present a challenge to the dispensing audiologist. The dispenser can choose a traditional dispensing model, which suggests providing extensive counseling on the communication problems likely to occur as a result of unilateral hearing loss, or recommend contralateral routing of the signal (CROS) amplification to the good ear. On the other hand, the dispenser could explore with the patient several other alternative fitting strategies.

This chapter will focus on the problems associated with unilateral hearing loss and provide information beneficial for dispensers who want to explore alternative fitting strategies for patients with unilateral hearing loss.

Definition of Unilateral Hearing Loss

For the purposes of this chapter, unilateral hearing loss is defined as unaidable hearing in one ear and normal hearing (15 dB hearing level [HL] or better at 250–8000 Hz) in the opposite ear. Unaidable hearing is defined as an ear having one or more of the following characteristics:

1. Profound sensorineural hearing loss so that amplified sound cannot be heard to any degree of usefulness
2. Very poor word recognition score
3. Marked intolerance for amplified sounds.

Incidence and Prevalence of Unilateral Hearing Loss

Although information is present regarding the incidence of unilateral hearing loss in children,[1-4] less information is present regarding the incidence of unilateral hearing loss in adults. Much of the information regarding the incidence of unilateral hearing loss in adults involves sudden hearing loss, often as a result of illness,[5,6] otologic surgery (acoustic neuroma), or nonotologic surgery.[7-10]

Rambur[11] reported that the incidence of sudden unilateral hearing loss in the United States was approximately 40,000 per year, equally distributed between males and females. Her report, as well as reports by Bye[12] and Berg and Pallasch,[13] indicate that sudden hearing loss usually occurs in adolescents or older adults, with the greatest incidence occurring between 30 and 60 years of age.[14] Hearing loss was usually unilateral, although she[11] and Megighian[15] found bilateral sudden hearing loss in up to 17% of the cases.

Bergenius[16] studied vestibular findings in sensorineural hearing loss. Of 1,635 patients undergoing audiologic evaluation from 1979 to 1982, 12.9% fulfilled the criteria for "pure unilateral sensorineural hearing loss or tinnitus alone." Noury and Katsarkas[17] quoted various references that stated that sudden hearing loss reveals no sexual predilection and has a mean age of occurrence between 40 and 47 years of age. It is usually unilateral, with bilateral involvement reported in 7% of the cases.

Although statistics related to children may not easily be generalized to adults, they may provide general trends. Oyler et al.[4] examined the incidence of unilateral hearing loss in a large school district of approximately 54,000 students, with a second part of the study looking at academic performance. The prevalence of unilateral sensorineural hearing loss was approximately 2 students per 1,000. In 106 children, there were slightly more males than females and almost twice as many children with hearing loss in the right ear as the left ear. Almost three-fourths of the hearing losses were sensorineural (N = 78).

Bess and Tharpe[3] estimated that nearly 7 million Americans have some degree of unilateral hearing loss. They quoted a prevalence rate for school-aged children of 3:1,000 in which hearing loss was 45 dB HL or greater, which increased to 13:1,000 if milder losses (26–45 dB HL) were included. They provided no information for children under age 3 years. The authors reported that Everberg[18] revealed a greater prevalence of unilateral deafness among males (62.3%) than females (37.7%); he also reported[18] a greater percentage of left ear impairment (52.5%). Of interest is that unilateral impairment is generally detected later in life, since speech and language skills appear to develop more normally. Of Everberg's 122 subjects,[18] 52.5% were identified after the first year in school. Bess and Tharpe[3] cited Tarkkanen and Aho[19] to collaborate these findings with an average identification age of 6 years. The hearing loss in 50% of the children was not detected until 7 years of age or older, which the authors find unacceptable in view of the deleterious effects unilateral hearing loss has on academic performance and will be discussed in another section of this chapter.[3]

Brookhouser et al.[2] investigated unilateral hearing loss in children, the results of which may lend information related to adult populations. Brookhouser et al.[2] also reported an incidence in unilateral hearing loss of 3:1,000 when including hearing loss greater than 45 dB HL or 13:1,000 when including hearing loss between 26 and 45 dB HL. They reported that Kinney[20] found 1,307 cases of sensorineural hearing loss in children, of which 48% were unilateral. Of 1,829 consecutive patients studied by the investigators,[2] (N = 690), 37.7% had asymmetrical hearing loss. Of those 690 cases, 391 (56.6%) were described as having isolated unilateral sensorineural hearing loss. When 67 of these 391 cases were deleted from the study (due to various factors, such as conductive component), they finally reported on the results of 324 children. Sixty-two percent were males and 38% were females, a statistically significant finding. The left ear was affected in 52%, while the right ear was affected in the remaining 48%. This finding was not statistically significant. The investigators felt their statistics were consistent with previous investigators' preponderance of males over females. However, previous findings of greater right-sided versus left sided hearing losses were not supported by this study.

Tieri et al.[21] observed 280 cases of unilateral sensorineural hearing loss from 1979 to 1986. The age range was 8 months to 12 years, with a mean age at diagnosis of 7.6 years. Approximately 62% were males and 37% females. They felt these findings were in agreement with those of Tarkkanen and Aho[19] and Hallmo et al.[22] The right ear was affected in 49.6% of cases and the left ear in 50.3% cases. Degree of hearing loss ranged from mild to profound, with 79.3% falling in the latter range. In addition, 250 audiograms revealed a flat configuration. The investigators,[21] noting that incidence is difficult to evaluate, cited the following statistics: Everberg,[18] an incidence rate of 0.06%; Tarkkanen and Aho,[19] 0.09%; and Kinney,[20] 8.5%. The investigators[21] noted that 24.7% of their children were diagnosed before the age of 6 years, as compared with the 47.5% under 7 years noted by Everberg[18] and the 7% before school age noted by Hallmo et al.[22] They concluded that school age diagnosis may be a result of critical teacher observation, older children's awareness of sensory skills, and exposure to a greater number of infectious diseases.

Although no clear-cut statistic is available regarding the incidence of unilateral sensorineural hearing loss in adults, perhaps the findings summarized earlier in this chapter may provide some insight. The incidence of unilateral hearing loss is of such significance that audiologists and otologists should be prepared to see such patients on a regular basis and plan rehabilitation programs to help maximize the residual hearing in both the affected and better ear.

Etiologies

Unilateral hearing loss can be present at birth (*congenital*) or at any time after birth (*acquired*). Congenital unilateral hearing loss can be *genetic* (dominant, recessive, or sex-linked) or *nongenetic* (cytomegalovirus [CMV], low birth weight, syphilis, mumps, or anoxia). In addition, unilateral hearing loss can be acquired at any age, and the resulting hearing loss may be progressive, fluctuating, or sudden.

Several investigators have examined the etiology of unilateral hearing loss in children. In each investigation, the cause of the unilateral hearing loss was unknown (*idiopathic*) in the majority of cases. Kinney[20] reported that of known causes in a series of 310 children, meningitis, measles, and mumps were the most common etiologies. Tieri et al.[21] examined 280 children between 1979 and 1986 and found that the etiologic factor was known in only 23% of the cases and that of the known factors mumps was predominant. Everberg[18] evaluated 122 children with unilateral hearing loss and noted that congenital factors are responsible for approximately 75% of the cases, with heredity being the major causal factor.

With the recent technologic advances in the treatment of neonates, additional risk factors for unilateral hearing loss have emerged. These include persistent pulmonary hypertension of the newborn (PPHN),[23] hyperbilirubinemia,[24] intraventricular hemorrhage,[25] and low birth weight.[26] Although these factors are most typically associated with bilateral hearing loss, unilateral hearing loss has also been reported.

Other less common causal agents have also been reported and include chicken

Table 11–1. Summary of Etiologies Resulting in Unilateral Hearing Loss

Study	N	Pathology	Percentage
Kinney[20]	310	meningitis measles mumps	
Tieri et al.[21]	280	mumps	23
Everberg[18]	122	congenital: heredity	75

		Other etiologies
		  Chicken pox
		  Cogan'a syndrome
		  Congenital cholesteatoma
		  Cytomegalovirus
		  Embolism
		  External ear deformities
		  Herpes zoster oticus
		  Hyperbilirubinemia
		  Intraventricular hemorrhage
		  Labyrinth membrane rupture
		  Low birth weight
		  Ménière's disease
		  Multiple sclerosis
		  Neoplasms
		  Otitis media
		  Perilymph fistula
		  Persistent pulmonary
		  Hypertension
		  Postotologic surgica!
		  Sludging of blood
		  Syphilis
		  Thrombosis
		  Trauma
		  Vascular pathologies
		  Viral labyrinthitis	

pox,[23] CMV,[27] Ménière's disease,[23] trauma,[23] and perilymphatic fistula.[28] Middle ear disease such as congenital cholesteatoma and otitis media have been known to cause unilateral hearing loss. Many external ear deformities such as congenital atresia of the external auditory canal are typically unilateral.

Many of the causes of childhood unilateral hearing loss can also cause adult-onset or acquired unilateral hearing loss. Mumps and other viral etiologies[29] such as viral labyrinthitis are well known causes of unilateral hearing loss in adults. Other well-documented etiologies include vascular pathologies (occlusion, emboli, hemorrhage),[9,10] neoplasms (acoustic neuroma), and labyrinth membrane ruptures (perilymphatic fistula).[28] Ménière's disease has been reported to cause unilateral hearing loss in approximately 50% of all cases.[30] Head trauma, leading to a transverse (sensorineural hearing loss) or longitudinal (conductive hearing loss) fracture of the temporal bone can precipitate a unilateral hearing loss. In addition, syphilis, Cogan's syndrome, postotologic surgical loss, multiple sclerosis, perilymphatic fistula, herpes zoster oticus, hemorrhage, thrombosis, embolism, spasms, aneurysm, and sludging of blood have been reported to cause unilateral hearing loss.[31] Table 11–1 summarizes many etiologies that have been reported to cause unilateral hearing loss in children and adults.

Problems Associated With Unilateral Hearing Loss

The individual with unilateral hearing loss can no longer enjoy the advantages of binaural hearing. For the interested reader, the advantages of binaural listening are covered in greater detail in Chapter 9 and by Valente.[32] These advantages include

1. Elimination of the head shadow effect
2. Presence of the squelch effect
3. Improved localization
4. Presence of binaural summation.

Head Shadow Effect

The "head shadow effect" for spondee words was initially described by Tillman et al.,[33] who reported that, as a spondee word arrives from one side of the head (*near ear or monaural direct*), the intensity of the signal is attenuated across the head by an average overall level of 6.4 dB before the signal reaches the opposite ear (*far ear or monaural indirect*). Furthermore, the head shadow effect increases as a function of frequency. For example, at frequencies above 2,000 Hz, the intensity level of the signal to the far ear can be as much as 15–20 dB less intense than the level of the signal at the near ear.[34,35]

The reduction in signal level in the higher frequencies at the far ear can have a significant impact on speech recognition. For example, if speech is delivered to the impaired ear side and noise directed to the good side (monaural indirect) at the same intensity level, the patient can experience great difficulties in communicating. In this situation, the speech signal is reduced overall by 6.4 dB to the good ear due to the head shadow effect, but the noise is unattenuated to the good ear. As a result, a −6.4 dB signal-to-noise (S/N) ratio is present at the good ear. Furthermore, a +6.4 dB S/N ratio is present at the impaired ear (monaural direct) because the noise is attenuated by 6.4 dB but the signal is unattenuated. In essence, the unilaterally impaired patient has a 13 dB deficit relative to the same listening situation for a normal hearing patient. Clearly, if this listening situation is reversed, then the unilaterally impaired patient is not at a disadvantage relative to the normal listener. Valente[32] summarized a series of studies concerning speech recognition for monaural direct versus monaural indirect listening. The advantage of monaural direct to monaural indirect word recognition can be as high as 20–50% depending on the type of signal, noise, azimuth, and S/N ratio.[32]

Squelch Effect

Giolas and Wark,[36] Koenig,[37] and others,[34,38,39] have described the advantages of binaural hearing to "squelch" or reduce the deleterious effects of background noise and/or reverberation on speech recognition. Gulick and colleagues[39] reported improved binaural "release from masking," particularly when time, intensity, or phase differences of the signal are present (i.e., signal presented at any azimuth in a sound field other than 0°), and these differences are not present for the masker (i.e., masker presented at 0° azimuth). That is, the presence of differences in time, intensity, and/or phase of the speech signal between the two ears will result in improved performance compared with the situation in which these differences are not present between the two ears.

Localization

Gulick et al.[39] devoted a section of their text to sound localization, describing various studies that have contributed to our knowledge. Explanations of directional hearing have centered about differences in stimulation between the two ears in time and intensity (i.e., duplex theory of localization) and the integration of this information for improved sound localization. In particular, the normal listener uses interaural time (low frequency cue) and intensity differences (high frequency cue) for improved localization in the horizontal plane. Obviously, if there is a large difference in hearing between the ears, localization skills would be reduced.

Binaural Summation

Brookhouser et al.[2] remind us that individuals with binaural hearing demonstrate improved thresholds for pure-tone and speech stimuli that are presented binaurally.[38,46] Gulick et al.[39] described this binaural summation phenomenon as an advantage in processing information (specifically, detecting threshold) with two ears over listening with one ear. They stated that if the ears are equally sensitive, the binaural threshold is about 3 dB better than the monaural threshold and the binaural advantage expands to 6 dB during suprathreshold listening (i.e., most comfortable loudness) and 10 dB at a 90 dB sensation level

(SL). This additional advantage may have significant effects on improved word recognition scores when listening binaurally in comparison to monaural listening. That is, if speech recognition increases at a rate of 5% per each additional decibel (i.e., articulation function), then the binaural advantage at suprathreshold levels could be 30% better (6 dB × 5%/dB) than the monaural score.

Performance in the Classroom

Several studies have described the deleterious effects of unilateral hearing loss on children. Bess and Tharpe[47] studied a group of 60 children with unilateral sensorineural hearing loss (greater than 45 dB HL in the speech frequencies). They felt that children would experience similar listening difficulties as adults, especially in the classroom and with language development. In their study, they found that 35% failed at least one grade (rate for general school population was 3.5%), and an additional 13.3% required resource assistance at school. A greater incidence of behavior problems was reported also. There seemed to be a correlation between early onset/severity of loss and risk for experiencing academic difficulties. Oyler et al.[4] reported a failure rate of 2% for grades Kindergarten through eighth, which is approximately ten times greater than in the normal-hearing population. Some children were even reported to have dropped out of school. Brookhouser et al.[2] reiterated that children with unilateral loss may be disadvantaged in the classroom, particularly if noise occurs close to the better ear. These children do not have the advantages of normal-hearing children in selecting meaningful signals mixed with background noise. Localizing a sound source in horizontal plane may also present difficulty. Brookhouser et al.[2] appear to corroborate reports of academic and behavioral difficulties. Suggestions for teachers and parents were listed, including careful audiologic/otologic monitoring and strategies to alleviate localization and auditory figure-ground difficulties.

Bess et al.[48] provide a profile of the unilaterally hearing impaired child who experienced academic difficulty:

1. Severe to profound sensorineural hearing loss
2. Early age of onset
3. Impairment in the right ear.

Culbertson and Gilbert[49] reported decreased performance in word recognition, language, and spelling. The investigators provided some useful suggestions for management strategies, especially within the classroom.

Bovo et al.[50] submitted a questionnaire to 115 unilaterally hearing impaired individuals who had become impaired during the first 12 years of life. Fifty-five males and 60 females were included in their study, with 62 having hearing loss in the left ear and 53 in the right ear. Seventy percent were over 6 years of age when diagnosed. Difficulties in speech recognition and localization were described, as well as feelings of embarrassment, passivity, and avoidance. Twenty-two percent failed at least one grade, 12% received special services in the area of learning disability, and 27% described embarrassment and a sense of inferiority. Fifty percent had not been provided preferential seating. The investigators recommended counseling classroom teachers in the areas of reducing environmental noise levels and reverberation in the classroom.

Patient's Perspective of Unilateral Hearing Loss

Giolas and Wark[36] stated that, although communication difficulties for patients with unilateral hearing loss have been minimized by some professionals in the past, the difficulties can be quite significant. A report by Harford and Barry[51] described some of the significant difficulties encountered by these patients. These investigators[51] interviewed 20 patients with unilateral hearing loss. An increased difficulty in recognizing speech in noise (i.e., reduction or elimination of the binaural squelch effect) was reported as the most adverse listening situation. The greatest difficulty appeared when the noise was directed to the better ear and speech was directed to the impaired ear (i.e., head shadow effect). However, speech recognition was reported "affected" regardless of location of the speech or noise to the "good" ear. Interviewees further reported difficulty with localization of the sound source, especially in noisy situations. In addition, there was difficulty receiving and understanding speech, even in quiet, when the sound source was some distance away. They expressed feelings of confusion, embarrassment, helplessness, and annoyance. On a final note, interviewees were interested in responding to the questions, because they felt professionals had not expressed concern regarding their communication difficulties.

From another patient's perspective, Bardon[52] described some of the detrimental physiologic effects accompanying unilateral hearing loss. Both dizziness and tinnitus, which can accompany unilateral hearing loss, are frightening and bothersome; in addition, if a hearing loss is sudden, it can be especially confusing and distressing. Bardon[52] felt that the extensive test batteries that patients undergo to diagnose etiology are time-consuming and may be somewhat stressful. He acknowledged that some literature describes unilaterally impaired children as having only minor communicative difficulties, if any. Adults were felt to have even fewer difficulties, especially if the loss developed later in life; these viewpoints were opposed by Bardon.[52]

Bardon went on to state that tinnitus was a "masker" that interfered with speech perception. Furthermore, it was harder to attend to tasks, and he found himself shifting his head to perform tasks better. Large rooms such as hallways, hotel lobbies, and airports created difficult listening environments where sounds appeared blended. Several talkers at the same time presented difficulty, as did competing conversation or music during dining conversation. There were difficulties outdoors, and in some situations (such as in traffic) there was a safety issue involved with reduced localization abilities. Additional listening difficulties were encountered when the sound source was behind, when visual cues were limited, and with children's voices. The quality of listening to music was affected with monaural listening, as was the ability to monitor the patient's own speaking voice. Feelings of fatigue and irritability seemed to accompany continual attempts to perceive conversations and other meaningful stimuli. Professionals were urged to take note of these deleterious effects in counseling their patients and helping them to recognize the need to change their listening situations and lifestyles.

Hearing Aid Fitting Process for Unilateral Hearing Loss

Case History and Referral

As mentioned earlier, the problems associated with unilateral hearing loss appear to have been largely ignored by hearing health care professionals. In addition, patients with unilateral hearing loss generally perform well in quiet or have the ability to rotate their head so that the good ear is directed toward the speech signal and therefore may not consider amplification to be required or beneficial. However, rotation of the head so that the good ear is directed toward the speech signal is not always possible. For example, if a patient has an anacusic right ear and is driving a car with a passenger on the right side, it would be very difficult, if not impossible, for the patient to rotate his head so his good left ear is facing the passenger!

When attempting to provide audiologic care for patients with unilateral hearing loss, the audiologist should seek answers to some important questions prior to considering amplification. Information should include the age of the patient, occupation, demands on listening, and indications of motivation toward amplification. Many authors[35,53–58] have stated that there is a greater likelihood of success with amplification in this group if (1) a high degree of motivation is present toward amplification; (2) the demands on listening are high because of lifestyle or occupation; and (3) if the patient is an adult. Several authors[35,53–58] report a higher rate of failure with CROS amplification when attempted to be fit to children. Kenworthy et al.[55] reported significantly greater success during monaural direct listening with an FM auditory trainer coupled to the better ear than with either CROS amplification or recommending preferential seating in children with unilateral hearing loss.

The patient history should include as much detail as possible regarding the duration and etiology of the hearing loss and any related symptoms such as tinnitus or dizziness. Like any other hearing aid fitting, the audiologist should require a medical clearance prior to dispensing a hearing aid. This is especially true in cases of unilateral hearing loss, because the hearing loss may be the result of a space-occupying lesion.

If the hearing loss is sudden, waiting several weeks before pursuing amplification is suggested because approximately 65% of cases of sudden hearing loss report complete or partial recovery.[11] Management of sudden unilateral hearing loss may include vasodilating drugs, anticoagulants, histamine, cervical ganglion blocks, steroids, inhalation therapy of 95% oxygen and 5% carbon dioxide, and calcium antagonists.[11]

Fitting Options

CROS

One of the most successful attempts in helping patients with unilateral hearing loss overcome the head shadow effect was the introduction of CROS (contralateral *routing of* the *signal*) in 1965.[51,53,58-60] In the earliest version, CROS amplification consisted of a microphone placed over or near the unaidable ear to pick up signals arriving at the side of the impaired ear. The output from the microphone was wired to an amplifier, receiver, and volume control, via a headband, and the amplified signal was delivered via tubing gently placed in the open ear canal of the good ear. Due to the presence of the open earmold, no gain was provided below 800 Hz and only marginal gain was provided between 800 and 1500 Hz. The greatest amount of gain was provided in the frequency region above 1500 Hz. Therefore, patients likely to receive the greatest benefit from CROS amplification were patients with no hearing loss in the good ear through 1500 Hz and a slight to mild hearing loss in the frequency region above 1500 Hz.

An eyeglass version of the CROS aid soon became available, with the wire running through the frames of eyeglasses. For those who did not wear glasses, the CROS was developed into behind-the-ear (BTE) hearing aids connected by a wire worn under the hairline. One of the major drawbacks of CROS amplification was the need for a wire to connect the output from the microphone on the impaired ear to the receiver on the good ear. To solve this problem, Telex introduced a wireless BTE CROS hearing aid in 1973. The wireless CROS uses an amplitude modulated carrier frequency to transmit signals from the microphone on the side of the impaired ear to the receiver placed in the good ear. Distance between the transmitter and receiver is critical (approximately 6.5 inches). For every half inch increase in distance between the transmitter and receiver, there is a 3–4 dB decrease in gain.[59] Today, the receiver portion placed into the good ear can be built into an in-the-ear (ITE) hearing aid with a wide vent. The most recent wireless CROS models also include adaptive compression.

While CROS amplification effectively eliminates the head shadow effect by amplifying signals from the hearing impaired side, localization and speech intelligibility in noise still remain a problem. Some CROS users report some improved localization based on differences of the quality of sounds from the two ears. If the signal appears "natural" it may be judged to be arriving from the good side. If the sound appears "tinny" or "metallic" it may be judged to be arriving from the impaired side.[53] Also, if the level of ambient noise is high, few users of CROS amplification report any significant benefit regardless of which side the signal or noise may be arising from. In these environments, it is best to counsel the patient to reduce the volume control setting or remove the hearing aids.[35,53,54,59]

One final point *must be emphasized* regarding CROS amplification. In the original report by Harford and Barry[51] and subsequent reports by Harford,[53] Harford and Dodds,[58] Courtois et al.,[57] and Punch,[59] there is a clear recommendation that success with CROS amplification is significantly related to the magnitude of hearing loss in the good ear. If hearing in the good ear is within normal limits, then the probability of success with CROS amplification will be minimal. On the other hand, if a mild hearing loss is present above 1500 Hz, then a greater probability of patient acceptance will be achieved. Our experience with CROS amplification over the past several years supports this recommendation. Very few (less than 10%) of our patients with normal hearing in the good ear reported that the benefits from CROS outweighed their perceptions of the presence of "harshness" or "tinniness" of the amplified sound heard in the good ear. Based on these findings, we have adopted a policy that CROS amplification is not our *primary* choice for unilaterally hearing impaired listeners *if* the patient has normal hearing in the good ear. On the other hand, CROS becomes our primary recommendation *if* a mild to moderate high frequency sensorineural hearing loss is present in the good ear above 1500 Hz.

TRANSCRANIAL CROS

Another approach to providing benefits of amplification to unilaterally hearing impaired has recently been advocated by several authors[62–66] who suggest placing a high gain–high output ITE or BTE hearing aid into the impaired ear to take advantage of the fact that the cochleas for each ear, which are contained within the temporal bone, are not acoustically isolated. That is, if a signal of increasing intensity is presented to the cochlea of an impaired ear, the signal will eventually be heard in the cochlea of the better ear because it will be intense enough to overcome the acoustic isolation (*interaural attenuation* [IA]) between the cochleas of the two ears. Because the signal picked up by a microphone placed in the impaired ear is transferred to the cochlea of the good ear through the cranial structures of the temporal bone, the authors referred to this type of fitting as a *transcranial CROS*.

The concept in developing the transcranial CROS is apparent to any audiologist who has experience in testing a patient via air conduction (earphone or insert receiver) who has normal hearing in one ear and a moderate-severe to severe hearing loss in the opposite ear. That is, the initial unmasked air conduction threshold for the impaired ear represents the magnitude of interaural attenuation (i.e., "shadow curve"). For this patient, this represents the lowest intensity at which stimuli (nonspeech or speech) will pass through the temporal bone and is heard by the cochlea of the normal ear. In much the same way, the output (input signal plus the gain of the hearing aid) from a strong BTE or ITE hearing aid placed on the impaired ear can deliver sound to the cochlea of the normal ear via bone conduction. Signals picked up by the microphone of a hearing aid placed over or in the impaired ear can be amplified and eventually cross through the head and be heard by the cochlea of the normal ear via bone conduction.[66]

One study[66] comparing conventional CROS with transcranial CROS amplification solicited the following comments from subjects. They noted that their subjects reported improved recognition of speech in "quiet" when the speech signal was presented to the impaired side, improved speech recognition in noise, and some improvement in the ability to localize. In addition, some subjects reported that the amplified sound presented through their transcranial CROS was more "natural" than the sound processed through their conventional CROS hearing aid. Other reports by McSpaden,[65] McSpaden and McSpaden,[62] and Sullivan[64] indicated that listeners found transcranial CROS fittings "more natural," provided improved localization via cues from a metallic sound from the aided side and a natural sound from the normal side, and improved listening in noise when the signal was from the impaired ear side. Patients did not report the harshness that some experience with CROS fittings.

In an effort to determine if transcranial fittings had merit, the authors recently evaluated 12 patients with an anacusic ear or profound sensorineural hearing loss in one ear and normal hearing in the opposite ear. For each patient, a strong ITE hearing aid (maximum saturation sound pressure level of 120 dB; full-on gain of 55–65 dB) with a long canal and pressure vent was fitted to the impaired ear. Four patients were experienced users of CROS amplification to the better ear. Two patients had experience with an eyeglass bone conduction hearing aid placed on the mastoid process of the impaired ear. Five patients had no experience with amplification, and one patient had experience with a mild ITE hearing aid coupled to the better ear. At the end of four weeks, half of the patients felt that the ITE transcranial CROS provided significant benefit, while the other half noted little additional benefit and decided to continue to utilize their current hearing aids or not pursue amplification.

It is important to remember that the acceptance rate at this facility for conventional CROS fittings for this population is 10%, while the acceptance rate for the transcranial CROS was 50%. It is interesting to note that the reasons for rejection of the transcranial CROS by many of the patients were related to feedback or to a sensation of vibration generated from the hearing aid. The results of this evaluation were encouraging, and we are currently in the process of directly comparing transcranial CROS BTE fittings (to eliminate, hopefully, the problems related to feedback and at the same time provide greater output) to traditional CROS fittings in a large sample of unilaterally hearing impaired adults.

CROS-PLUS

A modification of transcranial CROS was introduced by Hable et al.[67] This fitting system was coined "CROS-PLUS" by the authors because a traditional CROS is fitted to the better ear in the usual manner and is combined with a power ITE hearing aid placed in the unaidable ear. A recent modification of the eyeglass CROS version provides for the offside frame on the poorer ear to contain two microphones. One microphone is for the CROS or BICROS arrangement to forward the signal to the better ear. The second microphone is part of a separate hearing instrument (i.e., microphone, amplifier, and receiver with a closed mold) to forward the signal to the poorer ear. This effectively eliminated the need for a separate ITE to be placed in the unaidable ear. In addition, this arrangement can be modified for BTE fittings to both ears. According to the authors, the CROS-PLUS has been fitted to over 150 patients for whom many report improved clarity of speech, improved localization, and improved recognition of speech in noise.

BONE CONDUCTION

Whereas 30–50 dB or more of gain is necessary for the output from an air-conducted transcranial CROS fitting to reach the cochlea of the good ear, minimal gain is required for a signal delivered via bone conduction to reach the cochlea of the good ear. This is because interaural attenuation for a bone-conducted signal is virtually 0 dB. That is, as soon as a signal is transmitted by bone conduction to the cochlea embedded in the mastoid process of the temporal bone of one ear, it is instantaneously heard in the cochlea embedded in the temporal bone of the opposite ear. Therefore, the signal detected by the microphone placed over the anacusic ear and amplified by a bone conduction hearing aid is immediately heard in the cochlea of the good ear.

Fowler[68] appears to be the first to advocate placement of a bone conduction hearing aid over the mastoid process of the impaired ear for patients with unilateral hearing loss. Usually, bone conduction aids are advocated for ears with chronic middle ear drainage or an ear canal with atresia. Since interaural attenuation for a bone-conducted signal is negligible, only one ear is required to have normal hearing via bone conduction.

Bone conduction aids are currently available in eyeglasses (Fidelity F228 or F229). In addition, bone conduction aids are available in body aid or BTE configurations, with the bone vibrator tightly held in place on the mastoid process via a headband. Just like the transcranial CROS, a bone conduction eyeglass hearing aid has a microphone, amplifier, volume control, and bone conduction receiver mounted in the eyeglass temple behind the ear with a vibrating pad projecting slightly toward the mastoid process on the side of the impaired ear and delivers sound from that ear, routing it transcranially via bone conduction to the cochlea of the normal ear. For a patient with an anacusic ear and normal hearing in the opposite ear, the bone conduction aid can provide improved awareness and recognition of speech arriving on the side of the poor ear. However, like CROS and transcranial CROS amplification, bone conduction aids do not appear to improve localization significantly or the recognition of speech dramatically in high levels of background noise for most patients.

In an attempt to determine if fitting a bone conduction hearing aid had any merit, the authors recently evaluated seven patients with anacusic hearing on one side following surgical removal of an acoustic neuroma. Of the seven patients, six decided to purchase the hearing instrument (rejection rate of 14.3%) after a 30–60 day trial period. Interestingly, one patient who decided to purchase the bone conduction hearing aid had a long history of experience with CROS amplification. These seven patients reported similar improvements in communication that were described earlier for our patients using a transcranial CROS. Again, it is important to remember that the acceptance rate at this facility for conventional CROS fittings for this population is 10%, whereas the acceptance rate was 86% for an eyeglass bone conduction hearing aid.

Although this fitting was very successful with this small group of patients, a bone conduction eyeglass fitting is not without numerous obstacles. First, when the eyeglass is removed the patient will be without amplification. Second, not all unilaterally hearing impaired patients have visual impairments and therefore may not be interested in pursuing an eyeglass fitting. This problem was solved for two patients by having the optician fit ordinary glass into the eyeglass frame. Third, it is very important for the bone vibrator to fit directly on the mastoid with sufficient static pressure to deliver the amplified signal effectively to the mastoid process.

Each eyeglass bone conduction aid is available with a series of ten extension tips to place the bone vibrator directly on the mastoid. It is often necessary to make several trips to an experienced optician before the ideal placement and pressure are achieved. For some patients, the required pressure necessary for maximum benefit from this type of hearing instrument may cause irritability of the skin under the bone vibrator, discomfort, and headaches. In fact, these problems led to rejection by one of our patients, although he found the hearing aid fitting to be beneficial. In addition, audiologists tend to shy away from eyeglass fittings because they themselves assume the patient would not be interested in pursuing such a fitting. The findings of Hable et al.[67] clearly point to the fact that the need to place hearing instruments in an eyeglass is not the obstacle many audiologists believe it to be.

Verification Strategies

Sound Field Evaluation

Figure 11–1 illustrates a suggested procedure for evaluating sound field un-aided and aided speech recognition in noise for CROS, CROS-PLUS, and bone conduction hearing aids. Similar procedures have been suggested by Harford,[53] Skinner,[69] Pollack,[54] and Hodgson.[35] In Figure 11–1A, the signal (NU-6 word lists at 70 dB SPL on the C scale) is presented from a loudspeaker 90° azimuth on the side of the good ear, and multi-talker babble is presented at 64 dB SPL (C scale) from a loudspeaker 90° azimuth on the side of the unaidable ear. In

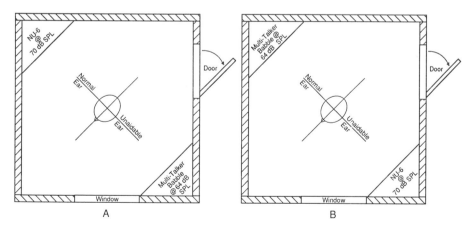

Figure 11–1. **(A)** Loudspeaker arrangements for measuring word recognition scores in a +6 dB S/N ratio. NU-6 word lists presented to the side of the normal ear, and multi-talker babble presented to the side of the unaidable ear. **(B)** Multi-talker babble presented to the side of the normal ear, and NU-6 word lists presented to the side of the unaidable ear.

this configuration, unaided and aided word recognition scores are determined with a calibrated +6 dB S/N ratio without the head present.

It should be anticipated that the results using the loudspeaker arrangement illustrated in Figure 11–1A will reveal the best unaided and the poorest aided scores and thus the smallest difference between unaided and aided performance. That is, in the unaided condition the good ear is directly receiving the NU-6 words (70 dB SPL). The intensity level of the multi-talker babble (64 dB SPL) presented from the side of the poor ear is reduced to the good ear by approximately 6.4 dB due to the head shadow effect.[33] This effectively reduces the noise level of the multi-talker babble to 57.6 dB at the side of the good ear. Therefore, the effective S/N ratio at the good ear has been improved to +12.4 dB (70/57.6), whereas without the presence of the head the S/N ratio was calibrated at +6 dB (70/64 dB SPL). For the aided condition, the multi-talker babble from the poor side is now amplified because a microphone is placed over or near the poor ear. Under this situation, the reduction of noise to the good ear has been eliminated and the noise is amplified and mixed at fairly high levels with the unamplified signal entering the good ear directly.

In Figure 11–1B, the position of the subject remains the same, but the loudspeaker output has been reversed so that the signal arrives at the side of the unaidable ear, while the multi-talker babble arrives at the side of the good ear. In the loudspeaker arrangement illustrated in Figure 11–1B, the audiologist should anticipate the poorest unaided and the best aided scores and thus the largest difference in aided versus unaided performance. In fact, it is not uncommon for the differences between unaided and aided performance to exceed 20%–30%. In the unaided condition, the speech signal is on the side of the poor ear and is attenuated by approximately 6.4 dB to the good ear, while the noise is unattenuated to the good ear. In this situation, the effective S/N ratio at the good ear is −12.4 dB for the same reasons described above and unaided performance should be rather poor. In the aided condition, a microphone is on the side of the poor ear to deliver the amplified signal (either by air or bone conduction) to the good ear. This effectively eliminates the head shadow effect and significantly improves speech recognition scores in comparison to the unaided condition in which the head shadow effect was present.

Although the results of the four unaided and aided comparisons are fairly predictable, it is important for the audiologist to complete these comparisons. These procedures clearly demonstrate to the listener the importance of placing the microphone on the impaired ear in a favorable position depending on of the origin of the signal or noise to the impaired ear. In essence, this verification process allows the patient to experience the full spectrum of listening situations in which unaided and aided performance will be markedly different. That is, the listening situation in which the patient had the greatest difficulty without amplification (i.e., speech on the poor side and noise on the good side) will now result in the best listening environment with the use of amplification. On the other hand, the listening situation that created the least difficulty without amplification (i.e., speech on the good side and noise on the poor side) will now result in the poorest listening environment with the use of amplification. The patient needs to experience and realize that situations will arise in which

Table 11–2. Speech Recognition Scores Measured in Sound Field as Illustrated in Figure 11–1

Aid	Unaided (%)	Aided (%)
Transcranial CROS		
NU-6 to good ear/multi-talker babble to the impaired ear (Fig. 11–1A)	92	94
NU-6 to impaired ear/multi-talker babble to the good ear (Fig. 11–1B)	74	92
Eyeglass bone conduction		
NU-6 to good ear/multi-talker babble to the impaired ear (Fig. 11–1A)	84	100
NU-6 to impaired ear/multi-talker babble to the good ear (Fig. 11–1B)	56	82

amplification will provide a poorer listening environment in comparison to when amplification is not used.

Table 11–2 provides the speech recognition results for two patients using the loudspeaker arrangements discussed in the previous section. The results are for one patient fitted with a transcranial ITE CROS on the impaired ear and for a second patient fitted with an eyeglass bone conduction aid with the bone vibrator placed on the mastoid process in the impaired ear. As can be seen for the transcranial CROS patient, the aided improvement was 2% for the condition described in Figure 11–1A where the NU-6 word lists were presented on the side of the good ear and the noise was presented on the side of the impaired ear. However, for the eyeglass bone conduction patient, the aided improvement was 16%, which is significant at the 0.01 confidence level.[70] When the listening situation was reversed as described in Figure 11–1B, the aided performance was 18% better than the unaided score for the ITE transcranial CROS and a 26% improvement for the eyeglass bone conduction fitting both of which were significant at the 0.01 confidence interval.[70]

Probe Measures for Traditional CROS Fittings

The method of choice today for verification of hearing aid fittings is real-ear probe tube measures. For an indepth description of real-ear probe tube measures the reader is referred to Chapter 5 and to Tecca[71] or Valente.[72]

Probe tube measures can be a very useful tool for measuring the performance of CROS, transcranial CROS, and CROS-PLUS fittings. Punch[59] suggested measuring the real-ear unaided response (REUR) and real-ear insertion response (REIR) at 250–6000 Hz for a CROS fitting with the probe tube placed at 4–6 mm from the tympanic membrane of the *good ear* with the loudspeaker at 45–90° azimuth to the impaired ear where the microphone for the various CROS fittings will reside. He suggested that the measured REIR will demonstrate if the CROS fitting eliminated the head shadow effect because the measured REIR should not exceed the magnitude of the head shadow (6–7 dB) plus an amount of gain appropriate for the magnitude of hearing loss in the good ear between 1500 and 6000 Hz. Punch[59] did not suggest a prescriptive procedure, but the NAL-R prescriptive procedure[73] appears to be an appropriate choice for the magnitude of loss in the good ear, which is appropriate for a CROS fitting. For fitting an ear with normal hearing in the good ear, less than 10 dB gain would be desired in the frequency region above 1500 Hz. For many CROS fittings measured at our facility, the measured REIR exceeds this goal, and this may be the major reason why many patients with normal hearing in the good ear reject CROS amplification.

Tecca[71] (Chapter 5) indicates that several real-ear probe tube measures should be made for CROS fittings. First, Tecca suggests measuring the REUR, real-ear aided response (REAR), and REIR with the loudspeaker at ±45° azimuth with the probe microphone in the better ear and the reference microphone placed over the poor ear. In this manner the audiologist first measures the REUR. Then the BTE or ITE CROS hearing aid is placed over or in the poorer ear, and the REAR is measured in the better ear. The REIR is calculated as the difference between the REAR and the REUR.

To determine the magnitude of the head shadow effect, the REUR can *initially* be measured with the loudspeaker at 45–90° azimuth to the good ear with the reference microphone over the good ear, but the probe microphone in the poor ear. The REUR is *repeated* with the loudspeaker relocated at 45–90° azimuth to the side of the poor ear with the reference microphone moved to the poor ear, but the probe microphone remaining in the poor ear. The difference in the REUR between these two measures represents the magnitude of the head shadow effect, and it can be on the order of approximately 6–7 dB. In addition, these measurements illustrate the effectiveness of the microphone placed on the poor ear when desired signals originate from the side of the poor ear.

Finally, the REAR is measured once with the loudspeaker located 45–90° on the *side of the better ear*. This REAR measure can be compared with either REUR mentioned in the previous paragraph. Comparison of the REAR to the REUR measured from the side of the poor ear determines the magnitude of the elimination of the head shadow effect. Comparison of the REAR to the REUR measured from the side of the good ear determines the "real" real-ear gain (REIR), and this should be compared with the prescribed REIR to verify if the patient is receiving adequate amplification.

Probe Measures for Transcranial CROS Fittings

The authors recently developed a procedure using the REAR that may be useful for the verification of transcranial CROS fittings. Using this procedure, the probe tube from the Frye 6500 real-ear analyzer is initially placed in the ear canal of the impaired ear at a distance of approximately 4–6 mm from the tympanic membrane, and the reference microphone is disenabled. An earphone (or ER-3A insert receiver) is placed over the ear canal of the poor ear and unmasked air conduction thresholds are determined at 250–4000 Hz. Because these patients have known profound sensorineural hearing loss in the poor ear and hearing is within normal limits in the good ear, the unmasked thresholds represent the interaural attenuation (IA) for the air conducted signal. These thresholds can range between 40 and 90 dB HL depending on test frequency and intersubject variability. The SPL measurements from the probe microphone placed in the ear canal of the poor ear correspond to the individual interaural attenuation at each test frequency.

Next, the good ear is plugged and muffed while an ITE or BTE transcranial CROS hearing aid is placed in the poor ear. The volume control is adjusted to where amplification is comfortably loud while the patient listens to 70 dB SPL of speech-weighted composite noise presented by the loudspeaker from the Frye 6500. Finally, 70 dB SPL of speech-weighted composite noise is presented to the listener, and the REAR is measured to determine if it exceeds the IA previously measured in SPL in the ear canal of the aided ear. This process verifies if the amplified signal is sufficiently loud to be heard in the cochlea of the good ear via bone conduction.

Thus, when using this procedure, the "prescriptive target" for a transcranial CROS fitting is the measured SPL in the canal of the impaired ear corresponding to the IA. The goal is for the REAR to exceed that target by approximately 15–20 dB so that the amplified speech signal would be at a sensation level (re: IA threshold) sufficient enough to make the amplified signal audible in the cochlea of the good ear.

Table 11–3 provides an example of this procedure in a patient in whom a transcranial ITE hearing aid was fitted. In this case, the unmasked air conduction thresholds representing the interaural attenuation ranged from 55 to 75 dB HL (column 2, Table 11–3). With the probe microphone in the ear canal of the poor ear, the measured SPL in the ear canal ranged from 66.5 dB SPL at 1500 Hz to 89.3 dB SPL at 4000 Hz. With the transcranial ITE CROS placed in the poor ear, the REAR for 70 dB SPL of speech-weighted composite noise ranged from 63 dB SPL at 4000 Hz to 96 dB SPL at 1000 Hz. More importantly, the aided REAR was below the measured earphone SPL response at 250 and 3000–4000 Hz (−6.6, −10.3, and −26.3 dB, respectively) and above the measured ear canal SPL response at 500–2000 Hz (+5.8, 16.5, 26.9, 19.5, and 2.7 dB, respectively). The goal for such a fitting would be that the aided REAR

Table 11–3. Measures of Interaural Attenuation (IA), IA Threshold, Measured REAR for Speech, Weighted Composite Noise, and Sensation Level

Frequency (Hz)	IA Threshold (dB Hearing Level)	IA Threshold (dB Sound Pressure Level)	Measured REAR (dB Sound Pressure Level)	Sensation Level (dB)
250	60	80.6	74.0	−6.6
500	65	78.2	84.0	+5.8
750	60	69.5	86.0	+16.5
1000	60	69.1	96.0	+26.9
1500	55	66.5	86.0	+19.5
2000	60	77.3	80.0	+2.7
3000	70	87.3	77.0	−10.3
4000	75	89.3	63.0	−26.3

measures would provide approximately 15 dB sensation level or greater at 1000–4000 Hz. If this goal could be achieved without feedback or a sensation of vibration, then the audiologist could be assured that the amplified signal reached the cochlea of the good ear. Of course, these measures would be supplemented by the sound field measures described above. It would be anticipated that the SPL of the REAR for this patient may have been greater if a BTE transcranial CROS had been fitted, because the appropriate volume control setting (i.e., adjusted to MCL) could not be achieved due to feedback.

In yet another approach for using real-ear probe tube measures to verify transcranial CROS fittings, Sullivan[64] measured the occluded transcranial REIR in the *good ear*. To do this, he placed the probe tube near the tympanic membrane of the good ear, placed a cotton block lateral to the end of the probe tip, and filled the ear canal with impression material. Warble tones were presented at 0° azimuth at 0.5 meters using an input level of 60 dB SPL. Measurements were made in the occluded good ear with the transcranial CROS off (REUR) and at full-on (REAR) in the impaired ear. He reported a median occluded REIR of 9.5 dB at 1500–3000 Hz. One patient revealed an REIR peak gain in the occluded good ear of almost 25 dB in the 3000 Hz region.

Conclusion

The primary goal of this chapter was to reinforce the idea that several fitting options are available for the sensorineural unilaterally hearing impaired patient. Hopefully, the ideas contained within this chapter will instill the concept that unilaterally hearing impaired patients experience significant communication problems, and suggesting "turning your head to the desired signal" or recommending CROS amplification to the good ear should not be the *exclusive* rehabilitative options for these patients.

We have gained considerable experience with the fitting strategies outlined in this chapter and urge the readers also to consider transcranial CROS, CROS-PLUS, or bone conduction amplification for unilateral hearing impaired patients. We believe, and have demonstrated on numerous patients, that one or more of these "nontraditional" fittings may be more beneficial in many cases than "traditional" fittings.

References

1. Kielmovitch IH, Friedman WH: Unilateral sensorineural deafness in children. *Otolaryngol Head Neck Surg* 1988; 99:548–551.
2. Brookhouser PE, Worthington DW, Kelly WJ: Unilateral hearing loss in children. *Laryngoscope* 1991; 101:1264–1272.
3. Bess FH, Tharpe AM: An introduction to unilateral sensorineural hearing loss in children. *Ear Hear* 1986; 7:3–13.
4. Oyler RF, Oyler AL, Matkin ND: Unilateral hearing loss: Demographics and educational impact. *Language Speech Hear Serv Schools* 1988; 19:201–209.
5. Petheram IS: Severe haemolysis and unilateral sensorineural deafness in infectious mononucleosis. *Practioner* 1976; 217:945–948.
6. Shanon E, Redianu C, Zikk D, et al.: Sudden deafness due to infection by *Mycoplasma pneumoniae. Ann Otol Rhinol Laryngol* 1982; 91:163–165.

7. Millen SJ, Toohill RJ, Lehman RH: Sudden sensorineural hearing loss: operative complication in non-otologic surgery. *Laryngoscope* 1982; 92:613–617.
8. Plasse HM, Spencer FC, Mittleman M, Frost JO: Unilateral sudden loss of hearing, an unusual complication of cardiac operation. *Thoracic Cardiol Surg* 1980; 79:822–826.
9. Arenberg IK, Allen GW, DeBoer A: Sudden deafness immediately following cardiopulmonary bypass surgery. *J Laryngol Otol* 1972; 86:73–77.
10. Wright JW, Saunders SH: Sudden deafness following cardiopulmonary surgery. *J Laryngol Otol* 1975; 89:757–759.
11. Rambur BA: Sudden hearing loss. *Nurse Pract* 1989; 14:8, 11, 14–19.
12. Bye F: Sudden hearing loss research clinic. *Otolaryngol Clin North Am* 1978; 11:71–79.
13. Berg M, Pallasch H: Sudden deafness and vertigo in children and juveniles. *Adv Otol Rhinol Laryngol* 1981; 27:70–82.
14. Megighian D: Epidemiological considerations in sudden hearing loss. *Arch Otol Rhinol Laryngol* 1986; 243:250–253.
15. Van Dishoeck HA, Bichman TA: Sudden perceptive deafness and viral infections. *Ann Otol Rinol Laryngol* 1957; 66:263–280.
16. Bergenius J: Vestibular findings in sensorineural hearing disorders. *Acta Otolaryngol* 1985; 99:83–94.
17. Noury KA, Katsarkas A: Sudden unilateral sensorineural hearing loss: A syndrome or a symptom? *J Otolaryngol* 1989; 18:274–278.
18. Everberg G: Etiology of unilateral total deafness. *Ann Otol Rhinol Laryngol* 1960; 69:711–713.
19. Tarkkanen J, Aho J: Unilateral deafness in children. *Otolarngology* 1966; 61:270–278.
20. Kinney CE: Hearing impairment in children. *Laryngoscope* 1953; 63:220–226.
21. Tieri L, Masi R, Ducci M, Marsella P: Unilateral hearing loss in children. *Scand Audiol Suppl* 1988; 30:33–36.
22. Hallmo P, Moller P, Lind O, et al.: Unilateral sensorineural hearing loss in children less than 15 years of age. *Scand Audiol* 1986; 15:131.
23. Hendricks-Munoz KD, Walton JP: Hearing loss in persistent fetal circulation. *Pediatrics* 1988; 81:650–656.
24. Bergman I, Hirsch RP, Fria TJ, et al.: Causes of hearing loss in the high-risk premature infant. *J Pediatr* 1985; 106:95–101.
25. Slack RWT, Wright A, Michaels L, et al.: Inner hair cell loss and intracochlear clot in the preterm infant. *Clin Otolaryngol* 1986; 11:443–446.
26. Clark BR, Conry RF: Hearing impairment in children of low birth weight. *J Audiol Res* 1979; 19:277–291.
27. Pass RF, Stagno S, Myers GJ, et al.: Outcome of symptomatic congenital cytomegalovirus infection: Results of long-term longitudinal follow-up. *Pediatrics* 1980; 66:758–765.
28. Goodhill V, Harris I, Brockman S, et al.: Sudden deafness and labyrinthine window ruptures. *Ann Otol Rhinol Laryngol* 1973; 82:2–12.
29. Wilson WR, Veltri RW, Laird N, et al.: Viral and epidemiologic studies of idiopathic sudden hearing loss. *Otolaryngol Head Neck Surg* 1983; 91:653–658.
30. Schuknecht HF: Meniere's syndrome, in Britton BH (ed): *Common Problems in Otology*. St. Louis: Mosby, 1991, pp 180–185.
31. Jerger S, Jerger J: *Auditory Disorders*. Boston: Little, Brown and Co., 1981.
32. Valente M: Binaural amplification. *Audiol J Contin Ed* 1982; 7:79–93.
33. Tillman TW, Kasten RN, Horner IS: Effect of head shadow on reception of speech. *ASHA* 1963; 5:778–779.
34. Markides A: Advantages of binaural over monaural hearing, in Markides A (ed): *Binaural Hearing Aids*. London: Academic Press, 1977.
35. Hodgson WR: Special cases of hearing aid assessment, in Hodgson WR (ed): *Hearing Aid Assessment and Use in Audiologic Habilitation*, ed 3. Baltimore: Williams and Wilkins, 1986, pp 191–216.
36. Giolas TG, Wark DJ: Communication problems associated with unilateral hearing loss. *J Speech Hear Dis* 1967; 32:336–43.
37. Koenig W: Subjective effects of binaural hearing. *J Acoust Soc Am* 1950; 22:61–62.
38. Keys JW: Binaural versus monaural hearing. *J Acoust Soc Am* 1947; 19:629–631.
39. Gulick WL, Gescheider GA, Frisina RD: *Hearing*. New York: Oxford University Press, 1989, pp 226–227, 317–343.
40. Lochner JP, Burger JF: The binaural summation of speech signals. *Acoustica* 1961; 9:313–317.
41. Pollack I: Monaural and binaural threshold sensitivity for tones and white noise. *J Acoust Soc Am* 1948; 20:52–58.
42. Pollack I, Pickett JM: Stereophonic listening and speech intelligibility against voice babble. *J Acoust Soc Am* 1958; 30:131–133.

43. Reynolds GS, Stevens SS: Binaural summation of loudness. *J Acoust Soc Am* 1960; 32:1337–1343.
44. Shaw WA, Newman GB, Hirsh IJ: The difference between monaural and binaural thresholds. *J Except Psychol* 1947; 37:229–242.
45. Bocca MR: Binaural hearing: Another approach. *Laryngoscope* 1955; 45:1164–1171.
46. Breaky MR, Davis H: Comparison of thresholds for speech. *Laryngoscope* 1949; 59:236–250.
47. Bess FH, Tharpe AM: Performance and management of children with unilateral sensorineural hearing loss. *Scand Audiol Suppl* 1988; 30:75–79.
48. Bess FH, Klee T, Culbertson JL: Identification, assessment and management of children with unilateral sensorineural hearing loss. *Ear Hear* 1986; 7:43–51.
49. Culbertson JL, Gilbert JE: Children with unilateral sensorineural hearing loss: Cognitive, academic and social development. *Ear Hear* 1986; 7:38–42.
50. Bovo R, Agnoletto M, Beghi A, et al.: Auditory and academic performance of children with unilateral hearing loss. *Scand Audiol Suppl* 1988; 30:71–74.
51. Harford E, Barry J: A rehabilitative approach to the problem of unilateral hearing impairment: Contralateral routing of signals (CROS). *J Speech Hear Dis* 1965; 30:121–138.
52. Bardon JI: Unilateral sensorineural hearing loss: From the inside out. *Hear J* 1986; 37:13–17.
53. Harford E: Is a hearing aid ever justified in unilateral hearing loss? in Boles L (ed): *Hearing Loss—Problems in Diagnosis and Treatment. Otolaryngol Clin North Am* 1969, pp 153–173.
54. Pollack MC: Special applications of amplification, in Pollack MC (ed): *Amplification for the Hearing Impaired*, ed 3. New York, Grune Stratton, 1988, pp 295–328.
55. Kenworthy OT, Klee T, Tharpe AM: Speech recognition ability of children with unilateral sensorineural hearing loss as a function of amplification, speech stimuli and listening condition. *Ear Hear* 1990; 11:264–270.
56. Matkin ND, Thomas J: The utilization of CROS hearing aids by children. *Maico Audio Lib Ser* 1972; 10.
57. Courtois J, Johansen PA, Larsen BV, et al.: Hearing Aid Fitting in Asymmetrical Hearing Loss, in Jensen JH (ed): *Hearing Aid Fitting: Theoretical and Practical Views*. 13th Danavox Symposium. Copenhagen: Stougaard Jenson, 1988, pp 243–255.
58. Harford E, Dodds, E: The clinical application of CROS. *Arch Otolaryngol* 1966; 83:73–82.
59. Punch JF: CROS revisited. *ASHA* 1988; 30:35–37.
60. Harford E, Musket C: Binaural hearing with one hearing aid. *J Speech Hear Disord* 1964; 29:133–146.
61. Tharpe AM, Bess FH: Identification and management of children with minimal hearing loss. *Int J Pediatr Otorhinolaryngol* 1991; 21:41–50.
62. McSpaden JB, McSpaden CH: A method for evaluating the efficacy and effectiveness of transcranial CROS fittings. *Audecibel* 1989; 38:10–14.
63. Chartrand MS: Transcranial or internal CROS fittings: Evaluation and validation protocol. *Hear J* 1991; 44:24–28.
64. Sullivan RF: Transcranial ITE CROS. *Hear Instrum* 1988; 39:11–12, 54.
65. McSpaden JB: One approach to a unilateral "dead" ear. *Audecibel* 1990; 39:32–34.
66. Miller AL: An alternative approach to CROS and Bi-CROS hearing aids: An internal CROS. *Audecibel* 1989; 39:20–21.
67. Hable LA, Brown KM, Gudmundsen GI: CROS-PLUS: A physical CROS system. *Hear Instrum* 1990; 41:27–30, 68.
68. Fowler EP; Bilateral hearing aids for monaural total deafness. *Arch Otolaryngol* 1960; 72:57–58.
69. Skinner MW: *Hearing Aid Evaluation*. Englewood Cliffs, NJ: Prentice Hall, 1988, pp 212–219.
70. Raffin MJM, Thornton AR: Confidence levels for differences between speech discrimination scores: A research tool. *J Speech Hear Res* 1980; 23:5–18.
71. Tecca J: Clinical application of real ear probe tube measurements, in Sandlin RE (ed): *Handbook of Hearing Aid Amplification*, vol II. Boston: College-Hill Press, 1990, pp 225–256.
72. Valente M (ed): Real ear measurements in hearing aid fittings. *Semin Hear* 1991; 12.
73. Byrne D, Dillon H: The National Acoustic Laboratories (NAL) new procedure for selecting the gain and frequency response of a hearing aid. *Ear Hear* 1986; 7:257–265.

12

Fitting Strategies for Patients With Conductive Hearing Loss

George A. Gates, Michael Valente

Introduction

Surgical correction of conductive hearing loss (CHL) is the principal and pre-ferred treatment by most patients. Surgical therapy is successful in the majority of cases, but not all patients are candidates for surgery because of medical, anatomic, or personal reasons. Although most who undergo an otologic opera-tion achieve socially adequate hearing (i.e., speech reception threshold [SRT] of 25 dB hearing level [HL] or less), some do not, and these patients can generally obtain additional benefit from amplification. In cases of CHL in the only hearing ear, the surgeon recommends amplification to avoid the risk of surgical complications that might increase the hearing loss, provided, of course, that the CHL is not the result of a progressive disorder, such as a cholesteatoma. Thus, amplification for CHL remains a topic of great interest to audiologists, otologists, and patients alike.

This chapter will discuss the types of CHL for which amplification is the primary treatment method, those for which amplification is fitted secondarily following recovery from surgery, and those for which combined surgical–audiologic treatment (i.e., implantable hearing device) is warranted. Bone conduction aids were once the mainstay of amplification technology for CHL. However, these devices may be superseded by newer technology. The use of conventional or programmable air conduction aids and the implantable electromagnetic bone conductor are emphasized in this chapter.

Background

CHL results from abnormalities in the structure of function of the sound conduction mechanism, which includes the external auditory canal, tympanic

249

membrane, ossicular chain, and middle ear space. In general terms, these abnormalities consist of mass lesions, which impede normal vibratory excursions by occluding the air-filled spaces, and structural abnormalities in which part or all of the substance of the conductive mechanism is absent or nonfunctional.

Mass Lesions

Any abnormality that occludes the normally air-filled spaces of the external auditory canal (EAC) or middle ear will decrease hearing sensitivity by impeding the normal transmission of vibratory energy to the inner ear. The magnitude of the loss is generally proportional to the degree of abnormality. In some cases the hearing loss is gradual in onset, while in others it may occur suddenly.

Cerumen Impaction

Cerumen often accumulates in the external ear canal. Outward growth of the skin of the canal normally carries the wax to the outside. This normal cleaning mechanism is thwarted by self-attempts to clean the ear with cotton swabs or other devices or by insertion of a hearing aid. Wax does not cause hearing loss until the canal is totally occluded. Sudden swelling of retained wax due to absorption of moisture is the most common precipitating event in adults. External otitis from excess moisture may produce swelling of the canal sufficient to block hearing, as well as to cause pain and discharge.

Otitis Media

Otitis media with effusion (OME) is the most common cause of hearing loss in children. The magnitude of the CHL depends more on the volume of effusion than on its consistency. The pure-tone average threshold ([PTA], average of 0.5, 1, 2 kHz) is slightly less than 30 dB, but there is considerable fluctuation in hearing. The variability in hearing level creates problems for the children in compensating for the decreased hearing. While there is considerable controversy about whether fluctuating CHL due to OME in childhood affects development, there is substantial evidence to suggest that OME does impose a risk of developmental delay. For example, Klein et al.[1] showed a modest but statistically significant retardation of language and intellectual development in children severely affected with OME.

Medical and surgical treatments of OME are generally satisfactory in restoring hearing, although a small number of children have such an intractable condition that amplification should be considered. The principal surgical treatment for OME in children is tympanostomy tube insertion. The tube keeps the middle ear ventilated and corrects the chronic negative middle ear pressure that is an important factor in the pathogenesis of OME and cholesteatoma. Adenoidectomy is also used in older children, and the reduction in subsequent OME appears to be the result of eliminating the source of infection rather than changing eustachian tube function per se.[2]

Otosclerosis

The most common cause of CHL in adults with a normal tympanic membrane is otosclerosis. New bone forms across the stapediovestibular joint, usually at its anterior edge, and limits the excursion of the stapes and thus attenuates the sound energy reaching the cochlear fluids. Because the stiffness of the ossicular chain is increased, there is often greater hearing loss in the low frequencies. The stapedius reflex is usually absent but in early cases it may be elicited; however, the on-effect is reversed in direction when the anterior footplate is the locus of the otosclerosis. In this case, the stapedius muscle contraction pulls the stapes inward (toward the vestibule) rather than outward (toward the tympanic membrane).

The results of stapes surgery are excellent: Over 90% of patients achieve socially adequate hearing. Nonetheless, there is a small risk (<1%) of hearing loss from stapes surgery, which may be total, and thus many patients choose amplification as the primary treatment. Amplification is presented as a treatment option by otologic surgeons because it is free of risk and the results are excellent. Otosclerosis may invade the otic capsule and produce a sensorineural loss secondary to distortion of the cochlea or from liberation of toxic materials into the perilymph. In far advanced cases, even when air conduction thresholds exceed the limit of the audiometer, stapes surgery may improve hearing to a level at which normal communication with amplification is possible. These are among the most grateful patients we see.

Stapes surgery may be considered in two general classes: total stapedectomy and partial stapedectomy (stapedotomy). Total removal of the stapes with insertion of a tissue seal of the oval window and reconstruction of the ossicular chain with a suitable prosthesis is the classic, time-honored procedure. Over the past decade many surgeons have turned to the small-fenestra stapedotomy procedure to minimize surgical trauma and preserve high frequency hearing. A stapedotomy is a circular opening created in the footplate with either the laser or specially designed instruments. Reconstruction is done with a small piston that fills the opening on one end and is crimped around the incus on the other end. Stapedotomy patients experience less vertigo and better high frequency thresholds postoperatively.[3] However, the differences between the two techniques in experienced hands are slight. Long-term results with either technique are well maintained.

Cholesteatoma

Cholesteatoma is a common mass lesion that affects hearing due to its effect on sound transfer and, in some cases, to disruption of the structures of the middle ear. Cholesteatoma results from ingrowth of squamous epithelium from the tympanic membrane retraction secondary to long-standing negative middle ear pressure or through an existing perforation. In either case, the cholesteatoma expands slowly over years to destroy the structures of the middle ear. Cholesteatoma appears to be less common in the United States, since pressure equalizing tubes have been used for over 40 years. Secondary infection is common in cholesteatoma. Early recognition of this disorder is vital to prevent further damage, and all professionals who care for patients with hearing loss should be alert to the possibility and ensure that patients with CHL receive expert evaluation by an otologist. Amplification is not an option until the cholesteatoma is removed or controlled.

Structural Pathology

Loss of structural integrity of the tympanic membrane or ossicular chain results in CHL, the degree of which varies with the type and extent of the defect. Small perforations of the tympanic membrane have little effect on pure-tone thresholds, while large perforations may produce up to a 30 dB hearing loss. The location of the perforation also influences the amount of hearing loss: Those in the center of the tympanic membrane cause more loss than those in the periphery. Ossicular discontinuity is most often the result of necrosis of the long process of the incus. Even a minuscule separation of the incus from the stapes results in a maximum conductive loss (60 dB air–bone gap) if the tympanic membrane is intact. Often, ossicular disruption and tympanic membrane perforation coexist with a hearing loss that is moderate (i.e., 45–55 dB HL).

The principal cause of these disorders is chronic infection, for which the generic term of *chronic suppruative otitis media* (CSOM) applies. CSOM may be inactive, in which case there is a tympanic membrane perforation and normal middle ear mucosa. In other cases the infection is recurrent, and the patient experiences intermittent aural discharge that would preclude the wearing of an air conduction hearing aid. Surgery is designed to eliminate any focus of infection in the middle ear and mastoid and to repair the structural defect. Serviceable hearing is restored in 75% of cases, and resolution of infection is achieved in over 90% of cases.[4] For those in whom scar tissue formation or other problem result in a permanent conductive loss, amplification is made possible through the control of infection and maintenance of a fittable ear canal.

Congenital Anomalies

Congenital absence or malformation of the conductive mechanism is uncommon. If the external auditory canal is open and of sufficient size, an air conduction aid may be fitted. In many cases, however, there is atresia of the ear canal and only a bone conduction aid or the implantable bone conductor will suffice. Reconstruction of congenital atresia cases is possible when there is sufficient development of the middle ear space and the facial nerve does not overlie the oval window. However, such reconstruction is difficult and technically complicated, and, although good results are obtainable in selected cases in expert hands,[5] amplification is necessary in many cases, even after reconstruction.

Neoplasm

The least common and most difficult hearing problem to correct follows the removal of neoplasms of the ear. In these instances much, if not all, of the external auditory canal and middle ear structures are removed, and conventional amplification is not possible. Fortunately, the implantable bone conductor offers an effective option, even when removal of the mastoid bone precludes a bone conduction amplifier.

Strategies for Amplification

From the foregoing it is clear that amplification plays an important role in rehabilitating many patients with CHL. Amplification is the primary treatment in certain disorders. In others it is reserved for secondary use depending on the results of surgery. In still other cases amplification and surgery are integrated into a unified treatment plan.

Primary

In certain cases amplification is the only treatment option. These include inoperable congenital atresia (type III), unilateral CHL with an anacusic contralateral ear, and patient's preference. For atresia, either a bone conduction aid or the implantable bone conductor (Audiant) may be used. The decision concerning surgery is based on the patient's age, degree of atresia (computed tomographic scans are essential), and preference.

Secondary

Air conduction aids are useful in patients who have less than optimal hearing following surgery and for whom further surgery is not an option. In the latter category are included cases of otosclerosis with an overhanging facial nerve, massively obliterative otosclerosis, or middle ear fibrosis. These patients often achieve excellent hearing with an air conduction aid.

Amplification is also a secondary treatment option for patients with surgically uncorrectable CHL who are unable to wear an air conduction aid. In this category are patients with a radical mastoidectomy with large meatoplasty or those with unrelenting otorrhea who are not candidates for surgical therapy for medical or social reasons. For these a conventional bone conduction aid or the implantable bone conductor is an appropriate option.

Amplification should be considered an option for older children with intractable OME. Although the number of children who fail medical and surgical therapy is small and the problems associated with use of an aid in patients with a fluctuating hearing loss are well known, there are cases in which OME has resulted in irreversible structural changes or intractable effusion for whom amplification and assistive listening devices are of benefit, particularly in the school setting.

Combined

Combined otologic–audiologic treatment should be considered for a number of clinical problems of CHL. These include advanced otosclerosis and advanced chronic suppurative otitis media.

Patients with far-advanced otosclerosis generally have both stapedial and cochlear otosclerosis. For these patients both stapedectomy and amplification are required. Even with complete closure of the air–bone gap, the elevated bone thresholds would not result in socially adequate hearing. Amplification alone is insufficient because of the limitations of output of even a body aid. The diagnosis of these cases is outside the scope of this discussion, but many patients have pure-tone thresholds above the limit of the audiometer. Stapedectomy followed by fitting of a power air-conduction hearing aid has been very successful in rehabilitating these profoundly impaired patients.

In some cases of advanced CSOM, reconstruction of the middle ear structures is not possible, and control of infection is the chief goal. The classic approach to this problem is to perform a radical mastoidectomy with a large meatoplasty. This is a satisfactory solution for most cases. However, when the mastoid is large and care of the cavity is a problem, an obliteration procedure may be warranted. Depending on the status of the eustachian tube, the mastoid and middle ear cavities are completely stripped of epithelial remnants and obliterated with abdominal fat. Then the ear canal is surgically closed, and the bone conductor is implanted. These patients are then freed of restrictions regarding swimming and diving and do not require once- or twice-yearly cavity cleaning, as do most patients. If the eustachian tube is patent, the above procedure can be modified by the use of musculoplastic techniques, and an air conduction aid may be fitted after healing is complete.

Surgery to Provide Amplification

Surgery for providing amplification is an emerging area of interest. Surgical modification of the external auditory canal for congenital or acquired atresia is a standard procedure. Devices under development include those that fit entirely in the external auditory canal and are coupled electromagnetically to the tympanic membrane or ossicular chain or can be surgically implanted within the temporal bone. Suffice it to say that these devices are in development, and it is likely that many will become available within this decade. For the moment, however, the implantable bone conductor is the only device for correction of CHL that is approved for use in the United States.

Implantable Bone Conductor (Audiant)

Patients eligible for the implantable bone conductor are those with (1) atresia not amenable to surgical reconstruction, (2) persistent otorrhea due to chronic suppurative otitis media resistant to medical and surgical therapy, (3) uncorrectable ossicular abnormalities, or (4) intolerance or allergy to earmolds. The audiologic criteria for the Audiant are listed in the next section. Suitable candidates meeting the medical and audiologic criteria should have realistic motivation and understanding of the benefits and limitations of the device. Contraindications include (1) the absence of suitable bone in which to place the device and lack of adequate skin cover, (2) active infection in the implantation site, and (3) systemic disease that might affect wound healing.

Advantages of the Audiant over a bone conduction hearing aid include the absence of pressure on the skin from the headband, elimination of feedback, reduced distortion, and improved high frequency hearing through more direct bone conduction.[6] Another advantage is stable bone vibrator placement through surgical implantation rather than external placement of the bone vibrator on the skin over the mastoid, which is subject to movement.

Surgical Considerations

The bone conductor may be implanted using local anesthesia on an outpatient basis.[7] A skin flap is elevated and thinned to the appropriate thickness as necessary. A suitable location on the skull above and behind the pinna is chosen, and small guide holes are made with a drill. A larger center hole is drilled, enlarged, and tapped using a mechanical system designed for this purpose that is stabilized by the guide holes. The internal device is a titanium-aluminum-vanadium cup-and-bone screw on which is mounted a rare earth permanent magnet encased in an inert polymer. The bone screw becomes osseo-integrated over several weeks and becomes rigidly coupled with the skull. The external processor is fitted 8–10 weeks postoperatively. The processor transforms vibrational energy into an electromagnetic field that passes through the skin, causing the magnet, skull, and cochlea to vibrate. Because of the rigid coupling, the sound transfer is excellent, especially at the higher frequencies, where speech understanding occurs.

Postoperative Care

Postoperative care is minimal. In the immediate postoperative period, antibiotic ointment and dressing changes are done. Once the sutures are removed and wound healing is complete, no continuing attention is necessary. Patients are advised to examine the area periodically for evidence of irritation. Routine assessment after healing is complete is unnecessary.

Complications from the Audiant have been few.[8] The chief early problem—skin loss and exposure of implant—was uncommon and is largely avoidable by proper planning of the skin flap. The implant should be placed where irritation from glasses or head gear is not a problem. Because of the small size of the implant, this is unusual.[8]

Hearing Aid Selection and Fitting

Options for selecting and fitting hearing aids for conductive or mixed hearing loss can generally be divided into three categories. As illustrated in Figure 12–1, patients can be fitted with *air conduction* in-the-canal (ITC, left), in-the-ear (ITE, center) or behind-the-ear (BTE, right) hearing aids. In addition, patients can be fit with eyeglass or body hearing aids. Second, patients can be fitted with *bone conduction* hearing aid(s). Finally, patients can receive an *implanted bone conduction* hearing device.

Air Conduction Hearing Aids

Determining which air conduction hearing aid is most appropriate is usually based on (1) the magnitude of hearing loss, (2) the magnitude of the air–bone

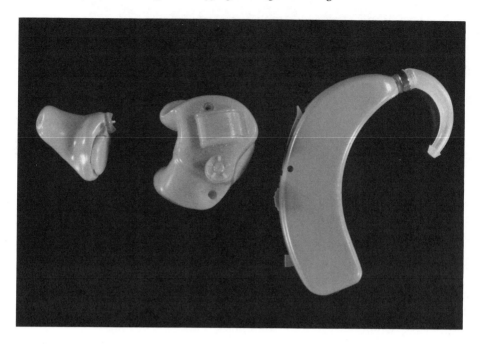

Figure 12–1. Examples of three air conduction hearing aids. To the left is an ITC hearing aid. In the middle is an ITE hearing aid. To the right is a BTE hearing aid.

gap, and (3) patient preference. As a general rule, as the hearing loss and magnitude of the air–bone gap increases, the need to fit a BTE or body hearing aid increases. Finally, air conduction hearing aids should be considered the most appropriate fitting for chronic conductive hearing loss when medical contraindications have been ruled out.

Fitting Strategies for Air Conduction Hearing Aids

Regardless of the type of air conduction hearing aid, the appropriate real-ear gain for patients with conductive or mixed hearing loss can be determined by using many of the prescriptive procedures reported in Chapters 1 and 2. That is, prescribed real-ear gain for hearing aids providing linear amplification is based on the air conduction threshold with additional gain prescribed to compensate for the magnitude of the air–bone gap. Lybarger,[9,10] Byrne,[11] and Byrne and Dillon[12] recommend that 25% of the air–bone gap should be added to the amplification requirements for patients with sensorineural hearing loss. On the other hand, Berger et al.[13] recommend that 20% of the air–bone gap should be added with the maximum additional gain limited to 8 dB at any frequency.

Other than those of Berger et al.[13] and Bryne and Dillon,[12] no prescriptive formulae described in Chapters 1 and 2 specify guidelines for providing additional gain to compensate for the air–bone gap. The authors feel that audiologists should always consider adding between 20% and 25% of the air–bone gap to the prescribed gain even if the selected prescriptive procedure[14-17] does not specifically provide such guidelines. For example, if a patient has a 65 dB sensorineural hearing loss at 2000 Hz, the NAL-R procedure advocated by Byrne and Dillon[12] prescribes 26 dB of real-ear gain. If the patient had a mixed hearing loss at 2000 Hz with an air–bone gap of 45 dB, the prescribed gain would be increased to 37 dB (i.e., 26 dB for the 65 dB sensorineural hearing loss and 11 dB to compensate for 25% of the 45 dB air–bone gap). However, if the audiologist were fitting to the Berger et al.[13] formula, the recommended gain would be 50 dB (i.e., 42 dB for the 65 dB sensorineural loss and 9 dB to compensate for 20% of the 45 dB air–bone gap with a maximum of 8 dB).

Verification Strategies for Air Conduction Hearing Aids

The verification process for air conduction hearing aids can either be real-ear gain using probe tube or functional gain measures (see Ch. 5), paired comparisons (see Ch. 6), and/or subjective evaluations (see Ch. 7).

Bone-Conduction Hearing Aid

Bone conduction hearing aids are available in BTE and in eyeglass (Fig. 12–2) and body (Fig. 12–3) configurations. Bone conduction aids are the most appropriate hearing aid fitting when it is physically impossible to use air conduction hearing aids. Examples of such circumstances may be atresia, severe stenosis of the ear canal, chronic middle ear drainage, or an allergic reaction to

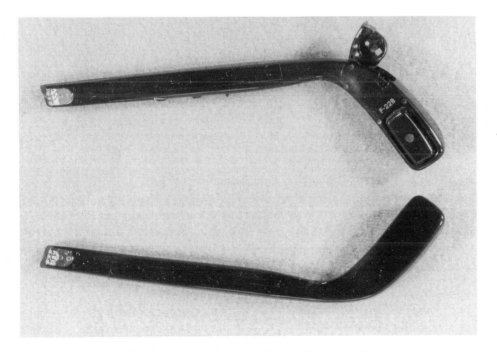

Figure 12–2. Example of a eyeglass bone conduction hearing aid.

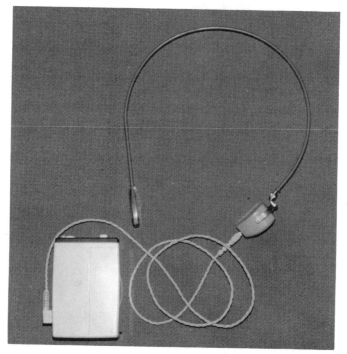

Figure 12–3.   Example of a bone conduction vibrator attached to a headband and body hearing aid.

the materials used to manufacture earmolds. In addition, it is important that bone conduction thresholds are within normal limits or only slightly impaired in order to achieve success with this type of amplification. Finally, *it is important to remember that conventional bone conduction hearing aids should be evaluated and fitted on at least a trial basis prior to fitting an implantable bone conduction hearing device.*

Bone conduction hearing aids deliver the amplified sound to a bone vibrator that is placed over the mastoid process. The vibrator is held in place by a headband or eyeglass frame. The most frequently used bone conduction hearing aids are eyeglass and body designs. The eyeglass arrangement is typically preferred for cosmetic reasons and should be initially recommended even if the patient has normal vision and will use non-prescription lenses. The use of bone conduction hearing aids is limited due to (1) minimal available gain at 3000–4000 Hz and (2) difficulties involved in achieving the precise placement and tension of the vibrator on the mastoid process. In addition, many patients using bone conduction hearing aids complain of headaches and soreness around the mastoid process due to the pressure of the bone vibrator on the mastoid process. Despite these "drawbacks," successful bone conduction fittings have been achieved by the authors because of our access to optometrists and opticians who have experience in the proper placement of the bone vibrator.

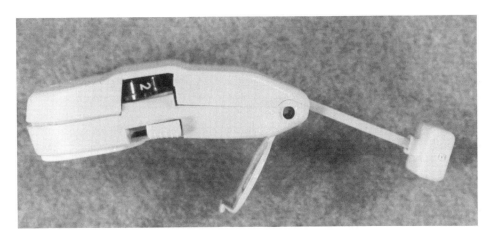

Figure 12–4. Audiant ATE implantable bone conductor hearing device.

FITTING STRATEGIES

Lybarger[9,10] provides guidelines that suggest that if the air–bone gap is <25 dB then a conventional air conduction hearing aid is the appropriate fitting. If the air–bone gap is between 25 and 40 dB, then either an air conduction or bone conduction fitting may be appropriate. Finally, if the air–bone gap is >40 dB, then a bone conduction fitting may be the most appropriate. However, to the authors' knowledge, Lybarger's recommendations have never been evaluated clinically, and the guidelines do not consider cases in which air–bone gap may be different at different frequencies within the *same ear*. In view of recent advances in earmold and hearing aid technology (improved isolation between transducers within the hearing aid case, for example), it is now possible to achieve greater gain without feedback. The dispenser is urged to view these previous guidelines with some skepticism and to evaluate, at least on a trial basis, air conduction hearing aids for patients in whom air–bone gaps exceed 40 dB.

As with air conduction hearing aids, the primary strategy for bone conduction hearing aids in cases of conductive hearing loss is to reduce or eliminate the air–bone gap. Again, the most appropriate fitting strategy is to determine the prescribed real-ear gain using many of the prescriptive procedures outlined in Chapters 1 and 2 with additional gain to compensate for the air–bone gap. Finally, like conventional air conduction hearing aids, bone conduction hearing aids should be fit bilaterally when appropriate.

VERIFICATION STRATEGIES

The verification process for bone conduction fittings is primarily limited to measures of functional gain (see Ch. 5). Recently, paired comparisons (see Ch. 6) and subjective evaluations (see Ch. 7) have become increasingly popular to verify the fitting of hearing aids for patients wtih sensorineural hearing loss.

The use of paired comparisons and subjective evaluations could be extended to fittings for patients with conductive or mixed hearing loss. Real-ear probe tube measures are not commonly used as a means to verify bone conduction fittings. However, Wade et al.[18] described a procedure in which the sound pressure level for both the unaided and aided thresholds can be measured with the probe tube from the real-ear analyzer placed at the position of the microphone of the Audiant bone conductor, with the patient absent, to determine more objectively the gain provided by this device. This procedure may be applied to measuring the real-ear gain of bone conduction hearing aids by placing the probe tube at the position of the microphone of the bone conduction hearing aid.

In 1986 the Food and Drug Administration (FDA) approved the Xomed Audiant implanted bone conductor for patients who are 3 years of age or older who cannot wear conventional air conduction hearing aids and who have a conductive hearing loss with normal cochlear reserve in at least one ear. This device consists of an external sound processor containing a microphone, an amplifier with input compression, adjustable tone control, volume control, and power source. The external sound processor is currently housed in at-the-ear (ATE), BTE, and body-type configurations.

The components within the processor convert the acoustic energy arriving at the microphone of the processor into electromagnetic vibrations. These vibrations are transmitted transcutaneously to an implanted rare earth magnet housed in a subcutaneously implanted hermetically sealed titanium alloy case. Recently, Xomed introduced the XA-II magnet, which has a broader surface area than the original magnet. This new magnet reportedly provides three times greater magnet strength and therefore greater gain. Wade et al.[18] reported equal performance between the body and ATE processors using the XA-II magnet in one patient having normal bone conduction sensitivity. However, a second patient, having a slight decrease in high frequency bone conduction sensitivity, reported dissatisfaction with the gain provided by the ATE processor coupled to the XA-II magnet.

The sealed internal magnet is coupled to a 3–4 mm titanium alloy cortical bone screw implanted in the lateral table of the skull. The internal magnet vibrates in unison with the audio signal and mechanically transmits this vibration to the skull. The vibration of the skull in turn stimulates the cochlea, causing the perception of sound. Currently, the 3 mm screw is typically used for patients between 3 and 7 years of age, while the 4 mm screw is used in patients over 7 years of age.

Audiant Bone Conductor

The Audiant is available in ATE (Fig. 12–4), BTE (Fig. 12–5), and in body-type configurations (Fig. 12–6). The body and BTE design include magnets that can be adjusted, via a turnscrew, in coil strength to ensure the proper placement of the coil to the implanted magnet at the time of the fitting. On the other hand, the ATE requires the selection of one of five available magnetic coil strengths that must be selected and ordered prior to the actual fitting.

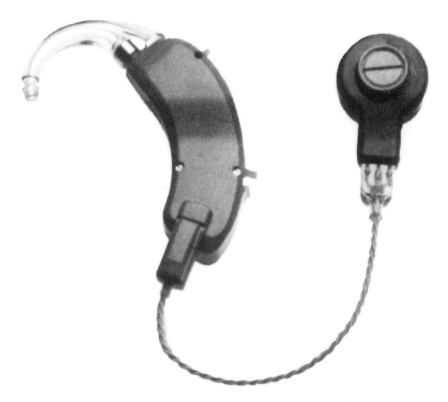

Figure 12–5. Audiant BTE implantable bone conductor hearing device.

The ATE is the smallest processor and is worn at ear level. It has a microphone arm that slides in and out approximately 1⅛″ of the ATE assembly for proper adjustment to the top of the pinna. The ATE processor contains several potentiometers for adjusting the low frequency gain and output.

The recently introduced BTE processor is a conventional BTE with a detachable adjustable magnetic coil and cord. It contains a two position "sensitivity" switch that determines the amount of gain required to provide maximum output. The BTE version also contains a three position (*t*reble, *b*ass, *n*ormal) low frequency tone control. The T position provides the greatest amount of low frequency attenuation, while the B position provides the greatest amount of low frequency amplification.

The body-type processor originally had the microphone placed on top of the processor case. Now the body processor can be purchased with a remote microphone. This remote microphone can be placed at ear level via a moveable wire hook to fit over the pinna or be placed on the shirt or hair via an alligator clip.

AUDIOLOGIC CRITERIA

Patients for whom *no bettter alternative treatment exists* may be considered candidates for this technology if the aided ear:

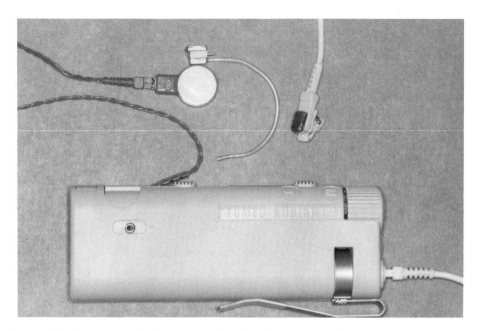

Figure 12–6. Audiant body processor implantable bone conductor hearing device.

1. Has a bone conduction PTA (500–1000–2000 Hz) no greater than 25 dB HL and no single frequency greater than 40 dB HL
2. Has an air conduction PTA (500–1000–2000 Hz) and speech reception threshold of 40 dB HL or poorer
3. Has an air conduction word recognition score in quiet (at 30 dB SL or at a most comfortable loudness level) between 80% and 100%
4. Is free from a generalized disease process that could result in poor wound healing
5. Is unwilling or unable to be a candidate for reconstructive surgery
6. Is unable or unwilling to use conventional air or bone conduction hearing aids
7. Is strongly motivated toward this surgical procedure
8. Is able to understand the objectives and expectations of this method of amplification
9. Is psycho-emotionally stable.

Examples of pathologies or conditions that may lend itself to the Audiant include

1. Congenital or acquired atresia of external canal or middle ear that is not amenable to surgical reconstruction[19]
2. Stenosis of the ear canal

3. Chronic suppurative otitis media that is resistant to medical–surgical therapy
4. Complications from radical mastoidectomies
5. Congenital or acquired ossicular malformations
6. Severe tympanosclerosis
7. Post operative mastoid cavity with chronic otorrhea
8. History of intolerance or allergy to ear molds.

ADVANTAGES

Advantages of the Audiant over conventional bone conduction amplification may include (1) absence of a headband and the associated sensation of pressure, (2) elimination of feedback, (3) reduced distortion, (4) improved high frequency amplification through more direct bone conduction,[6] and (5) stable bone vibrator placement through surgical implantation rather than external placement of the bone vibrator on the mastoid process and the resulting movement of the bone vibrator.

ATE VERSUS BODY PROCESSOR

Several reports have recently been published pertaining to the gain provided by the ATE and body processors. Scientific evaluation of the BTE processor is not available, because it was only recently introduced. Wade et al.[21] reported that 10–15 dB less overall gain was provided by the ATE when compared with the body processor. Due to the reduced gain provided by the ATE, Wade et al.,[21] as well as Browning,[22] recommend the ATE if the bone conduction thresholds are 15 dB HL or better and the body processor if bone conduction thresholds are poorer than 15 dB HL. Moreover, Wade et al.[21] suggested altering

Table 12–1. Mean warble tone thresholds (dB HL), spondee thresholds (ST, dB HL) and word recognition scores (WRS, %) for ten patients with conductive hearing loss with no device, the Audiant Body and ATE Processors, and the Oticon P11P Bone Conduction Hearing Aid*

Frequency (Hz)	No Device	BC Thresholds	Body Processor	ATE Processor	Oticon P11P
250	56.5	11.0	31.6	40.9	29.5
500	52.5	9.5	16.8	26.8	12.5
1000	58.5	12.5	17.5	25.5	18.5
2000	52.5	15.0	17.7	27.7	19.5
3000	58.0	20.0	19.8	33.8	27.5
4000	64.0	24.0	28.0	36.8	32.0
6000	68.5	DNT	36.4	39.4	41.5
8000	62.5	DNT	32.6	36.5	39.5
ST	56.0	DNT	19.4	29.3	17.5
WRS	DNT	DNT	93.4	87.7	93.6

* DNT, Did Not Test

(Data are from Johnson et al.[6])

the criteria of patient selection so that the bone conduction threshold is <25 dB HL at any frequency and not 40 dB HL at any single frequency as originally suggested by the manufacturer. Browning[22] went further to suggest that candidates for the body processor should have bone conduction thresholds between 5 to 49 dB HL at 250–4000 Hz, whereas candidates for the ATE processor should have bone conduction thresholds between −5 and 33 dB HL at the same frequencies. The findings of Wade et al.[21] and Browning [22] supported the findings of Johnson et al.,[6] who reported that a 3–20 dB greater gain was provided by the body processor for improving warble tone thresholds at 250–8000 Hz compared with the ATE processor (see Table 12–1). The results of these studies reveal that, while the Audiant body processor does provide substantial gain for the body processor (equal to or better than a conventional bone conduction hearing aid), the same benefit should not be expected when fitting the ATE processor. It should be noted that the results of these studies are in some disagreement with the findings reported Gates et al.,[8] who reported an average difference in gain of 5.1 dB between the two processor designs.

FITTING STRATEGY

If the results of the audiometric examination establish that a patient meets the selection criteria described above, then the patient would be counseled on the Audiant and referred to the otolaryngologist. Assuming that *all* criteria have been met, the audiologist and otolaryngologist would determine the processor (ATE, BTE, body) that appears to be the most appropriate. As discussed earlier, this decision would depend primarily on the bone conduction thresholds. Additional information may include onset of the hearing loss (i.e., congenital vs. acquired) and prior experience with amplification. Browning[22] reported greater patient acceptance (100%) of the Audiant if the patient had prior experience with a conventional bone conduction hearing aid, but less acceptance (36%) if the patient had prior experience with a conventional air conduction hearing aid. Wade et al.[21] reported greater success with the Audiant if a patient had congenital hearing loss with no prior experience with amplification than with patients who had acquired hearing loss and had prior experience with conventional hearing aids. Rejection of the Audiant by the latter group tended to be related to the perception of minimal gain when compared with their previous aided experiences.

At approximately 8–10 weeks after the implant, the audiologist would place the patient in a sound field at 1 m facing a loudspeaker at 0° azimuth. Measures would include

1. Unaided spondee and warble tone thresholds at 250–8000 Hz with the contralateral ear muffed or masking noise introduced in cases of unilateral hearing loss
2. Unaided word recognition score at 50 dB HL (70 dB SPL)
3. Aided warble tone (250–6000 Hz) and spondee thresholds
4. Aided word recognition scores at 50 dB HL (70 dB SPL).

VERIFICATION STRATEGY

Expected performance with the Audiant is improving the aided air conduction thresholds to within 10 dB of the bone conduction thresholds at 500–4000 Hz with the body processor[20] and within 13 dB for the ATE.[6] At 250 Hz, Johnson et al.[6] reported that the aided threshold should be within 21 dB of the bone threshold for the body processor and within 30 dB for the ATE processor. At 500 Hz, the aided threshold should be within 17 dB of the bone conduction threshold for the ATE processor. Additional improvements may be found in fidelity and in reduced feedback relative to the performance of a conventional bone conduction hearing aid. Wade et al.[18] reported that the ATE would require 10–15 dB greater gain at 4000 Hz in comparison to the performance of the body processor. Browning[22] reported that the body processor provided 8 dB greater overall gain than the ATE processor. Gates et al.[8] reported that the mean aided thresholds for the Audiant were within ±5 dB of the bone thresholds at 1000–4000 Hz and that the performance between the ATE and body processors were similar.

In a recent study, Wade et al.[18] evaluated the Nobel-Pharma percutaneous device available in Europe (N = 17) with the Audiant (N = 24). They reported that the percutaneous device provided 5–12dB greater gain at 250–4000 Hz. However, neither device successfully closed the air–bone gap at 250–500 Hz or 4000 Hz, whereas both were more effective in closing the air–bone gap at 2000–3000 Hz. Overall, the percutaneous device was more effective in providing greater gain than the Audiant at all test frequencies, but patients preferred the Audiant for cosmetic reasons if they had normal bone conduction thresholds.

While some studies[6,8,19,20] report positive results with the Audiant, several recent studies suggest that the anticipated performance of the Audiant may be limited. For example, Wade et al.[18] reported that only 29% of their patients used the Audiant regularly, whereas 42% used it occasionally and 21% do not use it at all. In addition, they reported that the Audiant would have to provide 45, 19, and 25 dB additional gains at 250–500, 1000–2000, and 4000 Hz, respectively, to close the air–bone gap. Browning[22] reported 39% of 18 patients did not use their Audiant and preferred to use their regular air conduction hearing aid. Roush and Rauch[23] reported that two of their four patients preferred to use their regular air conduction hearing aid, while the remaining two subjects enjoyed the benefit provided by the Audiant.

Summary

Surgical correction of most conditions causing conductive hearing loss provides satisfactory results. Amplification plays an important role in cases in which the postoperative hearing level is suboptimal and in cases in which surgery is not possible or appropriate. The various otologic conditions causing conductive hearing loss were reviewed, and the interaction of surgery and amplification were discussed.

Depending on the circumstances, air conduction aids, or the new Audiant bone conductor may be used. The indications, contraindications, and criteria for use were discussed.

References

1. Klein JO, Teel DW, Mannox R, et al.: Otitis media with effusion during the first three years of life and development of speech and language, in Lim DL, Bluestone CD, Klein JO, et al. (eds): *Recent Advances in Otitis Media With Effusion*. Philadelphia: BC Decker Inc, 1983, pp 332–334.
2. Gates GA, Avery CA, Cooper JC Jr, et al.: Effectiveness of adenoidectomy and tympanostomy tubes in the treatment of chronic otitis media with effusion. *N Engl J Med* 1987; 317:1444–1451.
3. McGee TM: Comparison of small fenestra and total stapedectomy. *Ann Otol Rhinol Laryngol* 1981; 90:633–636.
4. Glasscock ME: Tympanic membrane grafting. *Laryngoscope* 1973; 83:754.
5. Jahrsdoerfer RA: Surgical correction of congenital malformations of the sound-conducting mechanism, in Glasscock ME, Shambaugh GE Jr (eds): *Surgery of the Ear*. Philadelphia: WB Saunders, 1990.
6. Johnson R, Meikle M, Vernon J, et al.: An implantable bone-conduction hearing device. *Am J Otol* 1988; 9:93–100.
7. Hough J, Vernon J, Johnson B, et al.: Experiences with implantable hearing devices and a presentation of a new device. *Ann Otol Rhinol Laryngol* 1986; 95:60–65.
8. Gates GA, Hough JV, Gatti WM, et al.: The safety and effectiveness of an implanted electro-magnetic hearing device. *Arch Otolaryngol Head Neck Surg* 1989; 115:924–930.
9. Lybarger SF: *Basic Manual for Fitting Radioear Hearing Aids*. Pittsburg, PA: Radioear Corp, 1955.
10. Lybarger SF: *Simplified Fitting System for Hearing Aids*. Canonsburg, PA: Radioear Corp, 1963.
11. Byrne D: Theoretical prescriptive approaches to selecting the gain and frequency response of a hearing aid. *Monogr Contemp Audiol* 1983; 4:1–40.
12. Byrne D, Dillon H: The National Acoustics Laboratory (NAL) new procedure for selecting the gain and frequency response of a hearing aid. *Ear Hear* 1986; 7:257–265.
13. Berger K, Hagberg WN, Rane RL: *Prescription of Hearing Aids: Rationale, Procedures, and Results*, ed 4. Kent, OH: Herald Press, 1984.
14. McCandless GA, Lyregaard PE: Prescription of gain/output (POGO) for hearing aids. *Hear Instrum* 1983; 34:16–20.
15. Libby ER: The 1/3–2/3 insertion gain hearing aid selection guide. *Hear Instrum* 1986; 37:27–28.
16. Cox R: Using ULCL measures to find frequenc/gain and SSPL90. *Hear Instrum* 1983; 34:17–22.
17. Cox R: The MSU hearing instrument prescription procedure. *Hear Instrum* 1988; 39:6, 81.
18. Wade PS, Halik JJ, Chasin M: Bone-conduction implants: Transcutaneous vs. percutaneous. *Arch Otolaryngol Head Neck Surg* 1992; 106:68–74.
19. Dunham ME, Friedman HI: Audiologic management of bilateral external auditory canal atresia with the bone conducting implantable hearing device. *Cleft Palate J* 1990; 27:369–373.
20. Hough J, Himelick T, Johnson B: Implantable bone-conduction hearing device: Audiant bone conductor. *Ann Otol Rhinol Laryngol* 1986; 95:498–504.
21. Wade PS, Tollos SK, Olsa R, et al.: Clinical experience with the Xomed Audiant osteointegrated bone-conduction hearing device: A preliminary report of seven cases. *J Otolaryngol* 1989; 18:79–84.
22. Browning GG: The British experience of an implantable, subcutaneous bone-conduction hearing aid. *J Laryngol Otol* 1990; 104:534–538.
23. Roush J, Rauch SD: Clinical application of an implantable bone-conduction hearing device. *Laryngoscope* 1990; 100:281–285.

13

Aural Rehabilitation for Individuals With Severe and Profound Hearing Impairment: Hearing Aids, Cochlear Implants, Counseling, and Training

Margaret W. Skinner, Laura K. Holden, Susan M. Binzer

Introduction

Individuals with severe or profound hearing impairment using appropriately fitted hearing aids have more difficulty understanding speech in everyday life than do those with milder degrees of hearing impairment. Even with hearing aids, they cannot hear the full range of sounds in the world around them. Since they either do not hear or cannot correctly identify many speech sounds through hearing, they expend an extraordinary amount of energy determining what has been said. Speechreading must serve as an incomplete supplement to what little is received auditorily, and it is often difficult or impossible for such persons to carry on a fluent conversation. As a result, friends and family members often feel awkward and unsure of how to communicate with these individuals.

There are a number of devices and rehabilitative alternatives that can provide substantial benefit to those with severe or profound hearing impairment. Some of these include personal hearing aids; hand-held microphones with direct audio-input to the hearing aids; high gain telecoils; amplifiers and adapters for telephone use; Telecommunication Devices for the Deaf (TDD); FM, loop, and infrared systems for personal or wide area use; open and closed captioning; alerting systems; cochlear implantation; counseling; and aural rehabilitation therapy. These rehabilitative options are all designed to provide access to sound, particularly speech.

This chapter will focus on the selection of appropriate hearing aids or a cochlear implant for adults and on the rehabilitative services needed to ensure maximal use and benefit from these devices. Selection of hearing aids, determination of cochlear implant candidacy, and habilitation for children with severe and profound hearing loss are more complex than for adults; therefore, information on these topics will not be included in this chapter. The fitting goal for any aid is to match incoming sound with each person's residual hearing so that (1) the range of conversational speech and environmental sounds are comfortably loud, (2) speech is as clear as possible, and (3) loud sounds are not too loud.

Since a hearing aid does not require surgery and is less expensive than a cochlear implant, it is essential to evaluate an individual's ability to hear with well-fitted hearing aids. If hearing aids provide as good or better speech recognition scores (by sound alone) than the average score of adults with multi-electrode, intracochlear implants, then an implant should not be recommended. However, if performance is poorer than the average cochlear implant recipient, then evaluation for a cochlear implant should be considered provided the adult uses oral/aural communication.

In addition to optimizing the benefit provided by hearing aids or a cochlear implant, assistive listening device assessment, counseling, and aural rehabilitation therapy are crucial to the process of maximizing each person's ability to communicate in everyday life.

Severe and Profound Hearing Impairment

Degree of hearing impairment is often defined by the average hearing loss at 500, 1000, and 2000 Hz obtained with supra-aural earphones. For severe hearing impairment, this average is between 70 and 89 dB hearing level (HL, ANSI, 1989[1]), and for profound hearing impairment it is 90 dB HL or greater.[2]

This chapter will focus on individuals with these degrees of binaural hearing impairment. For evaluation of this hearing impaired population, it is important to use an audiometer with an output extending to 130 dB sound pressure level (SPL; in supra-aural earphones measured in a 6 cc coupler) to determine whether an individual can hear between 250 and 4000 Hz and, if so, at what threshold level. Many individuals with profound hearing loss have no hearing at some audiometric frequencies (most commonly at 1000 Hz and above), and some have no hearing at any frequency. Examples of four audiograms from individuals with severe and profound hearing impairment are shown in Figure 13–1; subject 1 uses hearing aids effectively and subjects 2–4 use multi-electrode, intracochlear implants.

Most people with severe or profound hearing impairment have *sensorineural* hearing loss. That is, there is significant loss or dysfunction of inner and outer hair cells and secondary degeneration of primary auditory neurons. Loudness recruitment is present that can be defined as the abnormally rapid growth of loudness above threshold as the physical intensity of sound increases. For these individuals, the range from threshold to uncomfortable loudness level (UCL) is small (e.g., 5–25 dB) and can vary at each frequency. For this reason, it is important to evaluate an individual's growth of loudness in specific

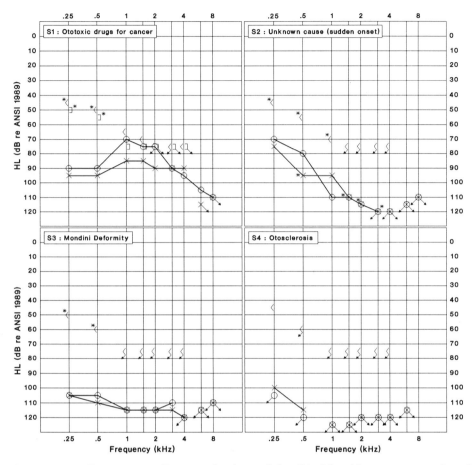

Figure 13–1. Pure-tone audiograms for four adults (S1–S4) with severe or profound hearing loss bilaterally; the presumed etiology is shown, and the asterisks denote responses to vibratory, not auditory, sensation. Subject 1 wears binaural hearing aids with good speech recognition; subjects 2 through 4 did not have open-set speech recognition with hearing aids at either ear and have been implanted with the Nucleus 22 Channel Cochlear Implant System. All have open-set speech recognition with the cochlear implant.

frequency regions. These data provide a basis for selecting the frequency response of a hearing aid. In addition to frequency specific growth of loudness, there is summation of loudness across frequencies. The amount of loudness summation varies among individuals and must be evaluated with broadband sounds to determine what overall use gain will make speech comfortably loud and what overall maximum output will prevent loud sound from being uncomfortable. Those with severe or profound sensorineural hearing impairment have decreased ability to detect changes in the intensity, frequency, and temporal aspects of sound as well as decreased ability to separate the frequency components of complex sounds that occur simultaneously (frequency selectivity). These decrements in auditory processing capability are associated with marked reduction in speech recognition, particularly in reverberant rooms and in the presence of noise.

Individuals with equivalent pure-tone thresholds can have very different auditory processing skills. Therefore, it is essential to recommend hearing aids or a cochlear implant based on an individual's ability to recognize speech. This ability cannot be adequately assessed with an audiometer because (1) the frequency response cannot be shaped so that amplified speech is matched to the individual's residual hearing, (2) speech often cannot be made loud enough to be comfortable, and (3) output limiting is not available for those with very small dynamic ranges. Consequently, speech recognition must be assessed with well fitted hearing aids.

Some people have a *mixed* hearing impairment in which there are conductive and sensorineural components. The most common etiology for the conductive component is otosclerosis; other etiologies are outer ear and/or ossicular malformation, disease, or surgical intervention in the middle ear that cause abnormal transmission of sound energy through the middle ear. This conductive component results in a decrease in the SPL reaching the inner ear. For this reason, these individuals often need hearing aids with greater gain and maximum output than those with the same degree of sensorineural hearing impairment. These issues are described by Gates and Valente in Chapter 12.

A few people have *neural* hearing impairment caused by loss or dysfunction of auditory neurons. This dysfunction can occur in the VIII cranial nerve or central auditory pathways. A bilateral, severe, or profound hearing impairment is usually caused by space-occupying lesions of both VIII cranial nerves or lesions of the brainstem at the level of the cochlear nucleus or superior olivary complex. Although a hearing aid is often useful until sound is no longer loud enough to be heard comfortably, a cochlear implant is not appropriate because the auditory pathways medial to the implant are severely compromised. The cochlear nucleus implant is an experimental device[3] that is appropriate for those with bilateral VIII cranial nerve neuromas.

Selection of Hearing Aids and Earmolds

Types of Hearing Aids

Individuals with severe or profound hearing impairment require hearing aids that provide high use gain (50–70 dB), output limiting that lies between approximately 120 and 142 dB SPL measured in a 2 cc coupler, tone controls, automatic gain control, and strong telecoils. Current hearing aids provide linear amplification; commercially available hearing aids with full dynamic range compression have not been designed to provide sufficient output for people with severe or profound hearing impairment. For those who use their hearing aids with the telephone and assistive listening devices (such as FM or infrared systems), a powerful telecoil is useful. Direct audio-input adapters are necessary for those who want to use hand-held microphones. Most people with severe to profound hearing impairment use behind-the-ear (BTE) hearing aids, but those with a conductive component often use body aids to obtain greater gain and output.

Earmolds

With severe or profound hearing impairment, it is essential to have tightly fitting, yet comfortable earmolds. Soft materials are often used because body heat causes the material to expand slightly and create a tight acoustic seal. For some people, a lucite shell earmold with a long bore is easier to insert than a soft earmold and therefore provides a better seal. Individuals with poorer hearing in the high (above 1500 Hz) than the low frequencies may be unable to utilize high frequency cues to recognize speech or other sounds; consequently, it is appropriate to use earmold tubing with a constant diameter (usually #13; 1.93 mm internal diameter) or reverse horn (stepped down diameter bore) that reduces the high frequency output as well as feedback. Those with the same or better hearing above 1500 Hz often use high frequency cues to recognize sounds; for this reason, it is important to make high frequency sound audible. The use of horn type tubing (e.g., 4 mm Libby horn), which provides up to 10 dB more gain between 3000 and 6000 Hz than #13 tubing, may be necessary to make these sounds audible.

The limiting factor in achieving the desired gain (especially in the high frequencies) is acoustic feedback from amplified sound in the ear canal reaching the hearing aid microphone and causing the familiar squeal. Acoustic feedback may make it impossible to use a horn earmold, and even when #13 tubing is used acoustic feedback often limits the maximum gain that can be obtained. That is, many people with severe or profound hearing impairment increase the volume control setting until feedback occurs and then turn it down slightly to prevent feedback and distortion.

Prescription of Real-Ear Gain

Several procedures have been developed for prescribing real-ear gain (actual gain provided by the hearing aid) in specific frequency regions for people with severe or profound hearing impairment. These procedures prescribe greater gain as a function of threshold level than the prescriptive procedures described in Chapter 1, which are adaptations of Lybarger's half-gain rule.[4]

The Libby[5] procedure prescribes real-ear gain that is two-thirds the air conduction threshold (dB HL) between 250 and 6000 Hz with the following adjustments: −5 dB at 250 Hz and 6000 Hz and −3 dB at 500 Hz. The Prescription of Gain and Output II (POGO II) procedure[6] prescribes real-ear gain based on air conduction thresholds (dB HL) as well. For thresholds that are less than or equal to 65 dB HL, the real-ear gain is one-half the threshold with the following adjustments: −10 dB at 250 Hz and −5 dB at 500 Hz. For thresholds that are greater than 65 dB HL, additional gain is added that is equal to the threshold minus 65 dB divided by two.

The Desired Sensation Level Method for Fitting Children, Version 3.0, (DSL) is applicable to adults.[7,8] Unlike the Libby and POGO II procedures, the DSL procedure specifies where an amplified long-term speech spectrum[8,9] (LTSS)

Table 13–1. The Desired Sensation Levels (dB)* as a Function of Threshold (dB HL) for the Audiometric Frequencies Prescribed by the DSL (Version 3.0[8]) Procedure

	Frequency (Hz)								
Threshold	*250*	*500*	*750*	*1000*	*1500*	*2000*	*3000*	*4000*	*6000*
0	47	54	53	48	46	46	43	41	30
5	41	48	49	44	43	43	40	38	27
10	36	44	44	41	40	40	37	35	24
15	32	40	41	38	37	38	35	33	22
20	28	36	37	35	35	35	33	31	20
25	25	33	34	33	32	33	31	29	19
30	23	30	32	31	31	32	30	28	17
35	20	28	30	30	29	30	28	26	16
40	19	26	28	28	27	28	27	24	15
45	17	24	26	26	26	27	25	23	14
50	16	22	24	25	25	25	24	22	13
55	14	21	23	24	24	24	23	21	12
60	13	19	22	22	22	23	22	19	11
65	13	18	20	21	21	21	21	18	10
70	12	17	19	20	20	20	19	17	9
75	11	16	18	18	19	18	18	15	8
80	10	14	17	17	17	17	16	14	7
85	8	13	15	15	16	15	15	12	5
90	7	12	14	13	14	13	13	11	3
95	5	10	12	11	12	11	11	9	0
100	3	8	10	9	10	8	8	7	—
105	—	6	7	7	7	5	5	5	—
110	—	4	5	4	4	2	2	3	—

*   The values presented assume a REUR approximating published[10] average adult values. Furthermore, if audiometric data have been collected using the Etymotic ER-3A insert earphone (in dB HL), the above values assume an average adult real-ear to coupler difference. (Reprinted with permission from the authors.)

should fall within an individual's residual hearing for the audiometric frequencies. The desired sensation levels (db above threshold) of third octave bands of amplified speech as a function of threshold (db HL) at the audiometric frequencies are given in Table 13–1. As the threshold increases, the sensation level decreases. For thresholds at 110 dB HL, sensation levels are only between 2 and 5 dB. Since the peaks of speech are approximately 12 dB above the long-term speech spectrum, it is important that the sensation levels be low so that the long-term speech spectrum levels as well as the peaks are amplified within the linear range of the hearing aid. The real-ear gain needed to amplify the long-term speech spectrum to the desired sensation levels (shown in Table 13–1) as a function of threshold (dB HL) and audiometric frequency is shown in Table 13–2.

The unamplified long-term speech spectrum used in the DSL procedure (see line 1, Table 13–3) is based on measurements of one-third octave band levels of (1) speech spoken by adult males, adult females, and children with the recording microphone in the unobstructed field, and (2) speech spoken by

Table 13–2.   The Desired Real Ear Gain (in dB)* as a Function of Threshold (dB HL) for the Audiometric Frequencies Prescribed by the DSL (Version 3.0[8]) Procedure

Threshold	Frequency (Hz)								
	250	500	750	1000	1500	2000	3000	4000	6000
0	0	0	0	0	0	0	0	0	0
5	0	0	0	1	2	2	2	2	2
10	0	0	1	3	4	4	4	5	4
15	0	1	2	5	6	6	7	8	7
20	2	3	4	8	9	9	10	11	10
25	4	5	6	11	12	12	13	14	13
30	6	7	9	14	15	15	17	17	17
35	9	9	11	17	18	18	20	20	21
40	12	12	14	20	21	22	24	24	25
45	15	15	18	24	25	25	27	28	29
50	19	19	21	27	29	29	31	31	33
55	23	22	25	31	33	33	35	35	37
60	27	26	28	35	36	36	39	39	41
65	31	30	32	38	40	40	43	43	45
70	35	33	36	42	44	43	46	46	49
75	39	37	40	46	48	47	50	50	53
80	43	41	43	49	51	50	53	54	56
85	47	45	47	53	55	53	57	57	60
90	50	48	50	56	58	56	60	60	63
95	54	52	53	59	61	59	63	64	65
100	57	55	56	62	64	62	65	67	—
105	—	58	59	64	66	64	67	69	—
110	—	60	61	66	68	66	69	72	—

* The values presented assume a REUR approximating published[10] average adult values. Furthermore, if audiometric data have been collected using the Etymotic ER-3A insert earphone (in dB HL), the above values assume an average adult real-ear to coupler difference. (Reprinted with permission from the authors.)

children with a second recording microphone at ear level to simulate the position of the hearing aid microphone. In the calculation of the DSL spectrum, equal weighting was given to (1) the combined measurements from males, females, and children in the unobstructed field, and (2) the measurements from children at ear level. The Cox and Moore[11] and Pascoe[12] unamplified long-term speech spectra (measured in the unobstructed field; adult males and females) are also used for prescribing real-ear gain; these spectra are shown in Table 13–3 (lines 2 and 3) for comparison. The overall level of the DSL and Cox and Moore spectra is 70 dB SPL. Since a speech-weighted composite noise signal[13,14] is often used for probe tube microphone measurements, its spectrum is also shown in Table 13–3 (line 4). For comparison of this spectrum with the others in Table 13–3, the overall level is 70 dB SPL; however, an overall level of 50 or 60 dB SPL is usually used to obtain insertion gain, because many hearing aids operate in their nonlinear range with a 70 dB SPL input level.

The National Acoustic Laboratories' procedure[15] (NAL) has been modified by Byrne et al.[16] for individuals with severe or profound hearing impairment

Table 13–3.   Unamplified Long-Term Speech Spectra

Spectra (dB SPL)	Frequency (Hz)								
	250	*500*	*750*	*1000*	*1500*	*2000*	*3000*	*4000*	*6000*
DSL (Version 3.0)[8,9]	63	64	60	56	52	51	45	42	42
Cox and Moore[11]	60	62	57	55	52	49	46	46	46
Pascoe[12]	62	67	—	56	55	57	50	49	46
Composite noise[13,14]	50	58	57	56	57	57	55	54	53

Table 13–4.   Formulas for Calculating Real-Ear Gain With the NAL Procedure[15] Modified for Severe/Profound Hearing Losses[16]

1. Calculate X_{dB} = 0.05 × (HTL$_{500}$ + HTL$_{1000}$ + HTL$_{2000}$ up to 180 dB) + 0.116 × combined HTL in excess of 180 dB

2. Calculate the prescribed real-ear gain (REG) at each frequency:
    REG$_{250}$ (dB) = X + 0.31 HTL$_{250}$ − 17
    REG$_{500}$ (dB) = X + 0.31 HTL$_{500}$ − 8
    REG$_{750}$ (dB) = X + 0.31 HTL$_{750}$ − 3
    REG$_{1.0k}$ (dB) = X + 0.31 HTL$_{1.0k}$ + 1
    REG$_{1.5k}$ (dB) = X + 0.31 HTL$_{1.5k}$ + 1
    REG$_{2.0k}$ (dB) = X + 0.31 HTL$_{2.0k}$ − 1
    REG$_{3.0k}$ (dB) = X + 0.31 HTL$_{3.0k}$ − 2
    REG$_{4.0k}$ (dB) = X + 0.31 HTL$_{4.0k}$ − 2
    REG$_{6.0k}$ (dB) = X + 0.31 HTL$_{6.0k}$ − 2

3. When the 2000 Hz HTL is 95 dB or greater, add the following gain (dB):

HTL 2 kHz	Frequency (Hz)								
	250	*500*	*750*	*1000*	*1500*	*2000*	*3000*	*4000*	*6000*
95	4	3	1	0	−1	−2	−2	−2	−2
100	6	4	2	0	−2	−3	−3	−3	−3
105	8	5	2	0	−3	−5	−5	−5	−5
110	11	7	3	0	−3	−6	−6	−6	−6
115	13	8	4	0	−4	−8	−8	−8	−8
120	15	9	4	0	−5	−9	−9	−9	−9

based on a study with 46 adults.[17] In this study, the optimal frequency response slope was estimated from intelligibility judgments, speech recognition scores, and real-ear gain measurements with the settings subjects preferred to use in everyday life. The results of this study indicate that more overall gain was needed than was prescribed by the original NAL procedure. For this reason, the calculation of X was modified (see line 1, Table 13–4) to provide more overall gain for mean thresholds over 60 dB HL. In addition, when the threshold at 2 kHz was 95 dB HL or greater, more gain was required in the low frequencies and less gain in the high frequencies than prescribed by the NAL procedure. The changes in gain as a function of frequency and hearing threshold at 2 kHz are shown in Table 13–4.

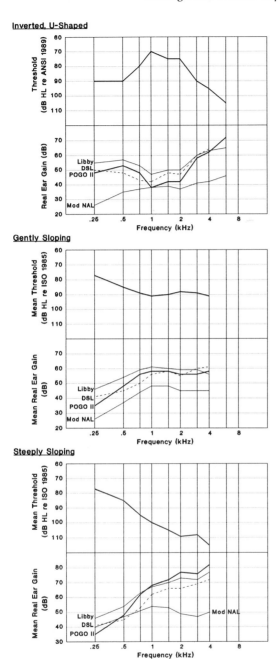

Figure 13–2. Thresholds (dB HL; supra-aural earphones; ANSI 1989[1] or ISO 1985[58]) and real-ear gain prescribed by the Libby, POGO II, DSL (Version 3.0), and modified NAL procedures for one individual with a severe, inverted U-shaped hearing loss (top), one group with a severe, gently sloping hearing loss (middle), and one group with a profound, steeply sloping hearing loss (bottom). Mean thresholds for the two groups are from those studied by Byrne et al.[17]

Figure 13–2 shows the real-ear gain prescribed by the four procedures for three threshold configurations: inverted U-shaped, severe hearing loss; gently sloping, severe hearing loss; and more steeply sloping, profound hearing loss. The first threshold configuration is from an individual who received ototoxic chemotherapy, and the next two configurations are the mean thresholds for

Table 13–5.   Comparison of Threshold Slope With Slope of Prescribed Real-Ear Gain Slope*

Threshold Configuration/Procedure	Slope (dB)
Inverted U-shaped	
Threshold	−15
Libby	−7
POGO II	−11
DSL	−1
Mod NAL	+2
Gently sloping	
Threshold	+3
Libby	+5
POGO II	+8
DSL	+10
Mod NAL	+8
Steeply sloping	
Threshold	+24
Libby	+19
POGO II	+29
DSL	+23
Mod NAL	+5

* Compared between 500 and 2000 Hz for the three threshold configurations in Figure 13–2 and the four prescriptive procedures (Libby, POGO II, DSL, and modified NAL).

two groups studied by Byrne et al.[17] The real-ear gain prescribed by the modified NAL procedure is substantially lower for all three threshold configurations except at 250–750 Hz for the steeply sloping, profound group. With this procedure, the 17 dB correction factor at 250 Hz causes the prescribed real-ear gain to be particularly low (26 dB) for the first two threshold configurations and degree of hearing impairment. When thresholds are relatively low (i.e., 70–77 dB HL), the Libby procedure prescribes substantially more real-ear gain at 250–1000 Hz than the other procedures. For thresholds that are 70–77 dB at 1500 and 2000 Hz, the DSL and Libby procedures prescribe approximately the same real-ear gain because the DSL procedure compensates for the lower long-term speech spectrum levels at these frequencies. For thresholds that are 89–95 dB HL at 3000 and 4000 Hz, the Libby, POGO II, and DSL procedures prescribe approximately the same real-ear gain.

Since hearing aid wearers have a range of overall gain settings from which to choose, the slope of the frequency response curve is a key factor to consider in comparing the real-ear gain prescribed by these procedures. For Table 13–5, the threshold or real-ear gain at 500 Hz has been substracted from the threshold or real-ear gain at 2000 Hz to calculate the slope. For the negative threshold slope of the inverted U-shaped configuration, the Libby and POGO II procedures prescribe real-ear gain slopes that are similar to, but less than, that of the threshold slope, whereas the DSL and modified NAL procedures prescribe real-ear gain slopes close to zero. For the +3 dB threshold slope of the gently sloping configuration, POGO II, DSL, and modified NAL prescribe real-ear gain slopes that are essentially the same and more than double the threshold slope. For the +24 dB threshold slope of the steeply sloping configuration, the +5 dB slope prescribed by the modified NAL procedure is less than one-fourth that prescribed by the other procedures.

However, maybe the most crucial factor in choosing a prescriptive procedure for a particular patient with a severe or profound hearing impairment is the frequency-gain response of the hearing aid in relation to residual hearing. For example, with the inverted U-shaped threshold configuration, it may be most beneficial to choose a frequency-gain response that optimizes amplification between 750 and 4000 Hz, whereas for the steeply sloping configuration it may be most beneficial to choose a frequency-gain response that optimizes amplification between 250 and 1500 Hz. These suggested differences in frequency-gain responses as a function of threshold configuration are supported by the results of Byrne and his colleagues.[16,17] Their results suggest that individuals with steeply sloping hearing losses and thresholds equal to or greater than 95 dB HL at 2000 Hz perform better with a hearing aid that has more real-ear gain between 250 and 750 Hz and less between 1500 and 6000 Hz than with the slope of gain as a function of frequency prescribed by the original NAL procedure. With this modified slope, speech may not be audible at 2000 Hz and above. In contrast, those with flat or gently sloping hearing losses seemed to benefit from more high frequency gain. Although these results reflect trends across subjects, the optimal frequency-gain response differed between some individuals with the same threshold configuration. Consequently, it is essential to consider any prescribed real-ear gain contour as a starting point and try different amounts of low versus high frequency real-ear gain to determine whether another frequency-gain response will be more beneficial to the individual in everyday life. It often requires some hearing aid experience to make reliable judgments of speech clarity and sound quality during this trial period.

Problems Measuring Real-Ear Gain With Severe/Profound Hearing Impairment

Real-ear gain is estimated by obtaining *functional* or *insertion gain* measurements. *Functional gain* is the difference between unaided and aided thresholds (for frequency-specific sounds) obtained in the same sound field conditions. *Insertion gain* is the difference between SPLs measured near the eardrum with a hearing aid (real-ear aided response [REAR]) and without a hearing aid (real-ear unaided response [REUR]). For both conditions, the same signals are presented and frequency-specific measurements are made. Functional and insertion gain measurements are made with the volume control setting used in everyday life (use gain) or the setting at which speech sounds clearest. Insertion gain measurements are often made with a broadband signal presented at 70 dB SPL (overall level) or a narrowband signal presented at 60 dB SPL (third-octave band level) to approximate the levels of conversational speech. In contrast, functional gain measurements are made with sounds at threshold that usually are at much lower levels. Since the measured output of hearing aids can be linear or nonlinear, it is essential to measure (either in a hearing aid test box or with a probe tube microphone) the output for a family of input levels (i.e., 50, 60, 70, 80, and 90 dB SPL) to determine at what level in each frequency region the hearing aid output becomes nonlinear at the use gain setting. The output needs to be linear through 70 dB SPL (broadband signal; overall level) for functional gain measurements to be an appropriate estimate of real-ear gain for conversational speech.[18] If the output is not linear through 70 dB SPL, functional gain measurements will overestimate the sensation level of conversational speech.

There are several limitations in determining real-ear gain with those who have severe or profound hearing impairment. For functional gain measurements, it is usually impossible to obtain unaided thresholds in the sound field. If unaided thresholds are obtained with earphones and a transfer function is used to estimate unaided sound field thresholds, these thresholds should be viewed as a rough approximation of the "true" unaided sound field thresholds.

For insertion gain measurements, it is often difficult to prevent acoustic feedback that occurs because the probe tube creates a small leak around the earmold that cannot be sealed with Oto-firm™ or other materials. To estimate the output in the ear canal (REAR) and insertion gain (REIR) at use gain, the following procedure can be carried out. The volume control setting must be reduced to eliminate acoustic feedback to make valid measurements. Then a family of output curves for inputs of 50, 60, 70, 80, and 90 dB SPL need to be obtained with a hearing aid test box at use gain and at the reduced volume control settings to determine the linearity of the output at both settings. When the output is linear for a 70 dB SPL composite noise input (or 60 dB SPL puretone input) at use gain, the difference in gain between the two volume control settings can be calculated by subtracting the 2 cc coupler output for the reduced setting (line 2 in Table 13–6) from the 2 cc coupler output at use gain (line 1) for a 70 dB SPL composite noise input. REAR at use gain can be estimated by adding the REAR obtained at the reduced setting (line 4) to the difference in gain between the two volume control settings (lines 3 or 5). The insertion gain associated with use gain can be estimated by adding the insertion gain obtained at the reduced setting (line 7) to the difference in gain between the reduced and use gain settings (lines 3, 5, or 8).

If unaided sound field thresholds cannot be obtained and aided probe tube measurements cannot be made even at a low volume control setting because of feedback, the only way to determine whether hearing aids make speech audible at use gain is to compare aided warble tone thresholds (for calibration of sound field stimuli, see Skinner[19]) with an unaided speech spectrum (see Table 13–3). That is, aided warble tone thresholds are subtracted from the unaided speech spectrum levels to estimate the sensation level of speech at each frequency. However, if the hearing aid output is nonlinear for inputs below the unaided speech spectrum levels (42–67 dB SPL, depending on the frequency and spectrum), then the actual gain of the hearing aid will cause speech to be at lower sensation levels than calculated above. For this reason, it is essential to determine whether the hearing aid output is linear for these input SPLs by measuring them in a hearing aid test box. For frequencies at

Table 13–6. Calculations for Estimating the Output in the Ear Canal (dB SPL; REAR) and Insertion Gain (dB)*

	Frequency (Hz)								
	250	500	750	1000	1500	2000	3000	4000	6000
2 cc coupler measurements									
1. Use gain VC	103	116	122	125	118	122	121	117	85
2. Reduced VC	85	98	105	108	101	106	106	102	70
3. Output diff	18	18	17	17	17	16	15	15	15
Probe tube microphone + 2 cc coupler measurements									
4. REAR-reduced VC	84	98	104	101	97	100	94	84	54
5. Output diff	18	18	17	17	17	16	15	15	15
6. Estimated REAR use gain VC	102	116	121	118	114	116	109	99	69
7. REIR-reduced VC	26	36	45	46	41	40	31	24	15
8. Output diff	18	18	17	17	17	16	15	15	15
9. Estimated REIR Reduced gain VC	44	54	62	63	58	56	46	39	30

* Calculated from 2 cc coupler measurements (dB SPL) at use gain and reduced volume control (VC) settings as well as the REAR and REIR obtained at the reduced setting. The input signal for all measurements was composite noise[13,14] presented at 70 dB SPL.

which the input–output function is nonlinear, the actual gain for the speech spectrum input level at each frequency should be determined by examining the family of input-output functions and then subtracting this gain at each frequency from the calculated linear gain. This difference between the linear and actual gains is the amount by which the sensation level of speech is lower.

Maximum Acoustic Output

The maximum acoustic output of a hearing aid should prevent loud sound from being amplified at uncomfortable loudness levels (UCLs). Since the maximum output can only be adjusted overall and not in specific frequency regions for most hearing aids, it is efficient to adjust the saturated sound pressure level (SSPL90) control so that loud broadband sounds are not uncomfortable for the individual. If there is a peak or peaks in the output (e.g., between 1000 and 3000 Hz), reducing the height of the peak with earmold modifications, a damper in the earhook, or a change in hearing aid may allow higher overall gain and output before reaching the individual's UCL. Use of an automatic gain control (AGC) circuit for high input levels (70 dB SPL and above) may also be helpful.

Optimization of a Hearing Aid Fitting for an Individual

Earmolds must be comfortable and provide a good seal without the presence of feedback. Tone controls of the hearing aids should be adjusted to a number of different settings to determine which setting causes conversational speech to be the clearest. In addition, the SSPL90 and AGC settings should be adjusted so that loud broadband sound is not uncomfortable. After these adjustments are made, the volume control should be adjusted so that feedback is not audible and conversational speech is comfortably loud.

Measurement of real-ear gain, the relation of the aided long-term speech spectrum to thresholds and UCLs, the relation of the maximum acoustic output to UCLs, and the relation of aided sound field thresholds to the unaided long-term speech spectrum are described in the next section. Based on these measurements, further adjustments in the hearing aid parameters may be needed. It is essential that the individual wear the hearing aids adjusted to these initial settings in everyday life and that subsequent adjustments be made to maximize comfort, clarity, and benefit.

Some individuals have never worn hearing aids or may not have worn hearing aids for a long time. If this is the case, hearing aids should be tried. However, if listening with hearing aids causes discomfort, such as dizziness or nausea, if the person perceives speech as a nonspeech-like sound, such as buzzing, or if the person cannot hear speech spoken at a normal level with the hearing aids, then it is not appropriate to encourage wearing hearing aids in everyday life or to proceed with the hearing aid evaluation outlined in the next section.

Evaluation of Hearing Aid Benefit: A Case Study

After an individual with severe or profound hearing impairment is fitted with hearing aids according to the principles outlined above, it is important to determine aided benefit. The evaluation should include probe tube microphone measurements (and hearing aid test box measurements, if necessary), aided sound field thresholds, and speech recognition tests.

Examples of measurements and test results included in an evaluation of hearing aid benefit will be based on data obtained from an individual with a severe sensorineural hearing impairment (subject 1 in Fig. 13–1). Although he wears binaural behind-the-ear (BTE) aids for sound localization, he only recognizes speech with the right ear; the data presented below are for the hearing aid he wears at this ear. Through an iterative procedure, he has tried a number of different earmolds, hearing aids, and hearing aid adjustments to determine what provides the most benefit in everyday life. The settings on the hearing aid he wears at the right ear include a low tone cut, SSPL90 of 134 dB, volume control setting of 3+ (out of 4+) in most listening situations, and a soft canal earmold with #13 tubing. It was possible to use the probe tube microphone system at these settings without audible feedback.

Probe Tube Microphone Measurements

Probe tube microphone systems enable clinicians to measure the SPL of sound near a person's eardrum. When all measurements are referenced to this measurement point, the relations between them can be compared directly. With a probe tube microphone placed near the eardrum, the SPL associated with threshold, UCL, REUR, and REAR for a number of input levels can be

Table 13–7. Unaided and Aided Data Obtained From the Individual With a Severe, Inverted U-Shaped Hearing Loss for Whom Prescribed, Real-Ear Gain is Shown in Figure 13–2*

	Frequency (Hz)								
	250	500	750	1000	1500	2000	3000	4000	6000
Unaided									
Pure tones									
1. Threshold (ER-3A) (dB SPL)	88	84	77	71	86	96	105	106	97
2. UCL (TDH-50) (dB SPL)	>105	>121	>124	121	>125	>134	>132	>127	—
Aided									
Composite noise									
3. 50-dB-SPL input	48	61	71	69	76	88	74	54	25
4. 60-dB-SPL input	57	71	80	79	86	98	84	64	35
5. 70-dB-SPL input	68	82	92	90	98	109	96	76	46
6. 80-dB-SPL input	75	84	99	100	108	117	106	86	55
Pure tones									
7. 90-dB-SPL input	99	114	124	126	132	132	124	114	93
Insertion gain									
8. REAR (SPL)	68	82	92	90	98	109	96	76	46
9. REUR (SPL)	47	60	62	52	52	66	61	39	28
10. Insertion gain	21	22	30	38	46	43	35	37	18
Aided long-term speech spectrum (LTSS)									
11. Unaided LTSS[8,9]	63	64	60	56	52	51	45	42	42
12. Diffuse field/BTE microphone[20]	0	1	2	2	3	3	3	3	3
13. In situ gain (70 dB input)	21	24	34	37	48	55	51	42	8
14. Aided LTSS (dB SPL)	84	89	96	95	103	109	99	87	53
SL Aided LTSS									
15. Aided LTSS (dB SPL; line 14)	84	89	96	94	103	109	99	87	53
16. Threshold (dB SPL; line 1)	88	84	77	71	86	96	105	106	97
17. SL aided LTSS	–4	+5	+19	+23	+17	+13	–6	–19	–44
18. Prescribed SL of aided LTSS	+7	+12	+17	+20	+19	+18	+13	+9	—

* Measurements were made with a probe tube microphone system. The stimuli were either pure tones or composite speech-weighted noise.

measured. An estimate of the amplified long-term spectrum of speech can be calculated and plotted in relation to residual hearing between threshold and UCL for the audiometric frequencies. The steps in this process are described in the following sections.

THRESHOLD/UCL

Pure-tone, air conduction thresholds were obtained with an ER-3A insert earphone, EAR™ foam tip, and audiometer. The SPL at threshold was measured with the probe tube placed in the same position used for insertion gain measurements in the ear canal (within 6 mm of the eardrum). Since the UCLs for pure tones were higher than the output of the insert earphone, TDH-50 earphones were used with the probe tube in the same position. As shown in line 2 of Table 13–7, except for 1000 Hz, UCLs exceeded the maximum output of the earphone.

AIDED OUTPUT OF THE HEARING AID

Speech-weighted composite noise[13] was presented at overall levels of 50, 60, 70, and 80 dB SPL to determine output linearity (dB SPL) measured with the probe tube tip placed near the eardrum. For these measurements, the volume control was adjusted to use gain (3+). With the exception of 250, 500, and 750 Hz, the output was linear for inputs up to 80 dB SPL (see lines 3–6 in Table 13–7).

An FM tonal sweep was presented at 90 dB SPL to estimate the maximum output of the hearing aid in the ear canal and to ensure that the amplified sound was not too loud. These levels are lower than the UCL levels at all audiometric frequencies except 1000 Hz (compare lines 2 and 7 in Table 13–7).

INSERTION GAIN

To obtain insertion gain for an overall input level of 70 dB SPL, speech-weighted composite noise was presented without and with the hearing aid to obtain REUR and REAR, respectively. The REUR values at each frequency were subtracted from the REAR values to obtain the insertion gain (see lines 8–10 in Table 13–7). The insertion gain values at 250–750 and 3000–6000 Hz were lower than any prescribed by the four prescriptive procedures described above (see data for the patient's inverted, U-shaped threshold configuration in Fig. 13–2), whereas insertion gain at 1000 Hz was the same as that prescribed by the modified NAL procedure and close to values prescribed by the DSL procedure at 1500 and 2000 Hz.

AIDED LONG-TERM SPECTRUM OF SPEECH

The aided long-term spectrum of speech (line 14, Table 13–7) can be calculated by choosing an unaided long-term spectrum (line 11; the DSL speech spectrum was chosen so that the sensation level at the audiometric frequencies could be compared with that prescribed), adding the diffuse field/BTE microphone transfer function[20] (line 12) and the in situ gain (line 13) for a 70 dB SPL input.

In situ gain is the difference between the SPL input at the reference micro-phone (placed close to the BTE microphone) and the SPL output near the eardrum.

SENSATION LEVEL OF THE AIDED LONG TERM SPECTRUM OF SPEECH

The sensation level of the aided long-term spectrum of speech can be calcu-lated by subtracting the thresholds from the aided long-term spectrum of speech at each audiometric frequency (lines 15–17 in Table 13–7). When the calculated sensation level was compared with that prescribed by the DSL procedure (lines 17 and 18), there was good agreement between 750 and 2000 Hz.

RELATION BETWEEN AMPLIFIED SPEECH AND RESIDUAL HEARING

Figure 13–3 shows the relation between the aided long-term speech spectrum (including the 30 dB range of momentary fluctuations denoted by the shading) and the range of residual hearing between threshold and UCL for the indi-vidual whose data are given in Table 13–7. The maximum output of the hearing aid is also shown and can be compared with the UCL data. UCL was obtained at 1000 Hz; at the other frequencies, UCL was higher than the maximum output of the earphone (denoted by the arrows). This comparison was confirmed by the aided 90 dB SPL tonal sweep, which was judged not too

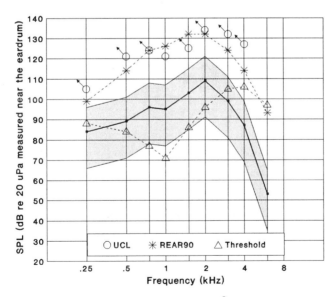

Figure 13–3. The aided long-term speech spectrum[8] (solid line curve) and maximum output of the hearing aid (REAR90) shown in relation to the thresholds and UCLs for subject 1 whose audiogram is shown in Figure 13–1. The shaded area around the long-term speech spectrum is the 30 dB range of momentary fluctuations for speech spoken at one vocal effort.

loud. This graph is very similar to that produced by the DSL Version 3.0 software.[8]

In everyday life, speech is spoken at many different levels and distances from the listener. Although speech at 70 dB SPL may be comfortably loud with a hearing aid, speech at soft levels (e.g., 55 dB SPL) or at distances of more than 3–5 feet may be inaudible for individuals with profound hearing impairment wearing linear hearing aids.

Sound Field Thresholds

Sound field thresholds were obtained from the individual described above, and the levels at threshold were measured with a sound level meter (Bruel and Kjaer, model 2230) and a microphone (Knowles No. 1785) adjacent to and in the same plane as the BTE microphone. These thresholds are shown in line 4 of Table 13–8 and are plotted in relation to the DSL long-term speech spectrum in Figure 13–4. Since the hearing aid output is linear for a 70 dB SPL input, the sensation level (dB) of the DSL long-term speech spectrum can be calculated by subtracting the aided thresholds from the long-term speech spectrum at the BTE microphone as shown in Table 13–8 and Figure 13–4. The values between 750 and 2000 Hz are in close agreement with those shown on line 17 of Table 13–7. If the hearing aid output had not been linear for a 70 dB SPL input, then a correction for nonlinearity at each audiometric frequency would have to be applied before subtracting the aided thresholds from the DSL long-term speech spectrum.

Ideally, an individual's aided sound field thresholds should fall at levels lower than the long-term spectrum of speech across the frequency range from 250 to 4000 Hz. However, this goal is rarely achieved with those with severe and profound hearing impairment. Often high frequency thresholds are so poor that hearing aid(s) provide no measurable benefit in this region. If the individual is to receive at least some benefit to speechreading from a hearing aid, the long-term speech spectrum should be audible at least at 250–500 Hz.

Table 13–8.   Calculation of the Sensation Level (dB) of the Aided Long-Term Speech Spectrum (LTSS)[8,9] for the Individual Whose BTE Data Are Shown in Table 13–7*

	Frequency (Hz)								
	250	500	750	1000	1500	2000	3000	4000	6000
1. Unaided LTSS	63	64	60	56	52	51	45	42	42
2. Diffuse field/ BTE microphone	0	1	2	2	3	3	3	3	3
3. LTSS at BTE microphone	63	65	62	58	55	54	48	45	45
4. Aided threshold at BTE microphone	73	52	43	33	36	39	50	70	—
5. SL of LTSS	−10	+13	+19	+25	+19	+15	−2	−25	—

* The unaided and aided LTSS and the aided threshold (re: the BTE microphone) are in dB SPL, and the diffuse field/BTE microphone transfer function and sensation level of the LTSS are in dB.

a)

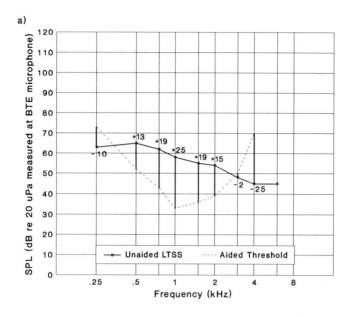

b)

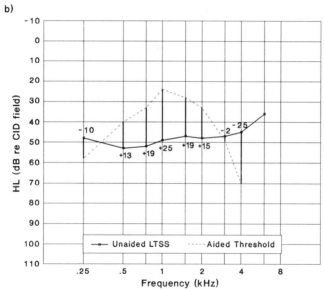

Figure 13–4. The unaided long-term speech spectrum[8,9] plotted in relation to subject 1's aided thresholds. (**A**) Graph plotted in dB SPL at the hearing aid microphone. (**B**) Graph plotted in dB HL (re: the CID sound field).

For a few individuals, it is impossible to make conversational speech loud enough to be heard.

Clinically, it is appropriate to use probe tube microphone measurements without aided sound field thresholds if the probe tube measurements can be obtained without feedback and if the individual can reliably indicate whether sound or a vibrotactile sensation is perceived for stimuli across the frequency range. Otherwise, it is essential to obtain aided sound field thresholds.

Speech Recognition

After verifying that the aided speech spectrum is audible over as much of the frequency range as is feasible, it is important to assess aided speech recognition with recorded speech tests at 70 dB SPL at each ear and binaurally. The most widely used test for adults is the NU-6 Monosyllabic Word Test[21] presented audition-only; since the person reports what is heard without any response alternatives given, this is called an *open-set test*. Of the 50 words on this test, the individual whose data are shown in Tables 13–7 and 13–8 recognized 66% of the words and 81% of the 150 phonemes with his hearing aid at the right ear; since he does not understand words at the left ear, his binaural score was the same. With this speech recognition capability, he can converse fluently on the telephone. Most adults who became severely or profoundly hearing impaired after learning language (postlinguistically deaf) get lower scores than this; some cannot understand words with their hearing aids. For those who get a score of 2% or more on the NU-6 test, one of two open-set sentence tests can be presented by audition-only. They are the Central Institute for the Deaf (CID) Everyday Sentence Test[22] or the Iowa Sentences Without Context Test.[23] For those who cannot understand NU-6 words, the Four Choice Spondee Test[24] consisting of 20 two syllable words is presented. Since the person is given responses from which to choose for each test word, this is called a *closed-set test*. An above-chance score (at the 0.05 confidence level) of 40% or more indicates that the individual can recognize some phonemes by sound alone. There are a number of recorded closed-set tests in the Minimal Auditory Capabilities Battery[24] and Iowa Cochlear Implant Test Battery.[23] These have been used to evaluate the aided sound recognition of individuals who became deaf before or around the time of learning language (prelinguistically or perilinguistically deaf) and do not have open-set speech recognition.

The CID Everyday Sentence Test has been recorded on videotape[25] and laser disc[26] so that it can be presented in three conditions (audition-only, vision-only, and audition + vision) with hearing aids worn binaurally, if feasible. For those with no open-set speech recognition, only the audition + vision and vision-only conditions are used. If the score for the audition + vision condition is higher than the score for the vision-only condition, the hearing aids are providing benefit to speechreading.

Criteria for Cochlear Implantation

If an individual with severe or profound hearing impairment has well-fitted hearing aids and cannot recognize speech by hearing alone as well as the average postlinguistically deaf cochlear implant recipient, then a cochlear implant should be considered. The following sections describe criteria for implantation and evaluation for cochlear implant candidacy.

There are three multi-channel intracochlear implant systems available for implantation in the United States. Since the Nucleus 22 Channel Cochlear Implant System[27] is the only multi-electrode, intracochlear device to date that has been approved by the Food and Drug Administration (FDA) for clinical use in children and postlinguistically deaf adults, the categories of implant candidates and recipients' performance will be described for this device. The Ineraid[28,29] and Clarion[30,31] Cochlear Implant Systems are under FDA approved clinical investigation and are described in other publications.

Criteria for Implantation

CATEGORIES OF IMPLANT CANDIDATES

Potential adult implant candidates can be categorized according to three protocols: profound, severe, or pre/perilinguistic. For patients to be placed in the profound protocol, they must be postlinguistically deaf; that is, deafness must have occurred after the age of 6 years. They must receive essentially no open-set speech recognition with well fitted hearing aids. However, it is possible that they may still receive a significant amount of benefit to speechreading with hearing aids.

The severe protocol has been approved by the FDA for clinical investigation at 24 centers in the United States. For this protocol, adults must be postlinguistically deaf with onset of severe hearing loss after age 12. For patients to be placed in the severe protocol, they must demonstrate open-set speech recognition with their hearing aids. Their scores on CID[22] and Iowa Sentence[23] tests need to be 25% or less bilaterally and 30% or less binaurally.[32] For individuals in this protocol, the Nucleus device is implanted in the ear with poorer speech recognition ability, and they are expected to wear a well fitted hearing aid on the opposite ear to take full advantage of speech recognition abilities.

The pre/perilinguistic protocol is approved by the FDA for clinical investigation at 20 centers in the United States. The adult protocol requires (1) candidates be at least 18 years of age, (2) onset of deafness before the age of 5, (3) spoken English as the primary mode of communication, and (4) little or no benefit from hearing aids.[33] However, in our experience with this population, other factors need to be considered, such as the individual's (1) past and present use of amplification, (2) social environment, (3) communication skills, (4) noise levels at work, (5) motivation to participate in at least 4 months of therapy after receiving the implant, and (6) expectations of benefit the implant can provide.

PERFORMANCE OF IMPLANT RECIPIENTS

Results with the cochlear implant vary from person to person; however, most recipients who had normal hearing and then lost their hearing as an adult can understand significant amounts of speech without speechreading when listening with the implant. Many can converse interactively on the telephone. Even individuals who had hearing loss as a child that progressed to profound

Table 13–9. Mean Scores (Percent Correct) and Standard Deviations on Three Speech Recognition Tests for Postlinguistically Deaf Cochlear Implant Recipients After 3–6 Months of Implant Use*

Speech Tests	N	Mean (%)	Range (%)	SD (%)
NU-6 Word Test	48	17.6	(0–58)	16.4
Iowa Sentence Test	50	42.6	(0–100)	31.7
CID Everyday Sentence Test	45	48.9	(0–100)	32.8

* All recipients wore the Mini Speech Processor (MSP) and used the Multi-Peak speech coding strategy (see section entitled Function for description of Multi-Peak speech coding strategy).[42]

loss as an adult are able to understand significant amounts of speech using the implant without speechreading. Table 13–9 shows the mean scores and standard deviations on three speech recognition tests for a group of postlinguistically deaf cochlear implant recipients after 3–6 months of implant use.[34]

On the average, postlinguistically deaf adults in the severe protocol understand speech as well as the group whose scores are shown in Table 13–9. However, when they use the implant and a hearing aid (at the contralateral ear), many are able to understand significantly more speech than with the implant alone.[35]

Unlike the postlinguistic population, adult pre/perilinguistic recipients do not understand speech by sound alone with their implants. Because deafness occurred at birth or around the time of learning language, the pre/perilinguistic population has very limited auditory memory. That is, they cannot effectively combine sound that the implant provides with sound they remember in order to recognize environmental sounds and understand speech. Pre/perilinguistic implant recipients learn to identify sounds much like a baby learns to identify sounds, by associating the sound with the object. Consequently, much work and commitment is required from the recipient for successful implant use.

Nevertheless, pre/perilinguistically deaf adults do enjoy some benefits that postlinguistically deaf adults enjoy with their implants. These include hearing sound from 250 to 6000 Hz at medium and even soft levels, recognition of many environmental sounds, improvement in the ease and accuracy of speechreading, improvement in monitoring the loudness of their voice, and feeling less isolated and more involved in daily life.

Evaluation for Cochlear Implant Candidacy

To determine whether a person is a cochlear implant candidate, the following tests need to be performed: an audiologic evaluation, evaluation of speech recognition skills, medical examination, computed tomographic (CT) scans of the temporal bone, electrical stimulation of the inner ear, vestibular function, and a psychological evaluation.

AUDIOLOGIC EVALUATION

The audiologic evaluation should include pure-tone air and bone conduction thresholds, speech reception or detection thresholds, speech recognition scores, and acoustic immittance. The typical audiogram for a cochlear implant candidate will show a severe or profound hearing loss with very poor speech recognition scores. The speech recognition score is often the most important factor in determining whether a person should be considered for an implant. If scores at both ears are 12% or less for NU-6 word lists, the person may be an implant candidate and should be referred for further evaluation. Many times, unaided speech recognition scores are not obtained because sound cannot be made loud enough. In this case, aided speech recognition testing should be performed in the sound field with well fitted hearing aids. If aided scores on NU-6 word lists presented at 70 dB SPL are 12% or less, a referral should be made for a cochlear implant evaluation.

EVALUATION OF AIDED SPEECH RECOGNITION SKILLS

Speech recognition skills are evaluated with well-fitted hearing aids (as described in the section on Evaluation of Hearing Aid Benefit) to determine the amount of benefit the person receives. At the present time, no one should be implanted who scores higher than the mean scores given in Table 13–9. The criteria for implantation may rise if future speech processing strategies and implant systems enable implant recipients to obtain higher scores than they can with present strategies and systems.

MEDICAL EXAMINATION

An examination by an implant team otolaryngologist is required to rule out any outer or middle ear pathology. It is important for the physician to have a complete history of past ear infections and surgeries. Active ear infections need to be resolved before an implant can be considered.[27] In addition, each candidates' general health must be sufficient to tolerate general anesthesia and the lengthy postoperative fitting and aural rehabilitation program.

EVALUATION WITH CT SCANS OF THE TEMPORAL BONE

CT scans are needed to rule out a space occupying lesion of the internal auditory canal and to evaluate patency of the cochleae especially at the first part of the basal turn where bone growth is most likely to occur.[27] Otosclerosis, temporal bone fracture, bacterial meningitis, and Mondini deformity all can affect insertion depth and/or placement of the electrode array. Information from the CT scan in conjunction with results from the electrical stimulation test and hearing aid history are used to determine ear of implantation.

Electrical Stimulation of the Inner Ear

Promontory stimulation testing is performed to determine if the individual can hear sound through electrical stimulation. The ear canal and eardrum are anesthetized; the physician places the active needle electrode transtympanically so that the uninsulated tip is in the mucosa on the inferior edge of the promontory near the round window. The ground electrode is placed on the person's cheek. The stimulus is a square wave (500 msec on/off). The person's ability to hear sound by electrical stimulation is evaluated for the following tests: threshold levels, growth of loudness, gap detection, frequency discrimination, and adaptation. Both ears are usually tested, allowing the person an opportunity to compare the sound quality at the two ears. The ear with the lowest threshold levels (μA), least adaptation, smallest gap detection thresholds, and best frequency discrimination is also identified; one ear may be better than the other on some or all of these measures. This information is considered in choosing the ear for implantation.

EVALUATION OF VESTIBULAR FUNCTION

Although most individuals who are profoundly hearing impaired have little, if any, vestibular function, it is important to evaluate the status of the vestibular system. Those with vestibular function may experience dizziness after surgery, and they need to be counseled appropriately prior to surgery.

PSYCHOLOGICAL EVALUATION

The psychological evaluation is an integral part of the evaluation process and should be conducted by a psychologist who has experience with severely and profoundly hearing impaired individuals. This evaluation should provide information on patients' feelings about and ability to cope with hearing loss, the kind of relationships they have with family, friends, and co-workers, their expectations for the implant, and their closure skills given incomplete information. Since cochlear implantation often causes marked changes in a recipient's life and in patterns of relating to family and friends, implantation can be stressful, especially if expectations are not met. Consequently, the psychological evaluation provides useful information for appropriately counseling the implant candidates and their families.

Factors Associated With Successful Implant Use

Certain factors contribute to successful implant use; consideration of these factors will assist the team in counseling candidates and preparing them for implantation. These factors include duration of deafness, hearing aid use, age at implantation, communication skills (including speech, language, speech-reading, and communicative assertiveness), motivation, support from family, friends, and co-workers, and the postoperative aural rehabilitation program.

Duration of Deafness, Hearing Aid Use, and Age at Implantation

The duration of deafness is usually defined as the length of time an implant recipient has been unable to understand speech with hearing aids. Several studies have shown that the shorter the duration of deafness the better the performance of postlinguistically deaf implant recipients on speech recognition tests presented audition-only.[27,36,37] These studies have also shown that the younger the age at implantation and the shorter the length of time between hearing aid use and implantation, the better will be performance on speech recognition tests.

Speech, Language, Speechreading, and Communicative Assertiveness Skills

The more adequate that implant recipients' speech, language, speechreading, and communicative assertiveness skills are, the more successful they will be with the implant. Almost all postlinguistically deaf adults have adequate speech and language skills, although their competence varies. Their speech-reading skills and communicative assertiveness skills vary from excellent to almost non-existent. Although some pre/perilinguistically deaf adults have excellent skills in all these areas, overall this population is much more likely to have poorly developed skills. Without intelligible speech, no amount of success with an implant will permit the interactive communication for which the implant was designed. Because all implant recipients use speechreading to enhance communication, the greater the ability to speechread, the more successful implant use will be.

Communicative assertiveness is a necessary skill. All implant recipients have times when they do not understand what is said and are required to respond. Recipients who have a knowledge of communication strategies and are able to employ them effectively will be more successful communicators.

Motivation

Motivation to be part of the hearing world is a necessary prerequisite to implantation. For the pre/perilinguistic candidate, motivation needs to be carefully assessed and separated from curiosity about what the implant may provide.

Another aspect of motivation is attitude. An open-minded approach to the process and to problem solving and a willingness to experience new situations and ways of managing them are likely to lead to more successful implant use. It is important to evaluate this attitude in older candidates because many tend to be less open-minded than younger candidates. Motivation to hear and to work at improving listening skills is necessary to complete the postoperative therapy program successfully.

Support From Family, Friends, and Co-workers

Support has been so important to the success of implant candidates that many programs require a "helper" to accompany the candidate through the process. This person is a friend or family member who provides moral support for the candidate, is a liaison between the candidate and other family members regarding the implantation process and expectations, and is someone with whom the candidate can practice the listening and communication skills that are being taught in the aural rehabilitation program.

If the candidate is employed, it is very important that a member of the cochlear implant team make a presentation to co-workers describing how the implant system works, emphasizing the need for patience as the recipient progresses through the therapy program, and describing ways in which they can improve their communication styles to assist their co-worker.

Postoperative Aural Rehabilitation Program

Many implant programs do not provide a therapy program despite the fact it has been shown that the greatest improvement in performance takes place in the first 9 months following initial stimulation[36] and that a therapy program initiated immediately following initial stimulation yields better performance scores than a delayed program conducted 9 months after initial stimulation with the implant.[38] A recent study suggests that, beyond the therapy program, recipients' progress needs to be carefully monitored because speech processor programs may not remain appropriate.[39]

Counseling Cochlear Implant Candidates

Candidates and family members should be thoroughly counseled regarding the benefits and limitations of a cochlear implant. Realization of the hard work, time, patience, and positive stress inherent in the process will ease some of the strain of the rehabilitation process. It is important for the candidate and helper to meet at least two implant recipients and their family members so that they can form more realistic expectations about implantation, benefits provided by an implant, and the rehabilitation process. Candidates may also want to wear a dummy processor and headset for several days to experience the day to day operational problems of being an implant user. Questionnaires, such as the Communication Profile for the Hearing Impaired (CPHI)[40] and the Performance Inventory for Profound and Severe Loss (PIPSL),[41] given both to the candidate and the significant other, can assist the team members in documenting perceived handicap and the use of positive and negative compensatory strategies that will need to be addressed during therapy.

Cochlear Implant

Description

The Nucleus 22 Channel Cochlear Implant System[27] consists of internal and external components (see Fig. 13–5). The internal components include the array (22 electrodes, 10 supporting rings and lead wires), the receiver/stimulator, and magnet. During surgery, the electrodes and ten supporting rings are placed in the scala tympani of the cochlea. The receiver/stimulator and magnet are seated behind the ear in the mastoid bone and completely covered by skin. Surgery usually lasts 2 to 3 hours and is done under general anesthesia. Patients spend 1.5–2 days in the hospital unless there are complications.

The external portion of the implant consists of the microphone, transmitter coil, and speech processor, which are connected by thin cables. The microphone is worn over the ear, similar to a BTE hearing aid, and the transmitter coil adheres to the skin over the site of the receiver/stimulator via a magnet. The speech processor is worn in a pocket, on a belt, or in a harness.

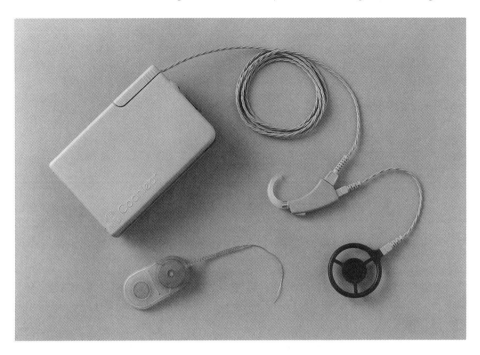

Figure 13–5. External and internal components of the Nucleus 22 Channel Cochlear Implant System. (Photograph courtesy of Cochlear Corporation, Englewood, CO.)

Function

Sound is detected by the microphone, amplified, and sent to the speech processor. The processor selects and codes important information from incoming sound and sends this information to the transmitter. The transmitter sends the coded sound through the skin to the receiver/stimulator. The receiver/stimulator decodes sound and causes appropriate electrodes to be successively stimulated with the correct current amplitude and pulse width. Electrical current from the electrodes stimulates the acoustic nerve. The nerve sends the signals to the brain, which interprets them as sound.

The speech-coding strategy determines what information the speech processor selects and codes. Nucleus speech processors are feature extractors that encode the fundamental frequency (F0) of speech, the frequency of spectral peaks in regions of the first and second formant (F1, F2) of speech, and the amplitude of these peaks.[27] In the most widely used speech-coding strategy, Multi-Peak, spectral energy is also detected by three high frequency bandpass filters. This strategy provides the person with high frequency information in addition to information from the first and second formants of speech.[42] Other speech-coding strategies currently available include F0F1F2, F0F2, F1F2, and F1F1F2.[43] Alternative speech-coding strategies are being evaluated, and the most promising will be available for future use.[44,45]

Fitting

The speech processor is programmed specifically for each person. Programming the speech processor occurs 4–6 weeks after surgery so that the incision site can heal, the swelling can recede, and the transmitter will adhere safely to the skin over the receiver/stimulator. At this time, the person receives the external components of the implant. To program the speech processor, the audiologist uses an IBM-compatible computer with a Dual Processor Interface (DPI). The speech processor is placed in the DPI, and the audiologist uses a control knob on the DPI and the computer keyboard to control the stimulus. The stimulus is a 250 Hz biphasic pulse (500 msec on/off). The audiologist obtains judgments from threshold to maximum comfortable listening levels for each electrode. To do this, the person rates the loudness of the stimulus on each electrode according to a loudness scale. The loudness of sound on all electrodes should be equal at the very soft, medium, and maximum loudness levels.

Differences in pitch throughout the electrode array should be apparent to postlinguistically deaf adults with stimulation on the most apical electrode (#22) perceived as low pitched and stimulation on the most basal electrode (#1) perceived as high pitched.

When an electrode is electrically stimulated, current flows from active to ground electrode. Choice of electrode pairing mode determines the number of electrodes between the active and ground electrodes and the number of electrodes available for programming. The Common Ground mode of electrode pairing is usually used to program children, and a Bipolar mode is usually used for adults. For Common Ground, when each of the 22 electrodes are active, the other 21 are coupled together as the common return or ground. This mode allows detection of faulty electrodes. For Bipolar pairing, one electrode is active and an adjacent apical electrode is the ground. For Bipolar + 1 to Bipolar + 3 pairings, one to three inactive electrodes are between the active and ground electrodes, respectively. With a wider pairing mode, less current is needed to reach very soft and maximum comfortable listening levels because a wider portion along the acoustic nerve is stimulated.[42]

The software used to program the speech processor allows for selection of speech-coding strategies (see description above), as well as many other parameters, to give the best sound quality and clarity to each patient. All parameters need to be examined to develop the clearest and most comfortable program for each person. The goal is for the speech processor program to provide sound so that in everyday life:

1. Conversational speech is comfortably loud
2. Sounds at normal levels are easily heard without visual cues
3. Very loud sounds are not uncomfortable
4. Medium soft and soft sounds can be heard
5. Pitch is balanced across the electrode array
6. Soft noise levels do not interfere with speech understanding.

After first stimulation with the implant system, the individual returns to the center either once or twice a week for adjustments in the speech processor program and aural rehabilitation therapy. Postlinguistically deaf adults return once a week for 10 weeks and pre/perilinguistically deaf adults return twice a week for 17 weeks and monthly thereafter for the remainder of the year. For pre/perilinguistic patients to reach their full potential with the implant, therapy beyond the required time is often necessary.

Aural Rehabilitation Therapy

A severe or profound hearing impairment causes a marked loss or distortion of auditory information which forces the person to use speechreading in an attempt to understand what other people say. Even with speechreading, the information received is incomplete; this results in a loss of the usual fluency of interactive conversation. Individuals vary in the degree to which they miss or misunderstand what is said as well as in their use of repair strategies to converse with other people. Disfluencies in this interactive process can make the person with hearing impairment self-conscious and resistant to working on maintaining relationships. New relationships are particularly difficult to form. A loss of interaction can result in irritability, anxiety, and depression and can negatively affect a person's sense of well-being. An appreciation of the complex nature of an individual's hearing impairment and its effect on that person's ability to communicate are a necessary prerequisite to setting goals for aural rehabilitation therapy.[46]

The effect of hearing impairment on communication, the paucity of aural rehabilitation services beyond the fitting of a hearing aid, and the hearing population's lack of knowledge of how to communicate with persons with hearing impairment contribute to the likelihood that some aural rehabilitation therapy will be necessary, especially for those with severe or profound hearing impairment. Aural rehabilitation therapy may take the form of speechreading auditory training, guidance in using assistive listening devices and hearing aids or a cochlear implant effectively, music therapy, communicative assertiveness (including development of effective communication strategies for the individual and family members), telephone training, environmental sound training, and counseling.

The goal of aural rehabilitation therapy is to provide clients and their families with strategies necessary for communicating effectively in situations encountered in everyday life and to practice the strategies so that they can be employed effectively. A detailed description of this therapy for individuals with hearing aids or cochlear implants is beyond the scope of this chapter and can be found in other publications.[46–53] However, it is important to describe a few central concepts.

An understanding of a family member's hearing loss and the resulting degree of disability can only contribute positively to improved communication between this person and the family. For this reason, it is very beneficial to include family members in as much of the rehabilitative process as is feasible, providing, of course, that the basic relationship between these family members is positive. Hearing loss simulation, administration of a speechreading test without sound, and visiting support groups for hearing impaired persons are just a few ideas that can assist families to understand better the impact of hearing loss on their family member.

Assistive listening devices are a much under-used option for people with all levels of hearing impairment. For those with severe and profound hearing loss, however, they may make the difference between functioning successfully or not. Alerting devices, TDDs, closed captioned decoders, and personal listening systems should be explored. For profoundly impaired hearing aid users, a personal listening system may need to be worn at all times, not just in typically difficult listening situations.

Another overlooked area of aural rehabilitation is communication strategies training. It cannot be assumed that compensatory strategies will emerge as needed, although some individuals may acquire them more easily than others. Without this training, few individuals will make full use of their available skills. Persons who successfully use communication strategies will be regarded by their communication partners as communicating more fluently and earnestly than those who pretend to understand.

For those hearing aid users who can still interact in groups and have never taken an aural rehabilitation class, the group setting is recommended instead of individual therapy. The opportunity to meet others in similar situations and to share with people who understand their concerns on a personal level can often move them toward healthy attitudes of self help. Individual therapy would be recommended for those who have already taken a group class or for those whose disability does not permit communication in group situations.

Aural rehabilitation therapy for cochlear implant recipients is recommended for several reasons: (1) Hearing via electrical stimulation is crude compared with the normal hearing mechanism, and the auditory information received is incomplete. Listening training with the implant can strengthen auditory skills and demonstrate to individuals their skills and limitations. (2) Observation of an individual's performance on auditory tasks and fluency of communication on speechreading plus audition tasks can assist the audiologist in adjusting the speech processor program for optimal reception of speech. (3) Counseling of the recipient and family members about operation of the implant, effective use of the implant and its accessories in various situations, and continued counseling about expectations for performance with the implant are all important for the recipient to be comfortable with this apparatus. (4) In the case of progressive loss, many ineffective communication strategies (e.g., saying "huh?" or pretending to understand) have been in use for many years by the time a person is a candidate for a cochlear implant. In the case of a sudden loss, the person may have not had the time or training to develop a working set of communication strategies.

Support groups can play a vital role in the continued rehabilitation of those with hearing aids or cochlear implants. Self Help for Hard of Hearing People (SHHH), Inc.,[54] is an international organization with hundreds of local chapters around the country. Both hearing aid users and cochlear implant recipients attend. The Cochlear Implant Club International (CICI)[55] is also an international group with local chapters, although smaller in size. Both organizations have newsletters and regular conventions for members.

Summary

The more auditory information individuals with severe or profound hearing impairment receive, the easier it is for them to communicate in everyday life. Consequently, it is very important to optimize the fitting of hearing aids or a cochlear implant to provide as much auditory information as possible given individuals' auditory processing capabilities.

The provision of well fitted hearing aids, a cochlear implant, and assistive listening devices must be incorporated into a comprehensive program of aural rehabilitation to maximize an individual's ability to communicate in everyday life. In this program, therapy is essential to develop effective communication strategies for the individual and the family and to provide guidance in using devices, auditory training for speech sounds, music and environmental sounds, training in use of the telephone, and counseling.

Results of recent research on new sound processing strategies for hearing aids and cochlear implants obtained from adults with profound hearing impairment[56,57] suggest that more auditory information may be provided by commercially available devices in the future. Since the processing will be nonlinear, new strategies for fitting these devices will have to be developed.

Acknowledgments

Preparation of this manuscript was funded by grant RO1-DC00581 from the National Institute on Deafness and Other Communication Disorders. We would like to express our gratitude to Lisa Potts and to our patients for their assistance in collecting the data for this chapter.

References

1. American National Standards Institute: *American National Standard Specifications for Audiometers,* ANSI S3.6-1989. New York: ANSI, 1989.
2. Katz J, White TP: Introduction to the handicap of hearing impairment in the adult: Auditory impairment versus hearing handicap, in Hull RH (ed): *Rehabilitative Audiology.* New York: Grune & Stratton, 1982, pp 13–25.
3. Shannon RV, Fayad J, Moore J, et al.: Auditory brainstem implant: II. Postsurgical issues and performance. *Otol Head Neck Surg* 1993; 168:634–642.
4. Lybarger SF: U.S. Patent application SN 543,278, 1944.
5. Libby ER: The 1/3–2/3 insertion gain hearing aid selection guide. *Hear Instrum* 1986; 37(3): 27–28.
6. Schwartz D, Lyregaard PE, Lundh P: Hearing aid selection for severe-to-profound hearing loss. *Hear J* 1988; 41(2):13–17.
7. Seewald RC: The Desired Sensation Level Method for fitting children: Version 3.0. *Hear J* 1992; 45(4):38–41.
8. Seewald RC, Zelisko RL, Ramji KV, et al.: *DSL 3.0 User's Manual.* London, Ontario, Canada: The University of Western Ontario, 1991.
9. Cornelisse LE, Gagne JP, Seewald RC: Ear level recordings of the long-term average spectrum of speech. *Ear Hear* 1991; 12:47–54.

10. Shaw EAG, Vaillancourt MM: Transformation of sound-pressure level from the free field to the eardrum presented in numerical form. *J Acoust Soc Am* 1985; 78:1120–1123.
11. Cox RM, Moore JN: Composite speech spectrum for hearing aid gain prescriptions. *J Speech Hear Res* 1988; 31:102–107.
12. Pascoe DP: An approach to hearing aid selection. *Hear Instrum* 1978; 29(6):12–16, 36.
13. Frye GJ: High-speech real-time hearing aid analysis. *Hear J* 1986; 39(6):21–36.
14. Revit L, Valente M: Personal communication, 1992.
15. Byrne D, Dillon H: Evaluation of the National Acoustic Laboratories' new hearing aid selection procedure. *Ear Hear* 1986; 7:257–265.
16. Byrne D, Parkinson A, Newall P: Modified hearing aid selection procedures for severe-profound hearing losses, in Studebaker G, Bess F, Beck L (eds): *The Vanderbilt Hearing-Aid Report II*. Baltimore, MD: York Press, 1991, pp 295–300.
17. Byrne D, Parkinson A, Newall P: Hearing aid gain and frequency response requirements for the severely/profoundly hearing impaired. *Ear Hear* 1990; 11:40–49.
18. Seewald RC, Hudson S, Gagne JP, Zelisko DL: Comparison of two methods for estimating the sensation level of amplified speech. *Ear Hear* 1992; 13:142–149.
19. Skinner MW: *Hearing Aid Evaluation*. Englewood-Cliffs, NJ: Prentice-Hall, 1988, pp 83–97.
20. Bentler RA, Pavlovic CV: Addendum to "Transfer functions and correction factors used in hearing aid evaluation and research." *Ear Hear* 1992; 13:284–286.
21. Tillman TW, Carhart R: An Expanded Test for Speech Discrimination Utilizing CNC Monosyllabic Words. *Northwestern University Auditory Test No. 6*. Technical Report No. SAM-TR-66-55. Brooks Air Force Base, Texas: USAF School of Aerospace Medicine, 1966.
22. Davis H, Silverman SR: *Hearing and Deafness*, ed 4. Baltimore: Holt, Rhinehart, and Winston, 1978, pp 537–538.
23. Tyler RS, Preece JP, Lowder MW: *The Iowa Cochlear Implant Tests*. Iowa City: University of Iowa, 1983 (addendum, 1985).
24. Owens E, Kessler DK, Raggio MW, et al.: Analysis and revision of the Minimal Auditory Capabilities (MAC) battery. *Ear Hear* 1985; 6:280–290.
25. Johnson DD: Communication characteristics of a young adult deaf population: Techniques for evaluating their communication skills. *Am Ann Deaf* 1974; 121:409–424.
26. Bernstein LE, Eberhardt SP: *Johns Hopkins Lipreading Corpus*. Baltimore: The Johns Hopkins University, 1986.
27. Clark GM, Blamey PJ, Brown AM, et al.: The University of Melbourne—Nucleus Multi-Electrode Cochlear Implant. *Adv Otorhinolaryngol* 1987; 38:1–189.
28. Dorman MF, Hannley MT, Dankowski K, et al.: Word recognition by 50 patients fitted with the Symbion multichannel cochlear implant. *Ear Hear* 1989; 10:44–49.
29. Dorman MF, Dankowski K, McCandless G, et al.: Longitudinal changes in word recognition by patients who use the Ineraid cochlear implant. *Ear Hear* 1990; 11:455–459.
30. Schindler RA, Kessler DA: State of the art cochlear implants: The UCSF experience. *Am J Otol* 1989; 10:79–83.
31. Schindler RA, Kessler DA: Preliminary results with the Clarion cochlear implant. *Laryngoscope* 1992; 102:1006–1013.
32. *Clinical Study for Severely Hearing Impaired Adults*. Englewood, CO: Cochlear Corporation, 1989.
33. *Prelingual/Perilingual Adult Clinical Study Protocol*. Englewood, CO: Cochlear Corporation, 1988.
34. Arndt PL: Data from Cochlear Corporation, 1992.
35. Arndt PL, Brimacombe JA, Staller SJ, et al.: Multichannel cochlear implantation in adults with residual hearing. Paper presented at the annual meeting of the American Academy of Otolaryngology—Head and Neck Surgery Foundation, Inc., Kansas City, MO, September 24, 1991.
36. Tye-Murray N, Tyler RS, Woodworth GG, et al.: Performance over time with a Nucleus or Ineraid cochlear implant. *Ear Hear* 1992; 13:200–209.
37. Blamey PJ, Pyman BC, Clark GM, et al.: Factors predicting postoperative sentence scores in postlinguistically deaf adult cochlear implant patients. *Ann Otol Rhinol Laryngol* 1992; 101:342–348.
38. Lansing C, Davis JM: Evaluating the relative contribution of aural rehabilitation and experience to the communication performance of adult cochlear implant users: Preliminary data, in Olswang LB, Thompson CK, Warren ST, et al. (eds): *Treatment Efficacy Research in Communication Disorders*. American Speech-Language-Hearing Foundation, 1990, pp 215–221.
39. Skinner MW, Holden LK, Demorest ME, et al.: Development of a protocol for monitoring performance of adults with cochlear implants. *Ear Hear* (in submission).
40. Demorest ME, Erdmann SA: Development of the Communication Profile for the Hearing Impaired. *J Speech Hear Dis* 1987; 52:129–143.
41. Owens E, Raggio M: Performance Inventory for Profound and Severe Loss (PIPSL). *J Speech Hear Dis* 1988; 53:42–56.

42. Skinner MW, Holden LK, Holden TA, et al.: Performance of postlinguistically deaf adults with the Wearable Speech Processor (WSP III) and Mini Speech Processor (MSP) of the Nucleus Multi-Electrode Cochlear Implant. *Ear Hear* 1991; 12:3–22.
43. *Audiologist's Handbook.* Englewood, CO: Cochlear Corporation, 1989.
44. Whitford LA, Seligman PM, Blamey PJ, et al.: Comparison of current speech coding strategies. Paper presented at the International Symposium on Cochlear Implants, Toulouse, France, June 2–3, 1992.
45. McDermott HJ, McKay CM, Bandali AE: A new portable sound processor for the University of Melbourne/Nucleus Limited multi-electrode cochlear implant. *J Acoust Soc Am* 1992; 91:3367–3371.
46. Erber NP: *Communication Therapy for Hearing-Impaired Adults.* Abbotsford, Victoria, Australia: Clavis Publishing, 1988.
47. Alpiner JG (ed): *Handbook of Adult Rehabilitative Audiology,* ed 2. Baltimore: Williams & Wilkins, 1982.
48. Eisenberg L: *Basic Guidance for Children With the Cochlear Implant,* rev ed. Los Angeles: House Ear Institute, 1983.
49. Eisenberg L: *Introduction to Sound: A Therapy Program Developed for the Prelingually Deaf Adult Using a Cochlear Implant.* Los Angeles: House Ear Institute, 1980.
50. Giolas TG: *Hearing-Handicapped Adults.* Englewood-Cliffs, NJ: Prentice-Hall, 1982.
51. Kienle M: *Adult Auditory Rehabilitation Manual.* St. Paul, MN: 3M Corp., 1987.
52. *Mini System 22 Rehabilitation Manual.* Englewood CO, Cochlear Corporation, January 1992.
53. Norton N, Eisenberg L, Berliner K, et al.: *Cochlear Implant Manual.* Los Angeles: House Ear Institute, 1980.
54. Self Help for Hard of Hearing People, Inc., 7800 Wisconsin Avenue, Bethesda, MD 20814.
55. Cochlear Implant Club International, P.O. Box 464, Buffalo, NY 14223-0464.
56. Faulkner A, Ball V, Rosen S, et al.: Speech pattern hearing aids for the profoundly hearing impaired: Speech perception and auditory abilities. *J Acoust Soc Am* 1992; 91:2136–2155.
57. Bimodal Speech Processor (Com-Bionic Aid)—Engineering and Speech Processing Studies, in *Annual Report of the Human Communication Research Centre, University of Melbourne.* East Melbourne, Australia, 1990, pp 18–19.
58. International Organization for Standardization: *Acoustics—Standard Reference Zero for the Calibration of Pure-Tone Air Conduction Audiometers,* ed 2. ISO 389. Geneva: International Organization for Standardization, 1985.

14

Future Trends in Hearing Aid Fitting Strategies: With A View Towards 2020

Barbara Kruger, Frederick M. Kruger

Introduction

This chapter is organized into four sections. The first section provides some brief comments on terminology. It will then look at (1) the cyclic pattern of progress from past to present and (2) the status of current fitting strategies as foundations for the future (see also Chs. 1 and 2). The second section considers the impact of evolving technologies on future fitting systems. The third section discusses fitting strategies for the next 5–10 years. It considers (1) prescriptive selection for linear and nonlinear circuitry, (2) predicting speech recognition ability of target hearing aid performance using the articulation index, (3) the projection of hearing aid performance measures into the individual's auditory area, and (4) the functions of the universal integrated hearing aid fitting systems. The fourth section speculates about fitting strategies with a view toward the year 2020. It considers (1) the evolution of a loudness-based hearing aid fitting system, (2) the articulation index, and (3) the modified speech transmission index.

Fitting strategies are presently defined as the a priori selection of the appropriate device and amplification requirements for a hearing impaired individual. They encompass the methods for measurement and specification of both the appropriate circuitry or electroacoustic characteristics (e.g., frequency response, gain, output, input–output function) and the appropriate type and/or size of the housing for the hearing aid(s).

Verification strategies encompass the methods by which one evaluates and *affirms* that what was selected and manufactured achieves the goals specified by the prescription. In the future, fitting and verification strategies will be

300

inseparable components of the hearing aid dispensing process, even more than they are today.

Cyclic Pattern of Progress

In each 10–20 year period of the past 60 years, there have been significant advances in hearing aid design and performance, as well as in the strategies involved for selecting and verifying hearing aid fittings. The changes of the past decade have been especially dramatic.

CLINICAL EVOLUTION

Historically, prescriptive methods and speech-based comparison methods have alternated as primary hearing aid fitting strategies.[1–3] Several key fitting strategies illustrate the early emergence of prescriptive or selective amplification methods.[4–6] At that time, the Harvard[7] and MedResCo[8] reports effectively eliminated the use of prescriptive methods by stating that one or two general frequency–response curves, which were not related to the audiogram or equal loudness contour, could adequately compensate for most hearing losses, despite the inaccuracies later illustrated by Resnick[9] and Killion and Monser.[10] Then, the evaluation and selection of hearing aids based on speech reception threshold, speech recognition score (historically and incorrectly called a *speech discrimination score*), and threshold of tolerance emerged.[11] This approach was practiced widely throughout the 1970s[12,13] and even into the mid-1980s.[14] Research as early as 1960[15,16] indicated that the resolution of speech recognition scores was far poorer than required by this fitting method. It was not until data from Thornton and Raffin[17] and Studebaker[18] more clearly illustrated the inadequate resolution of this technique that the direction changed back toward prescriptive methods.

Prescriptive methods began to reappear in the 1960s and early 1970s for adults[19–21] and for children.[22,23] It was not until the late 1970s and 1980s, however, that the direction of hearing aid fitting strategies again turned strongly toward prescriptive methods. They re-emerged with strength[1,24–39] and mushroomed in popularity in the late 1980s and early 1990s as prescription rules were implemented in real-ear probe tube microphone measurement instrumentation, thereby leading to the birth of contemporary "fitting systems."

Concurrent with the acceptance of prescriptive methods, there is now a re-emergence of the use of speech materials for (1) the selection and verification of optimal hearing aid response,[40,41] (2) the prediction of optimal speech recognition based on the articulation index,[2,42,43] and (3) the evaluation of hearing aid benefit and quality.[44–57]

TECHNOLOGICAL EVOLUTION

Technologic advances in instrumentation resulting from needs defined by research in auditory physiology, psychoacoustics, and physical acoustics during the period extending from the 1940s to the 1980s, have facilitated the strong resurgence of prescriptive methods in the 1980s and 1990s. The modeling of the middle ear and related research in the 1950s–1960s[58–61] led to the development of the impedance bridge. These data and those defining the sound pressure transformations from a free field, to various locations in the ear canal, to the eardrum,[62–66] led to the development of the Zwislocki coupler[67,68] or occluded ear simulator (ANSI S3.25[69]), which represents the median impedance of the human ear. This device allows direct estimates of average real-ear hearing aid performance previously only indirectly possible with the 2 cc coupler, which was intended to be a "temporary" device developed by Romanow.[70] The 2 cc coupler is used for reference calibrations and standardized electroacoustic performance measurements (ANSI S3.7,[71] ANSI S3.22[72]). These data, the data on the real-ear 2 cc coupler sound pressure differences (RECD),[73] and the data from the head and torso and the body baffle effects,[74,75] resulted in the development and standardization of the KEMAR (Knowles Electronics Manikin for Acoustic Research).[76,77]

In the 1960s and 1970s, the emphasis of basic research returned to the modeling and study of cochlear mechanics[78–81] and the psychoacoustics of perception.[82–83] The sense organ was viewed predominantly as a linear processor, but the nonlinearities of the ear began to be identified.[84] In the 1980s and 1990s, physiologic and psychoacoustic findings continued to provide evidence of cochlear nonlinearities.[85–87] The outer hair cells, with significant efferent innervation, were recognized for their involvement in controlling the intensity range from 0 to 70 dB sound pressure level (SPL), somewhat like an automatic gain control (AGC) system. At high levels, the cochlea functions more linearly. Cochlear modeling (of physiology and function) will play an increasing role in explaining cochlear nonlinearities[88] and will make significant contributions to future hearing aid design and hearing aid fitting strategies.

Concurrent developments in physics and electronics resulted in the invention of the transistor, changes in battery technologies, numerous types of semiconductors, CMOS logic, hybrid circuitry, integrated circuits, and more. These developments eventually led to the miniaturization of hearing aids and the creation (in the early 1970s) and the growth of the in-the-ear (ITE) and in-the-canal (ITC) market in the 1980s and 1990s. The expansion of the ITE market increased the desire to understand and specify (real-ear) hearing aid response characteristics on 2 cc couplers. The simulation of the human external ear, the understanding of ear canal resonance, and the relation of sound field pressures to eardrum pressures facilitated both the clarification of the Correction for Flat Insertion Gain (CORFIG)[10] *and* led to changes in microphone, amplifier, and receiver design. This has resulted in the smoother, more wideband frequency ranges found in many of today's hearing aids (promoted by Knowles and Killion,[89] Killion,[90,91] and others).

The development of high speed, microprocessor-based computers, with increased memory capacities and high speed math coprocessors, made it possible to obtain affordable fast-Fourier-transform (FFT) based real-time spectrum analyzers. The design of new, controlled frequency response, miniature microphones and related components helped to take probe microphone measurement out of the laboratories of the 1940s–1970s and into the clinical practice of the 1980s. Today's real-ear probe microphone measurement equipment will continue to advance in sophistication. It will not be just an appendage to hearing aid test box equipment, but will gain in importance as a significant component/subsystem of the future hearing aid fitting and verification systems that implement future fitting strategies. Prescriptive methods, speech-based comparative methods, and benefit determination methods all will be integrated into future hearing aid fitting and verification systems.

Current Fitting Strategies as a Foundation for the Future

Current hearing aid fitting strategies have, as their objective, the optimal audibility of speech sounds within the individual's dynamic range. The expectation is that this will maximize speech recognition and will produce amplification that is comfortably loud. Although all of today's fitting strategies were developed for fitting linear hearing aids, the more sophisticated methods provide a foundation for the strategy modifications needed to fit current nonlinear, multi-band and future digital hearing aids.

An overview, rationale, and comparison of threshold-based (see Ch. 1) and suprathreshold-based (see Ch. 2) gain-prescription hearing aid selection procedures was presented earlier. The reader is also directed elsewhere for information on hearing aid selection/fitting strategies[38,92] and for a "how-to" book on real-ear probe microphone measurements.[93]

With future hearing aid fitting strategies in mind, Hawkins[94] organized current fitting strategies into five categories that range from the very simple to the most sophisticated:

1. Pure-tone audiogram only
2. Pure-tone audiogram and prescription procedure for frequency-gain response with saturation sound pressure level (SSPL90) approximated
3. Pure-tone audiogram and prescription with customized values with a specified, loudness-based SSPL90
4. Pure-tone audiogram and a desired amplified speech spectrum
5. Threshold and suprathreshold measurements to define the dynamic range and amplify the speech spectrum to comfortable loudness.

Of these fitting strategies, the first is the most basic, least professionally responsible, but unfortunately most frequently used. It simply involves sending only the pure-tone audiogram (often only air conduction thresholds) to the manufacturer. Selection of the hearing aid electroacoustic characteristics and performance are entrusted to the manufacturer. At present, when 80% of the U.S. market is the dispensing of ITE and ITC hearing aids, this practice represents 80–90% of the U.S. ITE/ITC market.[93–95] This strategy may appear to be the most economical and most expedient method but, in reality, it does a disservice to the hearing impaired individual, the dispenser, and the manufacturer.

For the second category, the desired real-ear insertion response (REIR) is specified and converted, based on the *average adult CORFIG*, to a desired 2 cc coupler full-on gain (FOG) response for submission to the manufacturer.[25,27,31, 33–35,37,96,97] A dispenser selected matrix is based on the average adult ear.

A desired but non-individualized SSPL90 may be submitted, sometimes with unspecified test criteria, or test stimulus type. This procedure is popular (faster) and allows prescription for individuals from whom it is difficult to obtain loudness judgments.

In the third prescription procedure category, the desired REIR is specified and converted, based on a *customized CORFIG*, to a desired 2 cc coupler FOG response. The customized CORFIG may be derived from the real-ear unaided response (REUR)[98,99] and/or real-ear–coupler difference (RECD).[100–104] A dispenser selected matrix is corrected for the individual variation of the REUR and/or RECD. Calculation of the 2 cc FOG response, corrected for the individual REUR and/or RECD, is now available in software for real-ear hearing aid fitting equipment (e.g., Fonix 6500) and as an independent software pack-age.[105] A suggested SSPL90 response is more often based on loudness discomfort measures rather than remaining unspecified.[28,106] This approach reduces variability. The justification for customization of the REIR has been debated, since earphone or sound field thresholds are referenced to an *average* ear, not the individual ear.[98,99,106] Killion and Revit[104] suggest a compromise: half the customized CORFIG or GIFROC (the coupler response to insertion response transformation), depending on the direction of application of the conversion.

The fourth prescriptive procedure category assumes a strong (i.e., predictive) relationship between threshold and suprathreshold loudness levels, such that the desired sensation levels (DSLs) needed to amplify the long-term average speech spectrum (Western Ontario University WOU-LTASS) to comfort levels (MCL) and not exceed discomfort (UCL), are estimated from threshold and converted to 2 cc coupler FOG values. It is the most advanced strategy to date and provides a strong basis for future fitting systems. It, as future fitting systems will, references a large database for DSL calculations and permits direct customization via real-ear measures or indirectly via retrievable age-dependent REURs and RECDs. Furthermore, it anticipates future fitting systems by displaying, in dB SPL, amplified speech within the individual's (e.g., child's) dynamic range or residual auditory area.

The fifth prescriptive procedure category defines the relationship between threshold and suprathreshold loudness levels such that perceptual loudness judgments define the dynamic range ("quiet" to UCL). The resulting amplification raises the long-term average speech spectrum to the MCL without exceeding the UCL.[18,38] The auditory area can be displayed in dB HL on an audiogram or in dB SPL. This method remains the most theoretically appealing and comprehensive, but most cumbersome. Future fitting systems will simplify the implementation of this category of fitting strategy and provide displays that contrast these target responses with those targets generated by the fourth fitting strategy.

Despite advances in hearing aid circuitry, current knowledge, and technologies for hearing aid fitting, at present 90% of the market wears linear hearing aids, which use manufacturer applied fitting strategies. The hearing aid wearers are most satisfied in one-to-one communication (88%) and somewhat less so when watching TV (69%). Satisfaction drops sharply with increasingly complex listening environments. For example, in large group settings satisfaction was lowest (25%).[108] In the future, as hearing aid wearers become more aware of their hearing aid options, they will demand improved fit and all-environment performance.

Most of today's fitting strategies, although designed for use in prescribing gain versus frequency response for linear aids, can be modified for use in future fitting systems. Future prescriptive methods will also specify the electro-acoustics of software-driven digital circuitry that will be dynamic, environmentally responsive, and intelligently selective. They will also specify tomorrow's nonlinear analog compression circuits, digitally programmable analog (single and multiband) circuits, and digital circuits.

Evolving Technologies for Future Fitting Strategies

Audiologic test and fitting equipment manufacturers have endeavored to simplify their equipment–user interface to facilitate proper instrument operation with a minimum of formal training. In the past, each button and control on the panel did only one job and was adequately labeled. With the advent of microprocessor-based systems (and, more recently, desktop microcomputer-controlled "smart" systems), this picture has changed.

Technologic advances have facilitated the design and construction of new test and measurement instruments with cathode ray tube (CRT) or liquid crystal (LCD) displays. Each panel control may have a number of functions, according to which "operating mode" has been selected. The operator will have to learn to use an instrument that "doesn't necessarily *look* like its function." Even more than now, future fitting systems will be able to measure and display information that was not available to the dispenser just a few years ago. In the future, it will no longer be sufficient to open an office, buy an audiometer, and begin to dispense hearing aids.

The Evolving Hearing Aid

The contents of hearing aids have changed radically during the last decade or two. Moreover, these changes only hint at what is to be expected in the next decade or two. By the end of the 1980s, technologically advanced integrated circuits were being designed specifically for use in ITE and ITC hearing aids. Some of these circuits contained input and/or output AGC, filters with much sharper roll-off than previously available (switched capacitor filters), and integrated amplifiers with dynamically adjusted frequency and amplitude characteristics. Several of these latter units could be set to reduce low frequency sensitivity in the presence of steady noise levels, while other units changed their response shape and amount of amplification as the incoming signal level increased.[109–116] These advances in circuitry provide increased flexibility in fixed and level-dependent frequency response shaping.

Hearing Aid Size Versus Function

During all of these developments, hearing aid circuits operated from a single 1.4 V (nominal) "battery." The challenge for the manufacturer has been to synthesize new, more sophisticated integrated circuits that could still operate with a single 1.4 V cell for an extended time period. The marketplace made this a more daunting challenge by insisting on smaller hearing aids with "longer battery life." Of course, smaller hearing aids required smaller batteries. But smaller batteries have less power capacity. This defined, and continues to define, the need for very small, sophisticated, low-power-consumption, integrated circuits with even smaller microphones, receivers, controls, and switches. It has become a race for sophisticated miniaturization.

One glaring problem had been neglected during this period of miniaturization: *the human factor*. At the same time that people were being told that small is better and a canal hearing aid is just short of "invisible in the ear," power switches and batteries were still required. Moreover, many people still insist on having volume controls—even when they are not necessary. Peoples' fingers have not changed in size, but these components have gotten smaller. Many hearing aid candidates cannot manipulate these miniaturized marvels.

Electronic technology has already passed human development in some areas! What *good* prescription strategy would use these new technologies to yield an amplification system design that was truly optimized for the hearing aid candidate, but then specify that it be designed into a tiny canal aid when the intended recipient was 87 years old and arthritic? Clearly, modern prescription strategies must include the human factor as well as psychoacoustic and electroacoustic factors.

The Digital Period Begins—Programmable Analog Hearing Aids and Fitting Systems

As the 1990s began, new hearing aid and hearing aid fitting systems buzz-words were already in use. Some of these (e.g., digital signal processing, digital filtering, digital control, computerized) suggested a little more than reality could deliver at the time. Most of the more sophisticated aids were, at best, analog circuits with digitally based controls or digitally stored settings. This could be called the beginning of the "digital period," since it was during this period that digital computers and microprocessor-based test equipment moved into the clinic. The hearing aids, however, remained digitally programmable analog devices.

To add flexibility, manufacturers have introduced "user programmability" to some of their products. The hearing aid wearer is offered a device for which different operating modes (that is, sets of different functional characteristics for different environmental listening conditions) can be selected. Fitting strategies are needed to specify electroacoustic characteristics for each operational mode. While a few of these units use external "remote" controls to select a particular mode, others use faceplate-mounted selector switches to choose from the different options. These digitally programmed analog hearing aids permit the selection and setting of a myriad of electroacoustic parameters (e.g., gain, output, low frequency cut, slope, high frequency roll-off, compression and/or AGC threshold, attack and release time) in the office. Today, some of the more sophisticated hearing aids are programmed via ultrasonic, radio-frequency, or infrared wireless links or direct connection to an in-office programming device. Few of these hearing aids as yet interface with hearing aid fitting systems, although independent probe microphone measurement-fitting systems can be used to verify their performance.

At the time of this writing (late 1992), the most sophisticated of the available hearing aids can be programmed in the office to closely meet prescription target fitting requirements. If a particular hearing aid does not offer a required (set of) option(s), an alternative model (or manufacturer) must be selected. No single design offering "all" possible fitting/performance options is presently available. Given that limitation, however, greater flexibility is offered hearing aid candidates since they can be fitted with a single device that can be optimized for performance in multiple environments. Alternatively, a difficult fitting can be made possible through the use of a multiband in-office programmable device. (Sometimes, a simple linear hearing aid *will* be the best choice.)

Some of these devices are actually fitted on the patient's ear, using a removable cable connection to the computer-based fitting system, which includes a built-in probe microphone real-ear measurement system as an integral component. The real-ear responses are used directly as the system calculates the new "performance requirements" and then converts the results to control signals that program the digital control memory (EEPROM) of the appended hearing aid. As advanced technologies provide greater flexibility in fitting strategy and option selection, it will be necessary to allow more office time for adjusting or reprogramming hearing aids, with the patient present and connected to the computer-based fitting system or programming equipment. Also, more time will be required for patient judgments, counseling, and explanations.

Digital Hearing Aids and Fitting Systems in the Future

If the late 1980s and early 1990s can be called the "period of the digitally programmable (analog) hearing aid," the next few years will be called the "period of the digital hearing aid." This means that we expect many of the hearing aids of the near future to be truly digital devices. They will convert incoming audio to a digital format, process the signal as called for by the fitting prescription, and then convert it back to the analog domain. In many cases, the digital signal will not even be converted to analog. It will be fed directly to the wideband, low distortion, high output receiver via the Class D output stage. In the late summer of 1992, one company announced that they were marketing a true digital hearing aid: one with both A/D and D/A converters and both digital audio and digital control paths. (The hearing aid was designed to control feedback and thereby permit the wearer to set a higher output level than otherwise possible.) This is only the beginning!

Digital hearing aids and future fitting systems are significant. Even early "smart" digital hearing aids will be reconfigurable in the dispenser's office. These hearing aids will be programmed with the adaptable target frequency responses, amplitude dynamics, and special features (e.g., impulse blanking, input compression and output limiting) selected to meet the individual's

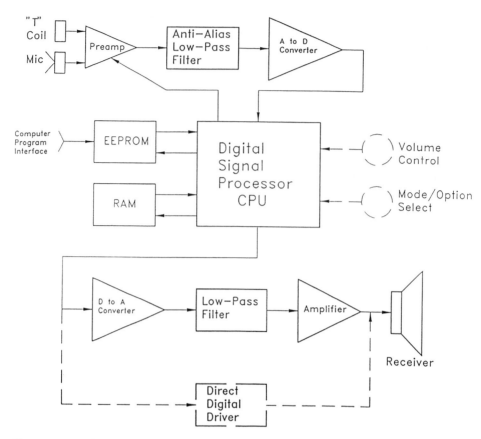

Figure 14–1. Diagram of a digital hearing aid.

needs. When they first appear, it is likely that these hearing aids will contain the following "building blocks," as illustrated in Figure 14–1: microphone preamplifier, anti-aliasing filter, analog-to-digital converter, microcontroller or microprocessor with separate random access and programmable read-only memory, and output direct drive circuits. If a more conventional output circuit is used, the circuit will contain a digital-to-analog converter, a low pass filter, and an output driver stage (which may be a high efficiency Class D converter-amplifier). Each evolving computer-based fitting and/or programming system will communicate with the hearing aids of different manufacturers via "daisy-chained" personality modules. These personality modules will link to the common computer interface at one end and provide the necessary programming, power, and acoustic measurement interfacing at the other.

In the present and near future, a basic digital fitting system will be supported by (if not be a part of) a high performance (e.g., a 33 MHz or faster) 80486-type computer, which will convert a variety of prescription information into programming data to be "down-loaded" (i.e., sent) to the hearing aid. In contrast to today's hearing aids, these new units will not contain any discrete component filters or other special dynamic components. The programmed read only memory (ROM) will contain the instructions (based on fitting decisions) telling the internal microprocessor how to operate on the digitized audio signal in the random access memory (RAM) to shape its frequency and dynamic characteristics. The computer will also accept and display the real-ear acoustic data.

DIGITAL HEARING AID FITTING WILL REQUIRE AN ITERATIVE
ADJUSTMENT PROCESS, WITH PATIENT INVOLVEMENT

In future fitting systems designs, the wearer's audiologic data, fitting information, acoustic environmental performance options, and wearer preferences also will be stored in the hearing aid's programmable ROM. When appropriately programmed by the fitting system, the neural network (or fuzzy logic)–based digital hearing aid will actually use this information to adjust dynamically its operational characteristics to maximize speech recognition ability and perceived sound quality in various types of noisy environments. Unlike recent attempts at special digital processor designs, this new approach will respond instantly to transients, but will adapt its characteristics and performance in a way, and at a rate, which will not be disturbing to the wearer. (A neural network design will permit the hearing aid to adapt to new noise environments even if the exact characteristics of the noise environment were not previously known. Moreover, as the system learns, it will alter the internal fitting data as appropriate. The use of fuzzy logic will permit important computer decisions to be made using indeterminate data.)

The reader may reasonably ask why, if high speed microprocessors and elegant digital signal processors (DSP) were available in 1991, are these true micro-processor and DSP-based digital hearing aids not available now? The answer is complex. First, the integrated circuit chips (i.e., ICs) in these devices contain the equivalent of hundreds of thousands of transistors and require more power, at a higher voltage, than is presently available even in a behind-the-ear (BTE) hearing aid (even with an internal voltage converter). Second, present chips are too large and require too many external connections to be of practical use. Third, the costs to manufacturer and support is high. Fourth, additional research is necessary to define and test potential algorithms for their performance before the hardware designs are perfected. Fifth, large fitting information databases to support the various emerging fitting strategies and computer-based fitting systems need to be defined and developed. Sixth, manufacturers must perceive a viable (and profitable) market before they commit their resources. Finally, new manufacturing technologies may have to be developed before these digital devices are manufactured. In other words, it does not make sense to manufacture a complex digital computer system for fitting a hearing aid until researchers know what algorithms and prescription strategies will work and how to enable the audiologist and dispenser to translate the desired hearing aid performance into firmware.

SOPHISTICATED FITTING SYSTEMS REQUIRE TECHNOLOGICAL
ADVANCES

Several recent developments in semiconductor technology have given us the
confidence to make the above projections. The demand for small, long running, notebook-sized portable computers has resulted in the production of
very small, low power, microprocessor chips that operate on 3 V or less. When
compared with present hearing aid power consumption, however, these
microprocessors still draw too much power. But this is changing almost daily,
as additional 3 V lower power support ICs become available. There are good
reasons why this 3 V operation is a significant milestone: First, reduction of the
operating voltage from 5 to 3 means a smaller chip size and a potential
reduction in power consumption of up to 70%. Second, this 3 V standard
works toward solving both technical and marketing demands. Lower power
means that parts can be packed closer together and battery operational life
is extended. Third, battery technology continues to advance. Newer battery
designs, with more advanced chemistries, will yield even higher power densi-
ties at the new 3 V level. This means that even the more sophisticated digitally
controlled hearing aids of today will be able to shed their battery charge-
pumps, or voltage "up-converters."

Mixed Signal Technology—Impact on Future Fitting Strategies

The concurrent evolution of mixed-signal technology (analog and digital circuits on a single integrated chip) to a present generation of application-specific
microcontrollers, which can interface directly with the analog world, process
information digitally, and then drive real-world analog components, provides
great encouragement regarding the hearing aids of the near future. This mixed-
signal approach will include total DSP applications in the single integrated chip
design. There are numerous examples of single chip mixed-signal designs in
automobiles: keyless entry, anti-skid brakes, and airbag systems. Their success
is likely due to an application-specific integrated circuit design approach that
built mixed-signal functionality around a DSP core.

   Each of these evolutionary steps brings us closer to the day of the custom
fitted, truly programmable, fully digital hearing aid. The fitting of these hearing aids will be enhanced through the application of smart, self-adjusting, and
algorithm remembering circuitry (fuzzy logic and neural network) approaches.
These ITE microprocessor (or DSP)-based hearing aids will even sense the
proximity of a telephone receiver and self-adjust to optimize the acoustic
characteristics of the (very variable) telephone link.

   Through smart circuit design, most of the computing circuitry of the future
microprocessor-based hearing aid will "go to sleep" (i.e., power down, or
turn itself off) when not needed. In a relatively stable acoustic environment,
the microprocessor may stop some functions, while the operational status is
maintained at minimum speed and minimum power. When the environment
becomes more dynamic, the microprocessor circuit will come alive, speed up as
required, and draw upon its internal database to calculate new operational
parameters, digital filter coefficients, gain settings, and so forth, to provide the
hearing aid wearer with optimized performance.

The clinician of the future will have to be more than a "device installer." When a fitting strategy for a particular client is developed, that strategy will include consideration of the client's lifestyle and personal counseling requirements.

Some possible digital hearing aid designs and design approaches are discussed at length, in Chapter 16 (this volume). The hearing aid functions described there will be implemented using very-large-scale integrated circuits and application-specific integrated circuits.

There is a real concern, however: As hearing aids and their programming or configuration hardware become more sophisticated, it will be necessary for key dispensing personnel to acquire advanced computer and electronics skills in addition to their clinical testing, prescribing, and fitting skills. Clinician training programs will have to teach technical as well as clinical skills, since the two are already becoming clinically inseparable. It will be the responsibility of the various certifying and licensing bodies to ensure that the clinicians will be able to prescribe, fit, and counsel adequately. It will be up to the hardware systems manufacturers to develop adequate user interfaces and training programs to ensure easy, yet correct system operation and maintenance.

Future Fitting in the "High-Tech" Office

Consideration must be given to the amount of dedicated equipment necessary to make the fitting of a specific manufacturer's hearing aid(s) possible. This issue becomes significant in an office in which the dispenser selects from a number of manufacturers' products as part of the prescribing activity and therefore requires more than one fitting system and multiple computers.

Most office computers have very few interface slots available. In the authors' offices, for example, five computer systems are linked together via a network based on the RS-422 standard. This standard provides for the "daisy-chaining" of a large number of computers or "smart" peripherals. Only one card slot is required in each computer. Any one computer can fully interact with and use the peripherals of any other, without affecting any of the local activities of the other computers. The computers and client test/evaluation equipment are integrated into one advanced prescribing and fitting system. The manufacturers of these systems can easily and relatively inexpensively include bus interfaces within their products. (A separate computer is, however, required at each test position. In some cases, the additional support computer[s] can be eliminated through the simple [and inexpensive] addition of a keyboard and data bus interface card to a fitting system, or programmer, which has its own internal CRT and microcomputer.)

Future Fitting Strategies in the Foreseeable Future: 5–10 Years

Future hearing aid fitting strategies should provide for the enhancement of audibility, of speech recognition, and of sound quality—for improved communication that is comfortably loud in real-world noise. When possible, the perception of music also should be improved. Future fitting strategies should strive to make amplified sounds comfortably loud. The "comfort" of the amplified sound will be integral to achieving satisfaction with the prescribed hearing aid "fit." Therefore, future fitting strategies will specify the desired nonlinearity of the hearing aid to match, at least, the loudness growth patterns of the listener's ear, especially for those listeners with sensorineural hearing impairment.

The goal of a useful and practical hearing aid fitting strategy is patient/client satisfaction. This should be accomplished efficiently, with a reasonable level of expertise and training, and with little or no patient training. Satisfaction is defined as a "good fit." A good fit will be physically comfortable and will provide optimal acoustic performance. Optimal acoustic performance can be defined as high fidelity compensation that optimizes speech recognition and with which the hearing impaired person is satisfied in situations they judge important, e.g., quiet, watching TV, in small-group and large group multi-listening noisy situations, and listening to music.

Designers and manufacturers of future fitting systems, real-ear probe microphone systems, software, and hearing aids need to note that a complicated, labor intensive, yet theoretically sound and sophisticated fitting method is not likely to be used (viable), even if the method yields consistent patient satisfaction. A sensible pragmatic approach must always consider the patient and the "time in the chair" necessary to get desired results.

Prescriptive Selection for Linear and Nonlinear Circuitry

Today's prescriptive procedures calculate the prescribed REIR from which a target 2 cc coupler FOG response can be derived that should yield the prescribed REIR for linear hearing aids. For each prescriptive target REIR, a different amount of 2 cc coupler FOG is necessary, according to the type of aid (i.e., greatest high frequency gain for BTE and least for ITC), to achieve the same REIR. There is little debate that different prescription rules result in somewhat similar, *but different*, target REIRs (e.g., for low, middle, or high frequencies).[117–123] It has been suggested by some that volume control setting can compensate for the differences across methods (see Ch. 2).[115,122,124–126] In the future, however, focusing on the accuracy of the match of the measured REIR to a target REIR, for a linear hearing and especially for a nonlinear hearing aid, will be less important than describing the desired dynamic performance characteristics in the real ear or 2 cc coupler.

The prescribed REIR for *linear* hearing aids was designed to amplify average conversational speech to the most comfortable loudness for a particular input level (e.g., 60, 65, 70 dB SPL); different speech spectra have been recommended. As the input level changes, the gain of a linear hearing aid remains the same until the hearing aid saturates and distorts at high input levels. For low input levels (i.e., quiet), the gain may be insufficient. For high input levels (even in quiet, without competing sources), the gain may be excessive. To maintain a comfortable listening level, frequent volume control adjustment is required. As a compromise, the typical "use" volume control position is often well below the prescribed REIR.[93,114–116,126,127]

To maintain amplified signals at comfortable levels, without the need for almost constant volume control adjustment, *nonlinear* circuitry is preferable for most sensorineural and even for many mixed hearing losses.[109–116,128] The ear with a sensorineural hearing loss—particularly for a first-time hearing aid user with "recruitment" (reduced dynamic range)—is typically more comfortable with a "smart" hearing aid, or with a "half-smart" hearing aid than with a "simple" linear aid. A smart hearing aid is one that processes sound adaptively with at least a level-dependent frequency response (LDFR). For example, the hearing aid circuitry may have bass increase at low levels (BILL) or treble increase at low levels (TILL).[129] In contrast, a half-smart hearing aid may have a frequency response that remains constant but whose overall gain increases or decreases in reaction to the level of the input signal (i.e., a fixed frequency response [FFR]). Selection of a different compression ratio, threshold knee-point, and/or attack-and-release times may require using a different manufacturer. This may also be true, to a lesser extent, for hearing aids incorporating output compression. In general, either input or output compression is preferred to linear amplification,[130] although the vast majority (80%–90%) of current fittings are still linear. In contrast, since 1989, about 90% of the devices dispensed in the clinical practice of one of the authors have contained nonlinear circuits. In the future, *a principal goal will be to control the type and magnitude of compression as a function of intensity and frequency (per band)*, while other goals will be met by providing additional individually unique capabilities.

EVOLVING FITTING STRATEGIES AS A FUNCTION OF INTENSITY
AND FREQUENCY

Current prescription rules provide a prescribed REIR that is most appropriate for listening in quiet. Prescriptive rules need to be established for reduction of low frequency (and/or midfrequency) gain for improved recognition of speech in environments in which the input level is louder than "average." The interaction of gain and frequency, as a function of the input signal type and level, needs further study to develop better fitting strategies. The rationale for selecting one of the above general types of nonlinear circuits should be based on information obtained (e.g., by report or by analysis of tape recordings) from the prospective hearing aid user about the types of environments (noises) they experience and on the philosophy and experience of the clinician. The digital hearing aid holds the promise of user–environment-dependent processing for any of the above LDFR circuit types, and more.

In the immediate future, prescription fitting software should generate target responses for various nonlinear circuit designs. The target REIR (with or without customization for the individual's REUR and RECD) should be calculated for input intensity levels of, for example, 50, 60, 70, 80, and 90 SPL. The 2 cc FOG response, or NSSPL90 (ANSI S3.42[131]) should be calculated for input intensity levels of, for example, 40, 50, 60, 70, 80, and 90 dB SPL. Both should be presented as a family of input intensity curves. The NSSPL90, or the SSPL90 for a hearing aid at reference test gain (RTG), measured with a composite speech signal, better represents the actual performance for some nonlinear circuits. Since the input speech signal spectra differ (e.g., NAL-R,[25] Cox and Moore[132] Frye, ANSI 3.42[131]), the software should allow correction for spectral differences and vocal effort.[133] At present, the desired level-dependent frequency response changes for the selection of available nonlinear circuitry can be drawn on a design-specification form and sent to a manufacturer, or the desired 2 cc coupler response and/or REIRs can be simply visualized in order to select the correct circuit. It is desirable to specify (and verify) performance for input levels below the kneepoint of some hearing aids (e.g. K-Amp, Ensoniq), that is, at 40 dB SPL in the 2 cc coupler and at 50 dB SPL for REIR. Performance verification is limited by the noise floors in rooms in which REIR measurements are made.

FAMILIES OF TARGET REIR CURVES AND 2 CC COUPLER GAIN CURVES

Examples of a family of prescribed "target" REIR and 2 cc coupler FOG frequency response curves, presented as functions of overall input intensity, for example, for REIR at 50, 60, 70, 80, and 90 dB SPL and for 2 cc coupler FOG at 40, 50, 60, 70, 80, and 90 dB SPL: for TILL and BILL-type LDFR circuits, and FFR-type input compression and output compression nonlinear circuits are illustrated in Figure 14–2 for the same hearing loss (i.e., pure-tone thresholds). Figure 14–2a,b presents a family of actual REIRs to illustrate prescribed REIR curves for input intensities of 50, 60, 70, 80, and 90 dB SPL and 2 cc coupler FOG curves for input intensities of 40, 50, 60, 70, 80, and 90 dB SPL for the TILL-type circuit (e.g., K-Amp). For example, for an individual with a mild to moderate, high frequency sensorineural hearing loss who experiences typical conversations in average environments, K-Amp circuitry will provide more gain and more high frequency boost for low and moderate input signals and

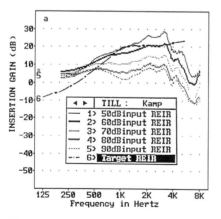
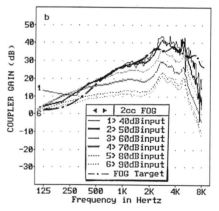

Figure 14–2. Family target REIR and 2 cc coupler FOG frequency response curves, presented as function of input intensity, e.g., 40, 50, 60, 70, 80, and 90 dB SPL, for TILL and BILL level dependent frequency response (LDFR) circuits, and for FFR type input and output compression nonlinear circuits.

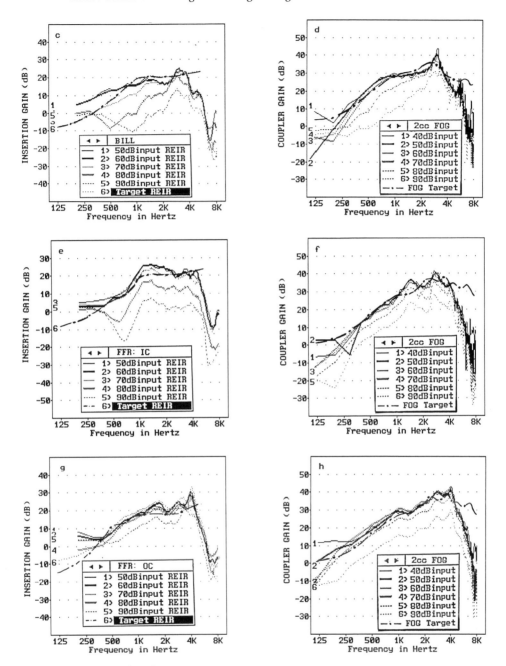

Figure 14–2. *Continued*

less overall gain for louder input signals (i.e., TILL processing). This may also be especially useful for someone with reduced dynamic range.

Figure 14–2c,d presents a family of actual REIRs to illustrate prescribed REIR curves for input intensities of 50, 60, 70, 80, and 90 dB SPL and 2 cc coupler FOG curves for input intensities of 40, 50, 60, 70, 80, and 90 dB SPL for the BILL-type circuit. This fitting approach may be required, for example, by an individual who is required to carry on conversations in the presence of loud low frequency sounds, such as noise from motors. In this case, reduction of the low frequency sound (hopefully noise and not desired signal), with continued amplification of the high frequencies, is often recommended. This has been more commonly referred to as automatic signal processing (ASP; i.e., BILL processing). This type of circuit also has been suggested for wearer comfort in noise, but conclusive evidence of improved speech recognition has not been shown.

Figure 14–2e,f presents a family of actual REIRs to illustrate prescribed REIR curves for input intensities of 50, 60, 70, 80, and 90 dB SPL and 2 cc coupler FOG curves for input intensity of 40, 50, 60, 70, 80, and 90 dB SPL for a device with a constant input compression (IC) ratio: a variant of FFR. This circuit may be recommended for an individual with a reduced dynamic range, whose listening environments include typical conversations and environmental noise, but who does not choose to purchase the more costly TILL or BILL circuitry. (High compression ratios, e.g., 3:1, or more, are especially relevant for individuals with significantly reduced dynamic range.)

Figure 14–2g,h presents a family of actual REIRs to illustrate prescribed REIR curves for input intensities of 50, 60, 70, 80, and 90 dB SPL and 2 cc coupler FOG curves for input intensities of 40, 50, 60, 70, 80, and 90 dB SPL for an output compression (OC) type circuit. This circuit may be recommended for an experienced hearing aid wearer who is exposed to typical conversations and environmental noise, is bothered by very loud sounds, and whose dynamic range is reduced by a sensorineural hearing loss. Wearer experience with linear hearing aids often results in the individual learning to "need" more gain at low and moderate input levels. They benefit from some restriction of peak output levels.

OPTIMIZING SPEECH RECOGNITION DURING HEARING AID FITTING

The AI has been used in hearing aid fitting to compare aided performance, as predicted by different prescriptive fitting methods.[105,150,151] Pavlovic[148] has presented and ranked a variety of AI methods from most accurate, A_1, recommended for computer calculations with visual displays; to A_d, an easy-to-use dot pattern; to the most simple, A_s. Simplified methods for deriving AI[148,151,152] use a count-the-dot pattern (100 dots) superimposed on an audiogram. The Mueller and Killion[154] method is based on the contribution of nonsense syllables. Pavlovic's methods are based on the contribution of average speech. AI for unaided and aided thresholds (for either REAR or REIR + unaided thresholds) can be used to indicate predicted improvement in speech recognition ability:[153] The number of dots included by the aided result, predicted by the fitting strategy compared with the unaided AI, is equivalent to the AI percentage change (i.e., improvement). Figure 14–3 illustrates two simplified count-the-dot methods. The same unaided thresholds, aided thresholds with a 60 dB SPL input composite speech signal, and target aided thresholds derived from

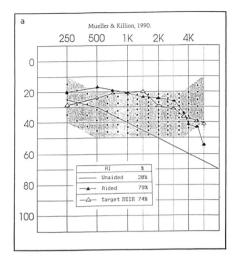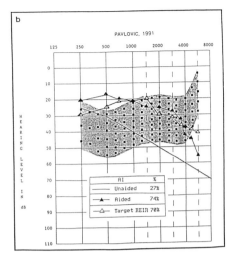

Figure 14–3. Simplified count-the-dot audiogram forms for calculation of the articulation index. (**A**) Illustration of the count-the-dot method of articulation index calculation proposed by Mueller and Killion.[152] (**B**) Illustration of the A_d count-the-dot method of articulation index calculation proposed by Pavlovic.[148] Both methods demonstrate the predicted improvement in speech recognition ability for target REIR versus unaided, and for aided versus unaided conditions.

NAL-R target REIR values are shown for the Mueller and Killion[152] method in Figure 14–3A and for the Pavlovic A_d method in Figure 14–3B.

Figure 14–3 demonstrates predicted improvement in speech recognition ability for the Mueller and Killion method and the Pavlovic count-the-dot methods, respectively: unaided, 20% and 27%; aided, 79% and 74%; and target REIR, 74% and 70%. Software packages[107,151,154] that calculate the AI for different hearing aid fitting strategies have incorporated different long-term average speech spectra, so there may be subtle differences in AI across the simplified methods available. To be user-friendly, software packages should provide a menu of possible AI calculation procedures and permit the selection and/or entry of different speech spectra. These options would facilitate clinical judgments about hearing aid selection and facilitate research on the utility of available procedures. The resultant graphic display of AI on an audiogram, or also on an SPL-o-gram, will be particularly useful for counseling.

THE DISPLAY OF AI FOR PREDICTING HEARING AID PERFORMANCE

Technically, the display of AI should add REIG to the speech spectrum—shifting the aided spectrum *down* into the individual's dynamic range when displayed on an audiogram[28,38,123,155,156] or *up* when displayed on an SPL-o-gram.[36,154] Clinically, when the display of the aided speech spectrum is projected down on an audiogram, things look worse even to the experienced clinician/scientist. Thus, it is a more common practice to add the REIG to the unaided thresholds so that the aided thresholds show improvement (lower, better thresholds). This clinical convention works well for the simplified AI methods, but the amplified speech at higher input levels can be neglected. Without visualizing the entire auditory area, including application of the REIR to the MCLs and UCLs, the SSPL90 could exceed the UCL. Thus, in the future, it will be important to develop software that enables both the clinician and the patient to visualize the *entire* auditory area in dB hearing level, as a function of frequency (e.g., on a audiogram) and in dB SPL (e.g., on an SPL-o-gram). In this way, the clinician can avoid SSPL90s that exceed discomfort levels.

The display of the aided spectrum on an SPL-o-gram,[2,36,157–160] projects the aided speech spectrum, or just the REAR, *up* into the residual dynamic range (threshold, MCL, UCL). *It looks like an improvement.* Thus, in the future, SPL-o-grams will likely gain in favor for the display and visualization of hearing aid performance. Simplified count-the-dot patterns for the determination of AI will be developed for displays of dB SPL as a function of frequency.

The recommendation to maintain the SSPL90 below the UCL is currently being debated. The recommendation may apply to linear hearing aids incorporating peak clipping as a method to reduce output. Exceeding UCL is more easily tolerated with compression, or with the clean undistorted high outputs achievable with Class D amplifiers.[130] For example, the K-Amp circuit with Class D output also has unity gain (e.g., 0 dB of gain, or reduced output) for higher input signals. Future fitting strategies will need to consider the type of amplifier, level at which saturation occurs, and the distortion/coherence of the output in terms of the criteria for satisfaction (above) and measurements describing the nonlinearity of the individual's ear.

Articulation Index as a Predictor of Speech Recognition Ability of Target REIR/REAR

The prescribed REIR (or desired functional gain) is the gain-as-a-function-of-frequency that the prescribed linear hearing aid should provide. It often becomes just a vehicle, or number in the sequence of calculations used, to obtain the desired 2 cc coupler response for communication with the manufacturer. However, when applied to the unaided thresholds, the prescribed REIR can be used to *predict the aided thresholds* for target use gain. With the modifications for nonlinear circuitry suggested above, the fitting strategy can prescribe a family of REIRs and/or REARs, or aided thresholds, as a function of overall input intensity. The professional must still select among the available electroacoustic characteristics of devices from different manufacturers, by using their preferred rule or by comparing responses predicted by different rules. The articulation index (AI) may be a useful tool to help in the selection of a response that is predicted to optimize speech recognition (ANSI S3.5[134]). The AI indicates audibility and may be used to predict recognition of the average speech signal as a proportion from 0.0 to 1.0.

The application of articulation theory[135–138] to the assessment of residual auditory function for sensorineural hearing loss[139–143] suggested that some modification to the AI procedure was necessary. The AI procedures for sensorineural hearing loss[144–148] provide more accurate predictions of speech recognition ability in a 30 dB dynamic range, with linear intensity weighting and consideration of the speech spectrum with natural pauses and peaks. The AI accounts for 90% or more of the variance associated with hearing aid performance.[149]

Just as traditional REIR prescriptions, developed for linear hearing aids, did not consider dynamic, nonlinear performance characteristics, neither does AI. It is, therefore, recommended that AI values be calculated for predicted aided performance using a family of intensity curves for the particular gain vs. frequency functions associated with the dynamic circuit selected. As noted above, the REIR/REAR should be derived as a function of intensity and as a function of the circuit dynamics, especially for nonlinear circuitry. When fitting strategies provide comfortably loud amplification, the AI can provide estimated speech recognition performance for the prescribed amplified response (via REAR or REIR) as a function of input intensity. There needs to be a balance in striving to achieve a higher AI without overamplifying. The individual's loudness growth and the frequency response and linearity/nonlinearity of the hearing aid circuit must be considered.

The AI is, however, only a guide to enhance a fitting strategy. If the selected fitting strategy has not adequately accounted for frequency shaping factors (e.g., venting, plumbing, microphone position, microphone and receiver characteristics), then the AI will not either. The AI correlates reasonably well with speech recognition performance, except for steep high frequency hearing losses.[38,161] It does not, however, account for hearing aid distortions, system noise, environmental signal-to-noise conditions, or the hearing aid.

In the future, with programmable digital hearing aids and with the advent of self-contained *environmental condition reference catalogs* (types, signal-to-noise ratios, and so forth), the differences in AI may play a larger part in fitting and for comparison with speech recognition performance for verification. AI will not, however, account for individual differences due to central processing ability, binaural processing, and/or recruitment and may not resolve differences in frequency response due to the degree of customization of the REIR/REAR based on the real ear unaided response and the real-ear–2 cc coupler-difference.

Projection of REIG/REAR into the Individual's Auditory Area

The auditory area, or dynamic range of hearing, for the individual with normal hearing is wider than for an individual with sensorineural hearing loss. Most threshold-based fitting strategies have some means for deriving an upper limit for amplified sound. This is described in psychoacoustic terms as the UCL or LDL. In electroacoustic terms, for the hearing aid it is referred to as SSPL90; and in the individual's ear it has been called RESR.[162] The output of a hearing aid will saturate at high input levels. The uncomfortable levels have been found by some to be higher for frequency-specific stimuli than for complex speech-like signals.[163,164] Both pure tones and speech-shaped noise (see Ch. 10) are recommended for future use and study. As hearing aids are manufactured to produce less distortion at high input signal levels (high coherence values), the SSPL$_{90}$ may be able to exceed UCL without rejection by the patient.[129] This will not be recommended as good practice. Since a recent study suggested that UCL may not be an accurate predictor of an individual's impression of loudness discomfort (memory dependent)[165] the accuracy and validity of UCL and MCL measures for real-life exposures warrant further study.

DEFINING THE INDIVIDUAL'S AUDITORY AREA

An individual's MCL falls within a somewhat wider comfort range, which falls within the even wider dynamic range. The location of MCL and UCL within the individual's auditory area depends on the methods used to assess MCL and UCL.[38,123,155,166,167] One of the most commonly recommended method scales categorizes the loudness of the sound:[1,106,123,155] Hawkins et al.[106] suggests the following nine categories: very soft; soft; comfortable but slightly soft; comfortable; comfortable but slightly loud; loud but O.K.; uncomfortably loud; extremely uncomfortable; painfully loud.

Pascoe[1,123,155] suggests the following ten categories: Nothing; too soft; very soft; soft; O.K. (softer); O.K.; O.K. (louder); loud; very loud; and too loud. Pascoe[123] has shown (N = 508) that average MCLs and UCLs, pooled across frequency (hearing levels did not show a significant frequency effect), are predicted reasonably well by most of the prescriptive formulae [6,21,27,29,31,37,168,169] for mild to moderate hearing levels. Thus, the amplified speech outputs recommended by target REIRs "fall" within or near the comfort range of the "mean listener."[123] However, the range of judgments is large enough (as much as 20 dB) that measures of individual loudness judgments are recommended.

Clinically, one of the authors has found that scaling with the six category ratings of quiet (Q), lower edge of comfort (LC), comfort (M or MCL), higher edge of comfort (HC), loud but tolerable for more than a second or two (L), and uncomfortable or not tolerable for more than a second or two (U or UCL) compares well with a forced-choice bracketing procedure for estimating a one level prediction of MCL. The bracketing procedure is a forced-choice method for selection of the most comfortable preferred-listening level of pairs of tones 10 dB apart (and then 5 dB apart for finer resolution) using a modified up-down procedure to change levels. Although the variabilities of MCL and UCL exceed those of threshold estimates, the reliability and validity of these measures[38,123,170] have been considered acceptable for *estimating* the SSPL$_{90}$ for future hearing aid selection; however, *individual* loudness judgments will continue to be recommended.

DISPLAYING THE AUDITORY AREA AND THE AMPLIFIED RESPONSE

A map of the individual's auditory area should provide information for the selection of optimal hearing aid responses. The amplified long-term average speech spectra (LTASS; range +12 to −18 dB) should be fitted, as well as possible, into the individual's residual auditory area. In theory, and in fact, the fitting strategies can derive a target REIR that places the speech spectrum into the hearing impaired individual's auditory area at about MCL. Mapping the individual's dynamic range allows the professional to visualize the optimization of amplified speech for a particular fitting stategy. Maps of the individual auditory area should be developed for linear circuits, and various types of nonlinear circuits, to provide visualizable options for consideration when selecting a desirable fitting for amplification. The mapped auditory area is useful both during specification of the desired hearing aid response characteristics and later during verification and counseling.

The auditory area can be displayed with intensity as a function of frequency, with dB HL on the ordinate, as on an audiogram, or with dB SPL on the ordinate (see Fig. 14–4). Both displays have been recommended.[1,38,123,155] The

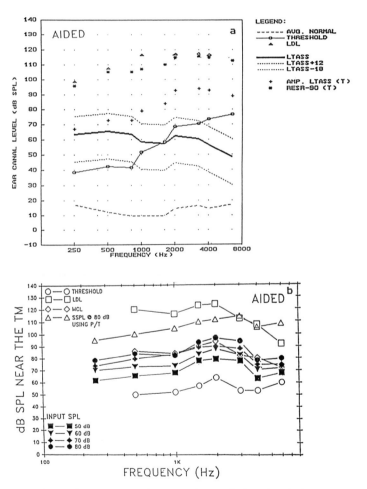

Figure 14–4. The auditory area, REAR, and unaided and aided speech spectrum are displayed on an SPL-o-gram. (**A**) Example an SPL-o-gram generated by the DSL method for the same hearing loss illustrated in Figures 14–2 and 14–3. (**B**) Example an SPL-o-gram generated by in situ ear canal SPL measurements. (From Valente, et al.[160])

latter has been recommended by others.[2,35,154,160] The REIR is preferably added to the speech spectrum (LTASS), shifting the aided spectrum down on the audiogram to fit within the threshold and the UCL and to align with the MCL. As a short cut, on an audiogram the REIR is often added to the unaided thresholds, and the aided thresholds show the audibility of the speech. However, the REIR should also be added to the MCL and UCL estimates by frequency, to indicate the entire dynamic range. If MCLs and UCLS were not obtained, derived DSLs should be displayed to account for the placement of aided dynamic range of speech (LTASS +12, −18 dB). The actual DSL method plots the thresholds and derived DSLs, for comfort and uncomfortable loudness in dB SPL as a function of frequency on a graph called an *SPL-o-gram*[38,154] (see Ch. 13). In Figure 14–4a, thresholds for the same hearing loss as illustrated in Figure 14–2 are converted to and displayed of dB SPL (in the ear canal). Amplified speech spectrum is well within the auditory area. The RESR of the hearing aid falls below the LDLs. The unamplified LTASS and the average normal hearing levels are also presented.

IN SITU AUDIOMETRY AND THE AUDITORY AREA

One way to define the auditory area and the hearing aid response on the individal's ear would be to measure, and/or derive, thresholds, MCLs, and UCLs in dB SPL in situ via probe microphone measurements.[2,160,171,172] Thus, in situ audiometry reduces the need for multiple conversions. The probe tube from the probe microphone is placed into the ear canal, either through an insert earphone or alongside the eartip of the insert phone, and extended beyond the eartip to a position near the tympanic membrane. Then, psycho-acoustic measurements, electroacoustic measurements, and hearing aid response measurements (both in the ear and on a 2 cc coupler) are all made in the same units. Figure 14–4b illustrates that the aided ear canal SPLs for a family of input levels (i.e., 50, 60, 70, 80, and 90 dB SPL)[160] fall within the auditory range, around MCL, and below both LDL and SSPL90 for an 80 dB swept pure tone signal.

Today, technology generally limits threshold measurements to those greater than 40 dB HL. It is typically necessary to derive (predict) in situ thresholds of less than 40 dB HL, which is possible when the insert receiver is coupled to an audiometer with a linear attenuator. For example, assume a measured MCL is 55 dB HL and the SPL measured via the in situ probe microphone is 59 dB SPL at 1,000 Hz. Therefore, the HL to real-ear SPL difference is 4 dB at this frequency. If the threshold measured using the same transducer were 15 dB HL, we could reasonably predict that the SPL near the eardrum would be 19 dB SPL for an in situ measure at threshold. The HL to real-ear SPL difference should be measured at each frequency.

In the future, however, technology will permit direct threshold measurements at low hearing levels (i.e., lower than 40 dB). Very narrowband tracking filter amplifiers and specialized digital signal analyzers will be used to reduce the effects of measuring system "front-end" noise to permit accurate in situ probe measurement of ear canal levels for thresholds as low as 15–20 dB SPL.

With this enhanced capability, it should be possible to determine *directly* the relationship between an individual's hearing threshold and the amplified speech output in the ear canal. *In situ audiometry* proposes the direct measurement of sound pressures in the ear canal for thresholds, for suprathreshold loudness estimates (e.g., MCL, UCL), and for aided speech spectra presented at overall levels of 50–90 dB SPL.

In the future, target REARs, derived as a function of input intensity (e.g., 50–90 dB SPL) for selected nonlinear devices (circuitry), will be projected into a software-generated display of the individual's auditory area. They will be displayed along with unaided threshold, MCL, and UCL values for comparison with prescribed target aided responses. The same display will indicate amplified speech spectra for quiet, moderate, and loud levels. Target REARs will be evaluated for predicted speech recognition ability (AI), for selectable input intensity levels (e.g., 50–90 dB SPL), and for predicted satisfaction or benefit and then compared with actual measured REARs. *For future digital devices, the time separation between the use of fitting strategy software for selection of hearing aid response characteristics and the verification of actual responses will be the time to "dial-in" and set the parameters of the digital hearing aid and then to measure and display the response characteristics on a map of the individual's auditory area.*

AUDITORY AREA IN dB HL OR dB SPL

The relative utility of measurements performed on the real ear, on a 2 cc coupler, or on an ear simulator and expressed in dB SPL or dB hearing level (HL), will continue to be debated. Today, most prescriptive fitting methods use thresholds measured in dB HL and converted to dB SPL on the 2 cc coupler. One method, used by the Cortiton Hearing Aid Company (Cortiton; G. Frye, Frye Electronics, personal communication), measures and expresses *all* relevant hearing aid fitting values in terms of dB SPL on the 2 cc coupler. All threshold and suprathreshold measures are obtained with insert earphones, *using audiometers calibrated in dB SPL on the 2 cc coupler*, and are displayed on the same graph (same units) as the hearing aid response in dB SPL, as determined on the 2 cc coupler in the hearing aid test box. Today, most recommend calculation of prescribed 2 cc coupler FOG responses. Some recommend prediction and/or measurement of the occluded ear simulator response.

Furthermore, now and in the future the entire mapped auditory area (e.g., threshold, MCL, and UCL), including the REAR, RESR, and normal and amplified speech spectra, will be useful, whether displayed in dB HL or dB SPL. Direct measurement and display of SPL (e.g., the SPL-o-gram) offers the advantage of eliminating many conversions. This direct SPL measure can be accomplished via in situ audiometry, with a probe microphone through an insert phone, or via direct measurement using an insert earphone and an audiometer calibrated in terms of 2 cc coupler dB SPL (Cortiton; G. Frye, Frye Electronics, personal communication).

The REIR will also remain a useful tool for some time, since the necessary calculations for different fitting strategies, with customization and necessary conversions, are easily performed by available software. It is desirable to have multiple window (1–4) displays on the monitor, where REIR is illustrated (in real time) in one window, REAR is illustrated in a second window (in real time), 2 cc coupler FOG (customized and/or average) is illustrated in a third window, and 2 cc coupler output dB SPL (customized or average) is illustrated in a fourth window. For the short-term, some software modification for nonlinear circuits will be simpler than starting over.

The audiogram, however, will likely remain in dB HL units for many years. Aside from the fact that it took many years to develop the conversions and to derive the audiogram format, there are international, as well as national, standards that establish the reference equivalent threshold sound pressure levels (RETSPLS) for each of the standard supra-aural and insert audiometric earphones (ANSI S3.6[173]). The entire professional community (audiologists, hearing aid dispensers, physicians, other related health professionals and non-health professionals [e.g., in the legal system]) expects to have a zero reference against which to compare the individual's hearing ability. It is simpler to see a 35 dB HL hearing loss on the present-day audiogram than on an SPL-o-gram, where the threshold, at 1,000 Hz, would be 42.5 dB SPL and the HL-to-SPL conversion (RETSPL) is 7.5 dB for a TDH 39 supra-aural earphone. In contrast, at 250 Hz the threshold would be 60 dB SPL and the HL-to-SPL conversion 25 dB SPL. Very few of even the mathematically facile professionals would want to take the time to do the necessary simple addition and subtraction. The use of SPL references would also make it harder to explain clinical findings to the person who needs the help the most: the patient with a hearing loss.

Universal Integrated Hearing Aid Fitting Systems

In the future, hearing aids will be fitted using systems that integrate software and hardware for real-ear measurements, software and hardware for coupler measurements, and various reference databases. Although a few manufacturers have fitting systems now, the future *universal integrated hearing aid fitting system* will permit the specification and fitting of many different types of hearing aids. Real-ear probe microphone measurement systems are typically controlled by stored software (i.e., firmware). Desirable features of future software programmed and controlled hearing aid fitting systems are listed.

1. Today, target REIR is (calculated and) displayed/printed. In the future, more emphasis will be placed on target REAR and on the residual auditory area (discussed above).

2. Various threshold and/or suprathreshold prescriptive fitting strategies are selectable by the audiologist. Clinicians should be able to inform the integrated fitting system whether they are interested in either REAR or REIR, or REAR and REIR measures. This will result in the display of the appropriate menus. Clinicians should have the ability to enter their own prescriptive formulae or to modify existing ones.

3. Thresholds, in dB HL or dB SPL, are entered in real-time as they are measured or at a later time. Whenever possible, measurements should be obtained in real-time.

4. The manner in which thresholds are obtained (e.g., earphone [including type of earphone: supra-aural or insert], sound field, or in situ probe measurement) should be selectable so the proper conversions to eardrum/ear canal SPL can be applied.[174–177] Insert earphones are recommended, since they better simulate the impedance of the hearing aid and allow direct measurement on the 2 cc coupler and the real ear (Cortiton; G. Frye, Frye Electronics, personal communication).[33,38,178,179] Although in situ probe microphone measurements reduce the need for conversions, there will continue to be instances when probe microphone measurements cannot be performed on some individuals or when data from other test methods or facilities will need to be considered and entered into the integrated fitting systems.

5. The REUR is obtained and then displayed. The measurement method is selected from a menu of sound source azimuths and elevations[180,181] probe microphone and reference microphone placements, and other options.[182] Sound pressure distributions around the head differ in the horizontal and vertical planes; a sound source location of 45° azimuth and 45° elevation is recommended for most reliable real-ear probe microphone measurements.[183] Furthermore, these options may eventually be relevant to the specification of binaural interaction with amplification and the *virtual environment* for the hearing aid.

6. RECD differences are optionally obtained[102] using an insert earphone with a probe tube through the eartip or alongside the eartip (extending at least 5 mm in front of the eartip[184,185] to a position near the eardrum) to measure the sound pressure in the ear and on the coupler. The real-ear insert receiver-to-coupler difference needs to be measured once and stored. The software will calculate the individual real-ear difference (i.e., the RECD).

7. The system will allow the user to retrieve appropriate database information for that individual or for average ears (e.g., by age or sex) for relevant information on REUR, RECD, various loudness judgments,[106,123,186] and binaural advantage.[187–189] The clinician may compare the individual's information to selected average data.

8. The clinician should be able to program the integrated fitting system to measure and display REIR, REAR, 2 cc coupler FOG, and/or 2 cc coupler dB SPL on single or multiple screen (i.e., windows) displays. The system will branch to the appropriate menus.

9. For the target REAR mode, the target REIR can be applied to either the unaided thresholds or to a menu of selectable speech spectra to

---

*Burnett and Beck[174] and Bentler and Pavlovic[175,176] have provided values for transformations that will be necessary for computer-based fittings and are of significant value in manual fittings: (1) free field to eardrum, (2) free field to BTE microphone location, (3) free field to ITE microphone location, (4) free field to ITC microphone location, (5) 6 cc to eardrum, (6) 2 cc to free field, (7) HL to SPL (2 cc), (8) CORFIG BTE, (9) CORFIG ITE, (10) CORFIG ITC, (11) MAF, (12) MAP, (13) MAPC (minimum audible field in a 6 cc coupler), (14) diffuse field to eardrum, (15) diffuse field to BTE, (16) diffuse field to ITE, (17) diffuse field to ITC, (18) 6 cc to eardrum, and (19) one-third octave levels of speech in free field to dB HL for one-third octaves and critical bands.

predict the target REAR. The unaided thresholds and the predicted aided responses/thresholds (derived from REIR and REAR) should be displayed. The choice of display format should include either, or both, the audiogram format and the SPL-o-gram format. In audiogram format, the REIR also will be applied to the obtained MCL and UCL values.

10. The target REAR at "comfort" differs from the 2 cc coupler's frequency response at FOG or at RTG, so proper labeling must be accomplished by default conditions and from menu selections in the software/firmware-based integrated fitting systems. For example, for the Frye 6400 and 6500, reserve gain and average, or customized, CORFIG calculations yield the target 2 cc coupler FOG response.

11. The target REIR should be prescribed and measured at a specificable "use" volume control position.

12. The calculation of target 2 cc coupler responses incorporates the proper transformations[175-177] and corrections (CORFIG[10]) to yield a flat insertion gain. Computer software will generate a selectable set of target 2 cc coupler responses (or gain curves) that are customized based on the individual's REUR and/or the individual's RECD, as well as a target based only on average transformations. It should then be possible to select the degree of customization.

13. The fitting system should request that the clinician specify the nature of the desired/prescribed REIR and/or REAR target responses as linear, nonlinear, or linear and nonlinear targets. The REIR and REAR (and 2 cc coupler FOG and/or SPL responses) will be displayed as a family of curves generated with different input intensity signals and levels. Nonlinear aids require multiple gain or dB SPL targets. The system will permit the clinician to select single or multiple screen displays of the same information. Linear aids, however, also should have multiple targets, not only for the typical "single" gain or SPL target prescribed as appropriate for "most" of the individual's dynamic range but also a saturation level target(s).

14. Speech composite signals, based on the desired (selected) speech spectra, should be able to be corrected for vocal effort. The clinician should be able to select the desired reference speech spectrum, apply default corrections, or modify the selected spectrum for both measurement and display. The clinician may apply corrections to use spectra with greater high frequency energy (e.g., Frye, NIST as standardized in ANSI S3.42[131]) resembling the long-term peak spectrum level or lower high frequency energy resembling the traditional LTASS (e.g., NAL-R,[37] Cox and Moore[132]). The spectral shape of the speech composite signal should change as input levels are varied.

15. Aided speech spectra are plotted in the auditory area with a family of the individual's loudness judgments and may be compared with reference data for loudness judgments and the unaided speech spectra.

16. An efficient integrated hearing aid fitting system would ask the user to press a button and the system would automatically present 50−60−70−80 dB

of speech-weighted noise. It would then allow the clinician to view the displayed result and determine if the prescribed family of REARs fits the individual's auditory area. The system would next automatically present 80–90 dB of either speech-weighted noise or pure tone stimuli and allow the user to view the display and determine if the prescribed REAR falls below the individual's UCL. A similar family of prescribed 2 cc coupler FOG and/or SPL curves would be displayed. All information would be stored in the system's databases (individual's files and group files) in forms that can be easily retrieved, manipulated, and restored. The individual's auditory area, described by the area between threshold and UCL, and further characterized by actual and/or derived loudness judgments, should be independently accessible for comparison with prescribed targets with aided responses measured in the verification stage.

EMERGING INTEGRATED HEARING AID FITTING SYSTEMS

The first available comprehensive software and database hearing aid fitting system is the "Desired Sensation Level (DSL) fitting strategy program for children and others who aren't able to make reliable judgments."[36,154–157] The software and database can derive (1) DSLs for amplified speech; (2) target in situ gain; (3) insertion gain; (4) $RESR_{90}$; (5) 2 cc coupler targets, converted by average, or custom, CORFIG; and (6) target sound field aided thresholds. The program can map the auditory area. Customization, via entry of the individual REUR and RECD, is available to modify the prescribed DSLs. If in situ probe microphone measurements and actual REUR and RECD are not obtained, default REUR values[190] and default RECDs for children[191] and for adults[192–194] are applied. A database of MCL and UCL measures has been compiled for computer access of retrievable values for adults[123,170] and children.[195]

The first integrated fitting systems began to appear during the middle of 1992. Emerging computer systems and software can be used to calculate prescribed REIG, estimated UCL, prescribed $SSPL_{90}$ to amplify below the UCL, and so forth, store volumes of electroacoustic response characteristics (FR, MPO, gain, tone control, vents effects, tubing options, options to avoid/reduce feedback, and occlusion effects), and even actually consider their interactions.[196] At present, however, the comparison of estimated values with direct measurements rely on the user.

One computer-based system, the Hearing Aid Selection Program (HASP)[196] is currently in use in Australia. It performs calculations for target REIG and SSPL90 for the average ear and searches a previously entered system database of available instruments. The dispenser selects the best combinations of control settings and options with consideration for conversion factors, venting, tubing, dampers, and batteries. The software reviews, and the fitter views and reviews, the possible characteristics for the best hearing aid selections and determines the "best" match to predicted REIG. That is, the fitting system software judges the closeness of fit.

Another reported, but not yet available commercial system, the Comprehensive Hearing Aid Selection and Evaluation System (CHASE),[2] is a modular software-based system that includes a real-ear test system. It reportedly will (1) perform and store a calibration sequence of measurements, (2) measure insertion gain, and (3) calculate and compare target REIG (for three fitting strategies [POGO-I,[31] NAL,[25] and MSU-v3[35]]) and target 2 cc coupler responses to the contents of a database for BTE, ITE, and ITC instruments, to be manually entered by the user. The database provides for (average) shell modifications, venting, horns, and cavities. It uses in situ probe microphone measurements to determine dB SPL judgments from "threshold" to "too loud" to define the auditory map for one-third octave bands of noise. It will be able to "position the aided speech spectrum at a specific location within the listener's dynamic range"[2] to determine optimal hearing aid fit. It also has a speech recognition testing module and a survey questionnaire module for verification. Reportedly, it will be an independent system that *will not* interface with other real-ear fitting systems, software, or databases.

FUTURE TRULY UNIVERSAL INTEGRATED HEARING AID FITTING SYSTEMS

Eventually, with future truly integrated fitting systems, it will be possible, with greater sophistication than with the early models, to compare the target REARs of various available hearing aid selections against the individual's auditory area, and so forth, in dB SPL and to select the hearing aid response characteristics most likely to optimize speech recognition while not being uncomfortably loud. Future interactive, computer-based, real-ear measurement and interactive hearing aid fitting systems should have large, easily accessible databases. The future systems should provide a much wider selection of existing prescriptions and provide for simple updating and/or insertion(s) of one's own prescription(s). The system should calculate all necessary target responses for hearing aids on appropriate couplers (menu selectable)—such as the 2 cc coupler, the occluded ear simulator (OES) (ANSI S3.25[69]), simpler versions of the OES that may replace the 2 cc coupler and KEMAR—and on an ear.

UNIVERSAL ACCEPTANCE OF MEASUREMENTS ACROSS FITTING SYSTEMS AND HEARING AIDS

The integrated hearing aid system *must* be able to accept measurements from independent real-ear probe tube systems universally, without requiring manual data entry. It is essential that present clinic equipment be able to be integrated with the new real-ear and coupler hearing aid measurement equipment and/or new digital hearing aid (manufacturers') fitting and verification systems. The real-ear probe response data should be transmitted between systems close to, if not actually in, real-time and should be readily convertible to human readable form (data tables and graphs). The data may be in one of the following forms: probe microphone REUR, REAR, REIR; directly measured sound pressures in the ear canal through insert earphones (with or without probe tube microphones); and for unaided and aided sound field responses that are either independent of, or associated with, threshold and/or loudness judgments.

It is imperative that both software and hardware manufacturers work together to permit data exchange between systems while not imposing unreasonable hardware requirements and excessive operator requirements. For example, some programmable digital hearing aid fitting systems will have their own probe subsystem. Yet the audiologist may want to make independent measurements on the clinic's main real-ear probe microphone spectrum analysis equipment, used for fitting all hearing aids, in order to evaluate the prescription from a particular fitting/programming system. Multiple probe systems will not all fit in the patient's ear simultaneously. Serial measurements for comparison is time consuming. The output of one probe-microphone measurement system should either provide data in a form that is compatible with all systems or provide simultaneous compatible (parallel) outputs.

INTERACTIVE DISPLAY OF SPECIFIED, ACTUAL, AND
CATALOGED PERFORMANCE

The fitting system should map the auditory area and display both the unamplified and amplified full speech spectra, corrected for vocal effort. It should be able to plot the individual's thresholds and auditory landmark loudness values, such as MCL and UCL, at least, with up to as many as seven delineations of loudness. It should compare these, in terms of sensation levels and in absolute values, against databases for adults and children compiled from existing research,[154] from one's own clinical database of patients, and from the individual's own database records. The system should contain a file of reference long-term average speech spectra used with various prescriptive formulae. It should be able to measure simply in one-third octave bands and to compare the office's own LTASS to these references and provide conversion for one-third octave band speech field to dB SPL on the 2 cc coupler. The system should also be able to store and/or link-up with stored hearing aid electroacoustic response data (from simple analog-linear to output SPL responses of nonlinear instruments, to true digital, and to digital with adaptive fuzzy logic/neural network and other signal processing capabilities) via peer-to-peer networks (e.g., Lantastic) that do not restrict the user to one or two data input–output ports. It should display a menu of various signal processing options whose functions can be assessed as a function of input signal level and as a function of type of signals: narrowband versus broadband noise, low frequency and high frequency speech-like stimuli, natural speech versus speech in noise, and, ultimately, even music and existing environment(s). The integrated fitting system should eventually define, specify, and, if desired, generate the virtual (test) environment for the individual wearing the hearing aid. In addition to a catalog of signals, the clinician should be able to generate, store, and use these stimuli "on the fly" during the operation of the fitting system. These future fitting strategies will be able to specify the desired auditory requirements of the hearing aid to match the individual's ears.

Manufacturers should strive to establish standards with which to guide contributions of such information to large, easily accessible databases. Each hearing aid manufacturer should be encouraged to supply this information in a standardized format (for a reasonable fee) with frequent updates to all dispensers on some common medium (e.g., CD ROM, computer floppy disc) or via a company BBS in a standard computer database language. Also, there should be standards for connecting different measurement systems and computers.

Future Hearing Aid Fitting Strategies: Speculation to 2020

In the distant future, some 20–30 years from now, most hearing aid designs will be based on true digital computer-controlled circuits. Virtually all of the hearing aid transducers will, however, remain quite similar to their present forms. In some of the devices, the output stage of the digital audio amplifier will directly drive the output transducer to the prescribed SPL. The microphone and preamplification stage will remain analog, or digitally controlled analog. There will always be different types of hearing aids and different manufacturers, despite speculation by some[197] that each manufacturer will have only three to four digital models that the audiologist will program in the office to meet the theoretical objectives of desired fitting strategies and then directly verify adequacy of fit. There will, however, still be simple analog hearing aids and reasonably simple "high tech" analog hearing aids with some digitally programmed and/or controlled features such as filters and level controllers. The hearing impaired person's desire for small, virtually invisible, ITC, *low cost* instruments and the low power requirement for device control and operation will maintain the demand for a wider variety of hearing aid types for at least the next 20–30 years.

Expanding the Capabilities of Earlier Integrated Hearing Aid Fitting Systems

Soon it will be possible to insert a laser optical probe into the ear canal and record the entire geometry of the ear canal. This recorded measurement data then will be available for three-dimensional display, transfer via network, or up-loading via modem, to the earmold or shell laboratory for production of the ear mold and/or hearing aid. This can revolutionize the present ear impression process. The resulting three-dimensional visualization of the ear canal (i.e., *the impression*) should provide a far more accurate "picture" of the ear canal than current impression techniques. However, it will be particularly important to capture accurately the pinna and transition to the canal as well as the ear canal (along a continuous reference plane) so that the lateral surface of the hearing instrument does not contact the pinna (e.g., the antitragus), leading to irritation, feedback, or a blocked microphone port. An accurate and precise specification of the external ear may significantly reduce the likelihood of feedback and discomfort. The earmold/shell laboratory, with input from the audiologist, will need to determine the tolerance applied to the earmold/shell production to ensure an easily insertable device with a comfortable fit and without feedback.

The concept of a computer-based integrated hearing aid fitting system with its extensive database, as developed in the previous section, will continue to evolve and expand as more sophisticated, microprocessor-based hearing aids appear. Hearing aid circuit design information also will be provided in forms well beyond today's fitting matrices. For microprocessor-based hearing aids, there will be references to different programmed digital filter options, to programmed gain functions, and to different real-time dynamic digital signal processing approaches. An option to reduce the occlusion effect[198,199] could be selected, for example.

In the future, options will be selected on the basis of rank, or some criteria table, to match a menu of patient needs, different environmental conditions, binaural capabilities and, possibly, different hearing loss etiologies. Psychoacoustic and/or physiological differences among types of hearing loss may be better understood, thus allowing more accurate testing, delineation, and compensation for different types of hearing loss (e.g., sensorineural hearing losses of viral, or traumatic origin, and so forth may have different functional characteristics).

Although speculative, the way in which people develop and then recognize their hearing loss may also suggest the need for different theoretical solutions and fitting strategies, requiring different hearing aid types and functions. The hearing aid of tomorrow may be able, for example, to identify the wearer's environment and remove environmental effects, such as reverberation. This could ultimately result in speech sounds spoken in a church being perceived as having been spoken in a quiet room. Further speculation suggests that many different digital processing options will become available as the various manufacturers compete in the marketplace.

Divergent Fitting Strategies

A dichotomy in fitting strategies will remain. Some threshold-based strategies will rely only, or mostly, on the auditory threshold to predict desired REIR and/or REAR and UCL to provide an indicator for $SSPL_{90}$. Other strategies will use a combination of threshold and suprathreshold measures using tonal and/or speech-weighted stimuli for predicted fitting responses that fall within the individual's auditory area. The dichotomy will remain because people will remain the same despite technological advances. Some people will have the ability and patience to make the judgments necessary for the more complex fitting methods; others (children; nervous, restless, or anxious adults; and those with limited mental capacity) will not.

The computer-based fitting and hearing aid programming system will contain all critical information regarding (1) the impedance of each ear; (2) its physical characteristics, size, ear canal dimensions; (3) distance from hearing aid sound output port to eardrum; and (4) the positioning of the hearing aid microphone within the ear to determine the most efficient direction of the sound path. It will contain all available information regarding the normal *modeled* functions of the ear and the modeled functions of the "pathologic" ear (different types of conductive and/or sensorineural ears). It will project the modeled area of basilar membrane excitation, the degree of inner versus outer hair cell function, and the degree of efferent control to predict auditory functions. It will model intensity, frequency, and temporal resolution for different types of input signals at different functional levels. Information regarding the individual's processing abilities and normal hearing function will be loaded into the microcomputer-based digital hearing aid. The hearing aid, then, through its fuzzy logic and/or neural network intelligence, will appropriately adjust its operational characteristics and output with changes in complex input signals. It will learn and "remember" how it adapted to enhance intelligibility and sound quality, in a particular environment, for the wearer.

Loudness With Sensorineural Hearing Loss

As cochlear modeling transitions from linear to nonlinear and signal processing strategies advance to compensate for cochlear function, models of the peripheral system will be incorporated into hearing aid fitting systems.

MODELING COCHLEAR NONLINEARITIES

Today, the modeling of cochlear mechanics recognizes cochlear nonlinearities, but still only uses two competing linear models.[200] The active cochlear amplifier model and the passive resonant tectorial membrane model are used to explain cochlear tuning (frequency selectivity–decreases at the higher intensities) and nonlinear compression (the ratio of dynamic range of the auditory area [10^5] to the dynamic range of the hair cell [10^3]).[200] Studies of the effects of outer hair cell damage help to explain a significant amount of observed cochlear dysfunction for mild to moderate sensorineural hearing loss. More recently, some nonlinear modeling has been applied to cochlear function. The multiple bandpass nonlinearity (MBPNL) model,[87,201,202] a cochlear model based on signal processing principles, accounts for input–output responses and cochlear nonlinearities seen in psychophysical data. It should be applied to the specification of future hearing aid capabilities. Furthermore, the compressive nonlinearity of a modified power law is able to explain nonlinearities of masking, temporal and spectral resolution and loudness growth, and summation for normal hearing and for sensorineural hearing loss.[203]

EVOLUTION OF LOUDNESS-BASED HEARING AID FITTING SYSTEMS

For the future, development of loudness-based hearing aid fitting systems may result from a revised excitation-pattern model (after Zwicker) based on a nonlinear modified power law model for modeling loudness with sensorineural hearing loss.[203] It assumes an internal noise source underlying the elevated thresholds associated with sensorineural hearing loss. This excitation pattern model for loudness has been applied to hearing aid fitting by Humes.[197]

The loudness pattern approach will examine the distribution of loudness across frequency in the auditory system, not just overall loudness. It will attempt to restore the excitation pattern of loudness.[197] Figure 14–5a illustrates excitation level (top) and specific loudness patterns (bottom) for a vowel /e/ presented at 77 dB SPL to an individual with normal hearing. Figure 14–5b illustrates differences in specific loudness patterns for a vowel /e/ presented at 77 dB SPL to an individual with normal hearing (nh) and for an individual with sensorineural hearing impairment (hi). Descendents of presently (1992)

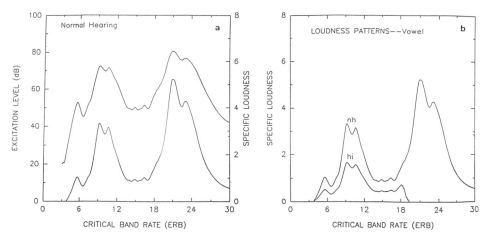

Figure 14–5.   Loudness patterns. (**A**) Illustration of the excitation pattern (top) and the specific-loudness pattern (bottom) for the vowel /e/ presented at 77 dB SPL to an individual with normal hearing. (**B**) Illustration of specific-loudness patterns for the vowel /e/ presented at 77 dB SPL to an individual with normal hearing (nh) and to an individual with sensorineural hearing impairment (hi). (From Humes.[197])

available software packages that define excitation level patterns and specific-loudness patterns in sones per Bark[204–205] for speech-like stimuli (from pure-tone thresholds and the amplitude spectrum of speech) will be used to develop target amplified responses. In the future, prescription methods based on this model could determine the recommended gain-by-frequency as a function of intensity "to restore"normal loudness patterns to the individual for different environments. The result is different gain values by frequency region and intensity level, for each speech sound selected to represent the necessary frequency distribution for amplification. Smart hearing aids that learn the individual's "success" with these signals will provide different responses/algorithms as needed by the situation.

There are, however, some factors that raise questions about the eventual applicability of the excitation pattern model in hearing aid fitting. A difficulty associated with the excitation pattern model is that excitation patterns are related to masking patterns and therefore have considerable variability.[197] Individual differences in masking and in loudness growth functions are most critical. Although the model appears generally applicable to the improvement of speech recognition ability, it must be refined further to reduce its sensitivity to individual variations before being used for individual hearing aid fitting. Considerable research remains to be done.

AI and Modified Speech Transmission Index

The AI, as described above, will continue in use as a part of hearing aid fitting systems through the next two decades. It also has been suggested that a modification of the speech transmission index (STI),[206] called the *modified speech transmission index* (mSTI) may be used to predict and thereby facilitate interpretation of speech recognition scores.[197,207] According to Humes,[197] the mSTI is obtained by placing a probe tube microphone in the ear canal and measuring the modulation transfer functions for modulation frequencies of 0.5–16 KHz, in octave steps, in each of 15 one-third octave bands from 250 to 6,300 Hz. The mSTI uses a 100% intensity-modulated, speech-shaped noise carrier. Subsequent analysis is done in one-third octave bands. If research proves that the mSTI (0.0–1.0) and speech recognition performance scores are strongly related for a wide set of listening conditions, then the mSTI could be used to predict a speech recognition score for a given hearing aid response and specific speech material/listening conditions. In the future, modulation transfer functions, established for a variety of environments, can be cataloged in the large computerized database system (above) and then be used to simulate performance in many different environments. It remains to be determined whether the application of the modulation transfer function can be used to estimate "expected" performance of individual listeners in aided and unaided conditions.

Continued Use of AI While the Search for Optimum Speech Recognition Signal Processing Proceeds

Research will continue to demonstrate the benefits of different signal processing methods for good speech recognition in varied listening conditions, especially at the moderate and high intensity levels to which most individuals with hearing loss typically listen. At high intensities, the normal ear loses its ability to fine tune. Basilar membrane tuning curves of normal ears show poorer frequency selectivity for high level signals. Recent evidence suggests that the poor frequency resolution[208] and temporal resolution[209,210] associated with sensorineural hearing loss is probably due to the high levels to which they are exposed. It appears now that it is not the sensation level but the actual intensity of the signal driving the cochlear that determines its response. It is probable that the ear with mild to moderate sensorineural hearing loss (due primarily to loss of outer hair cells) functions normally, i.e., linearly, at high input levels. However, further research is needed on cochlear and psychoacoustic function, and on speech signal processing strategies, both as a function of intensity levels and as a function of sensation level, in order to understand better their functional relation to improved speech recognition ability and to hearing aid satisfaction.

To date, many signal processing strategies/algorithms have been developed (e.g., multiband compression, orthogonal polynomial compression and principal component compression, digital signal processing methods for frequency domain-like Wiener filtering or spectral subtraction, the time–domain-like envelope filter, and a multiple microphone adaptive noise canceler), but none has significantly improved speech intelligibility[86] (see Ch. 16 for a discussion of these and other algorithms). Thus, at present, and for the near future, integrated hearing aid fitting systems incorporating the AI, and possibly the mSTI, will be used to predict speech recognition ability.

A Dream Sequence About a Future Hearing Aid Fitting System—Beyond 2020

An individual, in the office, has just had an audiologic evaluation and was identified as having a hearing loss with the audiometer section of the universal hearing evaluation/hearing aid design and fitting system. A special shielded "cap" is then placed on the individual's head. The system then generates complex auditory stimuli and, via the cap, picks up yet to be identified electrophysiologic responses with more subtle resolution than possible today. Some relevant physiologic and psychoacoustic factors concerning loudness and speech encoding are assessed and stored in the system. This integrated stimulus–response system is adaptive and eventually yields a fitting prescription that is optimized for the individual for a wide variety of stimulus sounds and environmental noise conditions. The computer processes the data; displays the appropriate target and actual loudness functions, predicted and actual speech recognition performance in quiet and noise; and benefit estimates, for the optimal hearing aid fitting, as a function of environment; and programs the selected hearing aid with all of the relevant configuration information. The system allows the audiologist, and the prospective user with the hearing aid, to experience *virtual* test environments.

Summary

In the future, hearing evaluation, the selection, fitting, and verification of hearing aid performance, determination of both short and long-term benefits, and counseling and rehabilitation (see Ch. 15) will be exciting, but will require greater expertise. Future fitting strategies will clearly make use of much more sophisticated devices and concepts. The "wish-list" for the universally interfaceable, computer-based, integrated hearing aid design and fitting system has been described above. There is a critical need for both agency and industry funding for clinical research regarding hearing aid technology. Research should include development and implementation of (1) expanded fitting and verification strategies for desired hearing aid performance, (2) improved hearing aid technology (e.g., circuitry appropriate for the many types of hearing impairments), (3) efficient universal integrated hearing aid fitting/verification systems, and (4) efficient, professional delivery of high quality hearing health care services.

The universal interfacing of equipment and software for fitting and verifying hearing aid programming and hearing aid performance, especially as device sophistication increases, will be critical to all: to the individuals who purchase and wear the hearing aids; to the audiologists and professionals who select, fit, evaluate, and dispense them; and to the industry that manufacturers the hearing aids and the equipment (hardware/firmware/software) for fitting and verification of hearing aid performance.

It is hoped that when we need these hearing aids in 20–40 years, they will meet our expectations. When the clinician of the future counsels us about realistic expectations for use of the hearing aids of the future, it will not mean accepting less than we really want and need to understand and function as active adults.

References

1. Pascoe DP: An approach to hearing aid selection. *Hear Instrum* 1978; 29(6):12–13, 36.
2. Humes LE, Houghton R: Beyond insertion gain. *Hear Instrum* 1992; 43(3):32–35.
3. Northern JL: Introduction to computerized probe-microphone real-ear measurements in hearing aid evaluation procedures, in Mueller HG, Hawkins DB, Northern JL (eds): *Probe Microphone Measurements: Hearing Aid Selection and Assessment*. San Diego: Singular Publishing Group, 1992, pp 1–19.
4. Knudsen VO, Jones IH: Artificial aids to hearing. *Laryngoscope* 1935; 45:48–69.
5. Watson N, Knudsen VO: Selective amplification in hearing aids. *J Acoust Soc Am* 1940; 11:406–419.
6. Lybarger SF: *Basic Manual for Fitting Radioear Hearing Aids*. Pittsburgh: Radio Ear Corp, 1955.
7. Davis H, Hudgins VC, Marquis RJ, et al.: The selection of hearing aids. *Laryngoscope* 1946; 56:85–115, 135–163.
8. Medical Research Council: *Hearing Aids and Audiometers*. Special Report Series 261. Report of the Committee on Electroacoustics. His Majesty's Stationery Office, London, 1947.
9. Resnick SB: A critical review of the Harvard and MedResCo studies on hearing aids. Communication Sciences Lab Report 10, City University of NY, Graduate School, 1977, reprinted in Levitt H, Pickett JM, Houde RA (eds): *Sensory Aids for the Hearing Impaired*. New York: John Wiley & Sons, 1980, pp 57–76.
10. Killion MC, Monser E: CORFIG: Coupler response for flat insertion gain, in Studebaker G, Hochberg I (eds): *Acoustical Factors Affecting Hearing Aid Performance*. Baltimore, MD: University Park Press, 1980, pp 149–168.
11. Carhart R: Tests for the selection of hearing aids. *Laryngoscope* 1946; 56:780–794.
12. Smaldino J, Hoene J: A view of the state of hearing aid fitting practices. *Hear Instrum* 1981; 32(1):14–15, 38.
13. Smaldino J, Hoene J: The nature of common hearing aid fitting practices, part II. *Hear Instrum* 1981; 32(2):8–11.
14. Martin FN, Morris LJ: Current audiologic practices in the United States. *Hear J* 1989; 4:25–44.
15. Shore I, Bilger RC, Hirsch I: Hearing aid evaluation: Reliability of repeated measurement. *J Speech Hear Dis* 1960; 25:152–167.
16. Resnick DM, Becker M: Hearing aid evaluation: A new approach. *ASHA* 1963; 5:695–699.
17. Thornton AR, Raffin MJM: Speech-discrimination scores modeled as a binomial variable. *J Speech Hear Res* 1978; 21:507–518.
18. Studebaker GA: Hearing aid selection: An overview, in Studebaker GA, Bess FH (eds): *The Vanderbilt Hearing-Aid Report*. Upper Darby, PA: Monographs in Contemporary Audiology, pp 147–55.
19. Victoreen JA: Equal loudness pressures determined with a decaying oscillatory wave form. *J Acoust Soc Am* 1974; 55:309–312.
20. Victoreen JA: *Hearing Enhancement*. Springfield, IL: Charles C Thomas, 1960.
21. Wallenfels HG: *Hearing Aids on Prescription*. Springfield, IL: Charles C Thomas, 1967.
22. Gengel RW: Acceptable speech-to-noise ratios for aided speech discrimination by the hearing impaired. *J Audiol Res* 1971; 11:219–222.
23. Gengel RW, Pascoe DP, Shore I: A frequency response procedure for evaluating and selecting hearing aids for severely hearing-impaired children. *J Speech Hear Dis* 1971; 36:341–353.
24. Shapiro I: Hearing aid fitting by prescription. *Audiology* 1976; 15:163–173.
25. Byrne D, Tonisson W: Selection the gain of hearing aids for persons with sensorineural impairments. *Scand Audiol* 1976; 5:51–59.
26. Byrne D: Selection of hearing aids for severely deaf children. *Br J Audiol* 1978; 12:9–22.
27. Berger KW, Hagberg EN, Rane RL: *Prescription of Hearing Aids: Rationale, Procedure, and Results*. Kent, OH: Herald Publishing House, 1977.
28. Pascoe DP: Frequency responses of hearing aids and their effects on the speech perception of hearing-impaired subjects. *Ann Otol Rhinol Laryngol* 1975; 82:(Suppl 23).
29. Libby ER: State-of-the-art hearing aid selection procedures. *Hear Instrum* 1985; 36:30–38, 62.
30. Libby ER: Hearing aid selection strategies and probe tube microphone measures. *Hear Instrum* 1988; 39(7):10–15.
31. McCandless G, Lyregaard P: Prescription of gain/output (POGO) for hearing aids. *Hear Instrum* 1983; 34:16–21.

32. Cox RM: Using LDLs to establish hearing aid limiting levels. *Hear Instrum* 1981; 32(5):16–20.
33. Cox RM: Using ULCL measures to find frequency-gain and SSPL90. *Hear Instrum* 1983; 34(7):17–21, 39.
34. Cox RM: A structured approach to hearing aid selection. *Ear Hear* 1985; 6:226–239.
35. Cox RM: The MSU hearing instrument prescription procedure. *Hear Instrum* 1988; 39(1):6–10.
36. Seewald RC, Ross M, Spiro M: Selecting amplification characteristics for young hearing impaired children. *Ear Hear* 1985; 6:48–53.
37. Byrne D, Dillon H: The National Acoustic Laboratories' (NAL) new procedure for selecting the gain and frequency response of a hearing aid. *Ear Hear* 1986; 7:257–265.
38. Skinner MW: *Hearing Aid Evaluation*. Englewood Cliffs, NJ: Prentice-Hall, 1988.
39. Byrne D, Parkinson A, Newall P: Hearing aid gain and frequency response requirements for the severely/profoundly hearing impaired (amplification for the severely hearing impaired). *Ear Hear* 1990; 11:40–49.
40. Cox RM, McDaniel DM: Intelligibility ratings of continuous discourse: Application to hearing aid slection. *J Acoust Soc Am* 1984; 76:758–766.
41. Cox RM, Alexander GC, Gilmore C: Development of the connected speech test (CST). *Ear Hear* 1987; 8(Suppl):119S–126S.
42. Pavlovic CV: Articulation index predictions of speech intelligibility in hearing aid selection. *ASHA* 1988; 7(8):63–65.
43. Pavlovic CV: Speech recognition and five articulation indexes. *Hear Instrum* 1991; 4(12):20–24.
44. Walden BE, Demorest ME, Helper EL: Self-report approach to assessing benefit derived form amplification. *J Speech Hear Res* 1984; 27:49–56.
45. Hagerman B, Gabrielsson A: Questionnaires on desirable properties of hearing aids. *Karolinska Ins Rep* TA109, 1984.
46. Leijon A, Lindkvist A, Ringdahl A, Israelsson B: Preferred hearing aid gain in everyday use after prescriptive fitting. *Ear Hearing* 1990; 11:299–305.
47. Leijon A, Lindkvist A, Ringdahl A, Israelsson B: Sound quality and speech reception for prescribed hearing aid frequency responses. *Ear Hearing* 1991; 12:251–260.
48. Gabrielsson A, Sjögren H: Perceived sound quality of hearing aids. *Scand Audiol* 1979; 8:159–169.
49. Gabrielsson A, Sjögren H: Perceived sound quality of sound reproducing systems. *J Acoust Soc Am* 1979; 65:1019–1033.
50. Gabrielsson A, Schenkman BN, Hagerman B: The effects of different frequency responses on sound quality judgments and speech intelligibility. *J Speech Hear Res* 1988; 31:166–177.
51. Gabrielsson A, Hagerman B, Bech-Kristensen T, Lundberg G: Perceived sound quality of reproductions with different frequency responses and sound levels. *J Acoust Soc Am* 1990; 88:1359–1366.
52. Cox RM, Alexander GC: Preferred hearing aid gain in everyday environments. *Ear Hear* 1991; 12:123–126.
53. Cox RM, Alexander GC: Hearing aid benefit in everyday environments. *Ear Hear* 1991; 1:127–139.
54. Cox RM, Alexander GC: Maturation of hearing aid benefit: Objective and subjective measurements (Maturation of Benefit). *Ear Hear* 1992; 13:131–141.
55. Cox RM, Rivera IM: Predictability and reliability of hearing aid benefit measured using the PHAB. *J Am Acad Audiol* 1992; 3:242–254.
56. Stone MA, Moore BCJ: Special feature enhancement for people with sensorineural hearing impairment: Effects on speech intelligibility and quality. *J Rehab Res* 1992; 29:39–56.
57. Thibodeau LM: Exploration of factors beyond audibility that may influences speech recognition. *Ear Hear* 1991; 12:109S–115S.
58. Wever EG, Lawrence M: The transmission properties of the middle ear. *Ann Otol Rhinol Laryngol* 1950; 59:5–18.
59. Wever EG, Lawrence M: *Physiological Acoustics*. Princeton, NJ: Princeton University Press, 1954.
60. Zwislocki JJ: Analysis of the middle-ear function. Part I. Input impedance. *J Acoust Soc Am* 1962; 34:1514–1523.
61. Zwislocki JJ: An acoustic method for clinical examination of the ear. *J Speech Hear Res* 1963; 6:860–864.
62. Weiner FM, Ross DA: The pressure distribution in the auditory canal in a progressive sound field. *J Acoust Soc Am* 1946; 18:401–420.
63. Shaw EAG, Teranishi R: Sound pressure generated in an external-ear replica and real human ears by a nearby point source. *J Acoust Soc Am* 1968; 44:240–249.
64. Shaw EAG: Transformation of sound pressure level from the free field to the eardrum in the horizontal plane. *J Acoust Soc Am* 1974; 56:1848–1861.

65. Shaw EAG: The external ear: New knowledge. *Scand Audiol* 1975; (Suppl 5):24–50.
66. Shaw EAG: The acoustics of the external ear, in Studebaker GA, Hochberg I (eds): *Acoustical Factors Affecting Hearing Aid Performance of Hearing Aid Performance.* Baltimore, MD: University Park Press, 1980, pp 109–125.
67. Zwislocki JJ: *An Acoustic Coupler for Earphone Calibration.* Report LSC-S-7. Syracuse, NY: Laboratory of Sensory Communication, Syracuse University, 1970.
68. Zwislocki JJ: *An Earlike Coupler for Earphone Calibration.* Report LSC S-9. Syracuse, NY: Laboratory of Sensory Communication, Syracuse University, 1971.
69. American National Standards Institute: *Occluded Ear Stimulator.* ANSI S3.25-1979, Revised 1989. New York: American National Standards Institute, Inc., 1989.
70. Romanow F: Methods for measuring the performance of hearing aids. *J Acoust Soc Am* 1942; 13:294–304.
71. American National Standards Institute: *Method for Coupler Calibration of Earphones.* ANSI S3.7-1973. New York: American National Standards Institute, Inc., 1973.
72. American National Standards Institute: *Specification of Hearing Aid Characteristics.* ANSI S3.22-1987. New York: American National Standards Institute, Inc., 1987.
73. Sachs RM, Burkhard MD: Zwislocki Coupler Evaluation With Insert Earphones. Report 20022-1. Franklin Part, IL: Knowles Electronics.
74. Kuhn G: The pressure transformation from a diffuse sound field to the external ear and to the body and head surface. *J Acoust Soc Am* 1979; 65:991–1000.
75. Kuhn G, Guernsey RF: The pressure distribution around the human head and torso. *J Acoust Soc Am* 1983; 73:95–105.
76. Burkhard MD, Sachs RM: Anthropometric manikin for acoustic research. *J Acoust Soc Am* 1975; 58:214–222.
77. American National Standards Institute: *Specification for a Manikin for Simulated In Situ–Airborne Acoustic Measurements.* ANSI S3.36-1985. New York: American National Standards Institute, Inc., 1985.
78. Tonndorf J: Cochlear mechanics and hydro-dynamics. *Found Mod Auditory Theory* 1970; 1:203–250.
79. Tonndorf J: Nonlinearities in cochlear hydrodynamics. *J Acoust Soc Am* 1969; 45:304–305.
80. Zwislocki JJ: A possible neuromechanical sound analysis. *Acoustica* 1974; 34:354–359.
81. Zwislocki JJ: Symposium on cochlear mechanics: Where do we stand after 50 years of research? *J Acoust Soc Am* 1980; 67:1679–1685.
82. Tobias JV (ed): *Foundations of Modern Auditory Theory,* vol 1. New York: Academic Press, 1970.
83. Tobias JV (ed): *Foundations of Modern Auditory Theroy,* vol 2. New York: Academic Press, 1971.
84. Rhode WS, Robles L: Evidence from Mössbauer experiments for nonlinear vibration in the cochlea. *J Acoust Soc Am* 1976; 54:588–596.
85. Johnstone BM, Patuzzi R, Yates GK: Basilar membrane measurements and the traveling wave. *Hear Res* 1986; 22:147–153.
86. Kemp DT: Development in cochlear mechanics and techniques for noninvasive evaluation. *Adv Audiol* 1988; 5:27–45.
87. Ludivgsen C: Processing for optimum speech intelligibility—measurements of hair cell function may have implications for hearing instrument design. *Hear Instrum* 1992; 43:22, 24–25, 28.
88. Goldstein JL: Modeling rapid waveform compression on the basilar membrane as multiple-bandpass-nonlinearity filtering. *Hear Res* 1990; 49, 39–60.
89. Knowles HS, Killon MC: Frequency characteristics of recent broadband receivers. *J Audiol Technol* 1978; 17:86–89.
90. Killion MC: *Design and Evaluation of High-Fidelity Hearing Aids.* Ph.D. thesis, Northwestern University. Ann Arbor, MI: University Microfilms, 1977.
91. Killion, MC: Problems in the application of broadband hearing aid earphones, in Studebaker G, Hochberg I (eds): *Acoustical Factors Affecting Hearing Aid Performance.* Baltimore, MD: University Park Press, 1980, pp 219–264.
92. Studebaker GS, Bess FH, Beck LB (eds): *The Vanderbilt hearing-aid report II,* Parkton, MD: York Press, 1991.
93. Mueller HG, Hawkins DB, Northern JL (eds): *Probe Microphone Measurements: Hearing Aid Selection and Assessment.* San Diego: Singular Publishing Group, 1992.
94. Hawkins DB: Current approaches to hearing aid selection. *Can J Speech–Language Pathology and Audiology.* In press.
95. Sammeth CA, Bess FH, Bratt GW, et al.: The Vanderbilt/Veterans Administration hearing aid selection study: Interim report. *ASHA* 1989; 31:131.
96. Bragg VC: Toward a more objective hearing aid fitting procedure. *Hear Instrum* 1977; 23(9):6–9.
97. Levitt H, Sullivan JA, Neuman AC, Rubin-Spitz JA: Experiments with a programmable master hearing aid. *J Rehab Res Dev* 1987; 24:29–54.

98. Skinner M, Pascoe D, Miller J, Popelka G: Measurements to determine the optimal placement of speech energy within the listener's auditory area: A basis for selection amplification characteristics, in Studebaker G, Bess F (eds): *The Vanderbilt Hearing-Aid Report.* Upper Darby, PA: Associated Hearing Instruments, 1982, pp 161–169.
99. Mueller HG: Individualizing the ordering and fitting procedure. *Hear Instrum* 1989; 40:18–22.
100. Punch J, Chi C, Patterson J: A recommended protocol for prescriptive use of target gain rules. *Hear Instrum* 1990; 41(4):12–19.
101. Revit LJ: *An Open Letter: New Thinking on the Proper Application of Real-Ear Unaided Measurements to Prescription and Fitting.* Tigard, OR: Frye Electronics, 20 March 1990.
102. Fikret-Passa S, Revit LJ: Individualized correction factors in the preselection of hearing aids. *J Speech Hear Res* 1992; 35:384–400.
103. Berninger E, Overgard A, Svard I: Coupler-related real-ear gain. *Scand Audiol* 1992; 211:15–22.
104. Killion MC, Revit L: CORFIG and GIFROG: Real ear to coupler, and back, in Studebaker GA, Hochberg I (eds): *Acoustical Factors Affecting Hearing Aid Performance,* ed 2. Needham Heights, MA: Allyn and Bacon, 1993, pp 65–85.
105. Valente M, Valente M, Vass W: Selecting an appropriate matrix for ITE/ITC hearing instruments. *Hear Instrum* 1990; 41:20–24.
106. Hawkins DB, Walden BE, Montgomery A, Prosek RA: Description and validation of an LDL procedure designed to select SSPL90. *Ear Hear* 1987; 8:162–169.
107. Byrne D, Upfold G: Implications of ear canal resonance for hearing aid fitting. *Semin Hear* 1991; 121:34–41.
108. Kochkin K: MarkeTrak III identifies key factors in determining consumer satifaction. *Hear J* 1992; 45(8):39–44.
109. Killion MC: An "acoustically invisible" hearing aid. *Hear Instrum* 1988; 39(10):39–44.
110. Killion MC: A high fidelity hearing aid. *Hear Instrum* 1990; 41(8):38–39.
111. Preves DA: The K-Amp circuit. *Am J Audiol* 1992; 1(2):15–16.
112. Fabry DA: Hearing aid compression. *Am J Audiol* 1991; 1:11–13.
113. Fabry DA: Programmable and automatic noise reduction in existing hearing aids, in Studebaker GA, Bess FH, Beck LB (eds): *The Vanderbilt Hearing-Aid Report II.* Pankton, MD: York Press, 1991, pp 65–75.
114. Kruger B, Kruger FM: The K-Amp[tm] hearing aid: A summary of features and benefits. *Hear Instrum* 1993; 44(1):20–21, 24.
115. Kruger B, Kruger FM: The K-Amp[tm] hearing aid: Clinical impressions with fittings. *Hear Instrum* 1993; 44(2):30–31, 35.
116. Kruger B, Kruger FM: K-Amp[tm] hearing aid: A wide range of fitting options impressions. *Hear Instrum* 1993; 44:26, 28.
117. Humes LE: An evaluation of several rationale for hearing aid gain. *J Speech Hear Dis* 1986; 51:272–281.
118. Dillon H, Murray N: Accuracy of twelve methods for estimating the real ear gain of hearing aids. *Ear Hear* 1987; 8:2–11.
119. Byrne D: Recent hearing instrument selection research suggests what? *Hear Instrum* 1988; 39(12):22–23.
120. Humes LE: And the winner is. . . . *Hear Instrum* 1988; 39(7):24–26.
121. Humes LE: Reply to Dennis Byrne. *Hear Instrum* 1988; 39(12):24–29.
122. Gauthier EA, Rapisardi DA: Does that target make sense? . . . With those thresholds? *Hear Instrum* 1988; 43(4):34–35.
123. Pascoe D: Clinical measurements of the auditory dynamic range and their relation to formulas for hearing aid gain. *Danavox Symp* 1989; 129–152.
124. Byrne D: Hearing aid selection formulae: Same or different. *Hear Instrum* 1987; 38(1):5–11.
125. Sullivan JA, Levitt H, Hwang JY, Hennessey AM: An experimental comparison of four hearing aid prescription methods. *Ear Hear* 1988; 9:22–32.
126. Valente M, Meister M, Valente M: Prescribed versus average used gain for experienced hearing aid users. *Aust J Audiol* 1990; 12(2):55–65.
127. Hawkins DB: Selection of a critical electroacoustic characteristic: SSPL90. *Hear Instrum* 1990; 41(8):24–26.
128. Van Tasell DJ, Crain TR: Noise reduction hearing aids: Release from masking and release from distortion. *Ear Hear* 1992; 13:114–121.
129. Killion MC, Staab W, Preves DA: Classifying automatic signal processors. *Hear Instrum* 1990; 41(8):24–26.
130. Hawkins DB, Naidoo S: The effect of peak clipping and compression limiting upon perceived sound clarity and quality. Paper presented at annual convention of American Academy of Audiology, Nashville, TN 1992.
131. American National Standards Institute: *Testing Hearing Aids With a Broad-Band Noise Signal.*

ANSI S3.42-1992. New York: American National Standards Institute, Inc., 1992.

132. Cox RM, Moore JN: Composite speech spectrum for hearing aid gain prescriptions. *J Speech Hear Res* 1988; 31:102–107.

133. Pearsons KS, Fidell S, Bennett RL: *Speech Levels in Various Environments*. Report No. 321. Canoga Park, CA: Bolt, Beranek and Newman, 1976.

134. American National Standards Institute: *American National Standards Methods for the Calculation of the Articulation Index*. ANSI S3.5-1969. New York, NY: American National Standards Institute, 1969.

135. French N, Steinberg J: Factors governing the intelligibility of speech sounds. *J Acoust Soc Am* 1947; 19:90–119.

136. Beranek LL: The design of speech communication systems. *Proc Inst Radio Engineers* 1947; 35:880–890.

137. Kryter KD: Methods for the calculation and use of the articulation index. *J Acoust Soc Am* 1962; 34:1689–1697.

138. Kryter KD: Validation of the articulation index. *J Acoust Soc Am* 1962; 34:1968–1702.

139. Fletcher H: The perception of speech sounds by deafened persons. *J Acoust Soc Am* 1952; 24:490–497.

140. Dugal RL, Bradia LD, Durlach NI: Implications of previous research for the selection of frequency gain characteristics, in Studebaker GA, Hochberg I (eds): *Acoustical Factors Affecting Hearing Aid Performance*. Baltimore, MD: University Park Press, 1980.

141. Skinner MW, Miller JD: Amplification bandwidth and intelligibility of speech in quiet and noise for listeners with sensorineural hearing loss. *Audiology* 1983; 22:253–279.

142. Pavlovic CV: Use of the articulation index for assessing residual auditory function in listeners with sensorineural hearing impairment. *J Acoust Soc Am* 1984; 75:1253–1257.

143. Kamm C, Dirks DD, Bell TS: Speech recognition and the articulation index for normal and hearing-impaired listeners. *J Acoust Soc Am* 1985; 77:281–288.

144. Pavlovic CV, Studebaker GA: An evaluation of some assumptions underlying the articulation index. *J Acoust Soc Am* 1984; 75:1606–1612.

145. Pavlovic CV, Studebaker GA, Sherbacoe RL: An articulation index based procedure for predicting the speech recognition performance of hearing impaired individuals. *J Acoust Soc Am* 1986; 80:50–57.

146. Pavlovic CV: Derivation of primary parameters and procedures for use in speech intelligibility predictions. *J Acoust Soc Am* 1987; 82:413–422.

147. Pavlovic CV: Speech spectrum considerations and speech intelligibility predictions in hearing aid evaluations. *J Speech Hear Disord* 1989; 54:3–8.

148. Pavlovic CV: Speech recognition and five articulation indexes. *Hear Instrum* 1991; 42:20–24.

149. Marincovich PJ: The articulation index and hearing aid selection. *Hear Instrum* 1987; 38(1):18, 58.

150. Rankovic CM: An application of the articulation index to hearing aid fitting. *J Speech Hear Res* 1991; 34:391–403.

151. Humes LE: *Selective Hearing Aids for Patients Effectively (SHAPE), Version 2.1*. 1987, pp 1–35.

152. Mueller HG, Killion M: An easy method for calculating the articulation index. *Hear J* 1990; 43:14–17.

153. Humes LE: Understanding the speech-understanding problems of the hearing impaired. *J Am Acad Audiol* 1991; 2:59–69.

154. Seewald RC: The desired sensation level method for fitting children: Version 3.0. *Hear J* 1992; 45(4):36–41.

155. Pascoe D: Hearing aid selection procedure used at Central Institute for the Deaf in Saint Louis. *Audiol Acoust* 1986; 29:12–16, 36.

156. Pascoe D: Hearing aid evaluation, in Katz J (ed): *Handbook of Clinical Audiology*, ed 3. 1985, pp 936–948.

157. Seewald RC: The desired sensation level approach for children: Selection and verification. *Hear Instrum* 1988; 39(7):18–20.

158. Seewald RC, Zelisko DL, Ramji KV, Jamieson DG: *DSL 3.0 Users Manual: A Computer Assisted Implementation of The Desired Sensation Level Method for Electroacoustic Selection and Fitting in Children*. 1991, pp 1–75.

159. Seewald RC, Hudson SP, Gagné JP, Zelisko DLC: Comparison of two methods for estimating the sensation level of amplified speech. *Ear Hear* 1992; 13:142–149.

160. Valente M, Skinner MW, Valente ML, et al.: Clinical comparisons of digitally programmable hearing aids, in Sandlin R (ed): *Digital Technology and Hearing Aid Amplification* Needhan Heights, MA: Allyn and Bacon, 1993.

161. Byrne D: Key issues in hearing aid selection and evaluation. *J Am Acad Audiol* 1992; 3:67–80.

162. Sullivan RF: Aided SSPL 90 response in the real ear: A safe estimate. *Hear Instrum* 1987; 38, 36.

163. Stelmachowicz P: Clinical issues related to hearing aid maximum output, in Studebaker G, Bess F, Beck L (eds): *The Vanderbilt Hearing-Aid Report II*. Parkton, MD: York Press, 1991, pp 141–148.
164. Stelmachowicz P, Lewis D, Seewald R, Hawkins D: Complex and pure-tone signals in the evaluation of hearing-aid characteristics. *J Speech Hear Res* 1990; 33:380–385.
165. Filion PR, Margolis RH: Comparison of clinical and real-life judgments of loudness discomfort. *J Am Acad Audiol* 1992; 3:193–199.
166. Hawkins DB, Ball TL, Beasley HE, Cooper WA: Comparison of SSPL90 selection procedures. *J Am Acad Audiol* 1992; 3:46–50.
167. Gottermeier L, DeFilippo CL, Block MG: Loudness judgment procedures for evaluating hearing aid preselection decisions for severely and profoundly hearing-impaired listeners (loudness procedures). *Ear Hear* 1991; 12:261–267.
168. Lybarger SFP: Selective amplification-a review and evaluation. *J Am Audiol Soc* 1978; 3:258–266.
169. Wallenfels HG: The "unfittables." *Hear Instrum* 1979; 30(10):14–116, 36.
170. Kamm C, Dirks DD, Mickey MR: Effects of sensorineural hearing loss on loudness discomfort level and most comfortable judgments. *J Speech Hear Res* 1978; 21:668–681.
171. Kiessling J: In situ audiometry (ISA). *Hear Instrum* 1987; 38(1):28–29.
172. Cox RM, Alexander GC: Evaluation of an in-situ output probe-microphone method for hearing aid fitting verification. *Ear Hearing* 1990; 11:31–39.
173. American National Standards Institute: *Specification for Audiometers*. ANSI S3.6-1969. revised 1989, New York: American National Standards Institute, Inc., 1989.
174. Burnett E, Beck L: A correction for converting $2\,cm^3$ coupler responses to insertion responses for custom in-the-ear non-directional hearing aids. *Ear Hear* 1987; 8(Suppl 5): 89S–94S.
175. Bentler RA, Pavlovic CV: Transfer functions and correction factors used in hearing aid evaluation and research. *Ear Hear* 1989; 10:58–63.
176. Bentler RA, Pavlovic CV: Addendum to "transfer functions and correction factors used in hearing aid evaluation and research." *Ear Hear* 1992; 13:255–262.
177. Killion MC: Revised estimate of minimum audible pressure: Where is the "missing" 6 dB. *J Acoust Soc Am* 1978; 63;1501–1508.
178. Dillon H, Chew R, Deans M: Loudness discomfort level measurements and their implications for the design and fitting of hearing aids. *Aust J Audiol* 1984; 6:73–79.
179. Wilber LA, Kruger B, Killion MC: Reference thresholds for the ER-3A insert earphone. *J Acoust Soc Am* 1988; 83:669–676.
180. Butler RA: The effect of hearing impairment on locating sound in the vertical plane. *Int Audiol* 1970; 9:117–126.
181. Butler RA, Belendivk K: Spectral cues utilized in the localization of sound in the median sagittal plane. *J Acoust Soc Am* 1977; 61:1264–1269.
182. Preves DA, Sullivan RF: Sound field equalization for real ear measurements with probe microphones. *Hear Instrum* 1987; 38(1):20–26, 64.
183. Killion MC, Revit L: Insertion gain repeatability versus loudspeaker location: You want me to put my loudspeaker W-H-E-R-E? *Ear Hear* 1987; 8:68S–73S.
184. Sachs RM, Burkhard MD: Insert earphone pressure response in ear and couplers. *J Acoust Soc Am* 1972; 52:183(A).
185. Sachs RM, Burkhard MD: Making pressure measurements in insert earphones, couplers, and real ears. *J Acoust Soc Am* 1972; 51:140(A).
186. Fortune TW, Preves DA: Hearing aid saturation and aided loudness discomfort. *J Speech Hear Res* 1992; 35:175–185.
187. Cox RM, Bisset JD: Relationship between two measures of aided binaural advantage. *J Speech Hear Disord* 1984; 49:399–408.
188. Feuerstein JF: Monural versus binaural hearing: Ease of listening, word recognition, and attentional effort. *Ear Hear* 1992; 13:80–85.
189. McCullough JA, Abbas PJ: Effects of interaural speech-recognition differences on binaural advantage for speech in noise. *J Am Acad Audiol* 1992; 3;255–261.
190. Kruger B: An update on the external ear resonance in infants and young children. *Ear Hear* 1987; 8:333–336.
191. Feigin J, Kopun J, Stelmachowitz P, Gorga M: Probe-tube microphone measures of ear-canal sound pressure levels in infants and children. *Ear Hear* 1989; 10:254–258.
192. Hawkins DB, Cooper WA, Thompson DJ: Comparisons among SPLs in real ears, $2\,cm^3$, and 6-cm^3 couplers. *J Am Acad Audiol* 1990; 1:154–161.
193. Hawkins DB: Clinical ear canal probe microphone measurements. *Hear Instrum* 1987; 8(Suppl 5):74–81.

194. Hawkins DB: Variability in clinical ear canal probe microphone measurements. *Hear Instrum* 1987; 38:30–32.
195. Cornelisse LE, Gagné JP, Seewald RC: Ear level recordings of the long-term average spectrum of speech. *Ear Hear* 1991; 12:47–54.
196. Dillon H, Byrne D, Battaglia J: Hearing instrument selection: By dispenser or by computer? *Hear Instrum* 1992; 43:18, 20–21.
197. Humes LE: Hearing aid selection and evaluation in the year 2000. *Can J Speech–Language Pathol Audiol* (in press).
198. Kuk FK, Plager A, Pape NML: Hollowness perception with noise-reduction hearing aids. *J Am Acad Audiol* 1992; 3:39–45.
199. Schweitzer C, Smith DA: Solving the "occlusion effect" electronically. *Hear Instrum* 1992; 43:30–33.
200. Allen JB, Neely ST: Micromechanical models of the cochlea. *Physics Today* July 1992: 40–47.
201. Goldstein JL: Modeling the nonlinear cochlear mechanical basis of psychophysical tuning. *J Acoust Soc Am* 1991; 2267–268.
202. Goldstein JL: Changing roles in the cochlea: Bandpass filtering by the organ of Corti and additive amplification on the basilar membrane. *J Acoust Soc Am* 1992; 2407.
203. Humes LE, Jesteadt W, Lee LW: Modeling the effects of sensorineural hearing loss on auditory perception. *Aud Physiol Percept* 1992; 617–624.
204. Glasberg BR, Moore BCJ: Derivation of auditory filter shapes from notched-noise data. *Hear Res* 1990; 47:103–138.
205. Moore BCJ, Glasberg BR: Formulae describing frequency selectivity as a function of frequency and level, and their use in calculating exciting patterns. *Hear Res* 1987; 28:209–225.
206. Steeneken HJM, Houtgast T: A physical method for measuring speech transmission quality. *J Acoust Soc Am* 1980; 67:318–326.
207. Humes LE, Dirks DD, Bell TS, et al.: Application of articulation index and the speech transmission index to the recognition of speech by normal-hearing and hearing-impaired listeners. *J Speech Hear Res* 1986; 29:447–462.
208. Dubno JR, Schaefer AB: Comparison of frequency selectivity and consonant recognition among hearing impaired and masked normal-hearing listeners. *J Acoust Soc Am* 1992; 91:2110–2121.
209. Florentine M, Buus S: Temporal gap detection in sensorineural and simulated hearing instruments. *J Speech Hear Res* 1984; 27:449–455.
210. Florentine M, Fastl H, Buus S: Temporal integration in normal hearing, cochlear impairment, and impairment simulated by masking. *J Acoust Soc Am* 1988; 84:195–203.

15

Future Trends
in Verification Strategies

RUTH A. BENTLER

Introduction

Complete textbooks have been written on how to fit hearing aids. Diagnostic tools continue to be developed, circuitry continues to become more sophisticated and complex, and the hearing impaired population continues to grow! Verification that the hearing aid chosen for a particular individual has the appropriate (1) frequency response; and (2) signal processing strategy, including (3) compression parameters, (4) bandpass cross-over points, (5) number of memories, and so on, becomes increasingly more complex as the options become more numerous. Audiologists may spend an indeterminate amount of time adjusting tone and output parameters, modifying the "plumbing," and calculating the difference in gain that may be obtained by moving a microphone a few millimeters. Once satisfied with the measures obtained with whatever tools are at hand, little further verification of the appropriateness of the fit may be carried out. If the primary goal in amplification is to provide an audible speech signal that is comfortably loud and free of distortion and is qualitatively pleasing to listen to, then additional (perhaps longer term) verification of the fit must be considered. The purpose of this chapter is to describe and discuss some approaches and issues that may be part of the verification process of the future. While technology continues to change dramatically, verifying that our fitting protocols have produced successful users of that technology may require a little reflection.

Many of the current fitting protocols include objective measures (e.g., electroacoustic measures done in situ and in 2 cc couplers, speech recognition tasks, articulation index calculations, response time measures) and subjective measures (e.g., expectations, self-report inventories, satisfaction questionnaires, qualitative judgments). A number of these fitting tools could be considered verification tools as well. Regardless of the technology employed, verification or outcome measures should confirm:

1.   High fidelity reproduction of sound
2.   Improved speech recognition performance
3.   Enhanced self-perception of communication ability.

Relative to the first goal, one might argue that newer technology may allow for some synthesis rather than reproduction of a speech signal; yet *high fidelity* must remain a goal. Others may argue that the expansion, compression, and other strategies discussed in Chapter 14 will inherently restrict the fidelity of the signal. If the output signal is free of distortion products and extraneous circuit-produced noise, it can be considered high fidelity regardless of the signal processing strategy employed.

While the second and third goals may seem closely related, objective measures of improved communication skills do not ensure or predict enhancement of self-perceived benefit and vice versa.[1-6] As a result, future outcome measures must consider both improved speech recognition and enhanced self-perception of communication ability as measures of effectiveness. Each of the three goals will be discussed, and possible future verification tools will be presented.

High Fidelity Reproduction of Sound

While high fidelity in hearing aids has been a technical goal for many years, it is only with the introduction of current transducers that this potential is finally being realized. Early instruments had technical limitations that resulted in limited bandwidth and excessive distortion that resulted in poor sound quality. Relative to current technology, Killion[7] contends that "problems of size, response of smoothness, bandwidth limitations, and noise level have now been completely solved" (p. 31). Problems in achieving high fidelity still exist in amplified signals due to distortion products as a result of the aid operating in saturation, amplifier nonlinearities and other sources that are not yet completely understood. Quantifying the impact of reduced fidelity as a result of distortion remains an elusive goal.

The use of coherence measures has been suggested as a verification of high fidelity.[8] Coherence is defined as that portion of the output signal that is directly related to the input signal (discussed in greater detail in Ch. 16). Coherence measures indicate the total distortion and noise measured at the output of a hearing aid (harmonic and intermodulation distortion as well as circuit noise). The distortion measurement currently specified in the ANSI S3.22[9] hearing aid standard is a measure of total harmonic distortion using pure tones of 500, 800, and 1600 Hz (assuming a "standard" instrument). Coherence measures are typically obtained using a steady-state signal such as a speech-weighted noise. Coherence values across the entire frequency range can vary from 0 to 1.0, and the graphic representation is referred to as a coherence function. At low inputs a hearing aid may show coherence values around 1.0, indicating that it is relatively free of noise and distortion. At higher input levels (and particularly dependent on the type of output limitation used) the coherence values may be considerably reduced. Much remains to be clarified in the use of coherence measures. At present, there are several known means of maximizing coherence:

1. Operating circuits below saturation: The input level plus the gain provided by the hearing aid produce an output that is below the selected saturation sound pressure level (SSPL90)
2. Using a hearing aid containing a Class B or Class D amplifier: By increasing "headroom," the output of the hearing aid is less likely to saturate with a typical input level than with a Class A amplifier.

The relationship between coherence values and subjective estimates of sound quality or speech recognition measures is unclear. It seems logical to suggest that the higher the coherence, the higher will be the judged quality and clarity of the amplified sound.[10,11] It has been acknowledged, however, that coherence functions may not be valid measures for instruments with automatic signal processing.[12,13]

More recently, Tyler et al.[14] have proposed that "true" speech sounds should be used in the electroacoustic evaluation of hearing aids as a measurement of performance. Other investigators have used true speech sounds to measure the effect of spectral and durational enhancement on the processed waveform.[15] Many current hearing aids are nonlinear, and it is expected that nonlinear circuitry will dominate the market in the near future. As a result it is difficult to specify the response characteristics of many of the current processing schemes using any of the current standardized stimulus types.[9] The stimuli currently implemented in electroacoustic measurements do not provide performance characteristics that can be generalized to the more dynamic speech sounds. Current measures of distortion do not differentiate among hearing aids, even though subjectively the circuits may sound very different. Many hearing aids of the future will continue to have multi-channel compression, and any adjustment of those compression parameters (e.g., kneepoint, compression ratio, attack and release times) in any of the available channels may impact the processed signal depending on its spectral content and, for true speech sounds, the formants and their transitions.

Tyler et al.[14] measured the output of a two-channel compression hearing aid for digitized "naturally produced" words. The words *observations, corresponding, telephoned,* and *gateways* were chosen to represent a wide range of phonemic sounds. Each word was processed through a commercially available two-channel compression hearing aid for which compression threshold and release time could be adjusted. The intent of these investigators was to obtain waveform and spectrograph information that current electroacoustic measures do not provide. As shown in Figure 15–1, the waveform for the word *observations* from the two-channel processor (cross-over frequency set to 1240 Hz) reveals the impact of altering the release time in the high pass channel. The spectrogram obtained from the total output shown in Figure 15–2 provides additional information. The ouput does not contain the energy above 5000 Hz that is present in the input; coupler measures of frequency response would indicate the same bandwidth effect. What is apparent in the spectrogram in

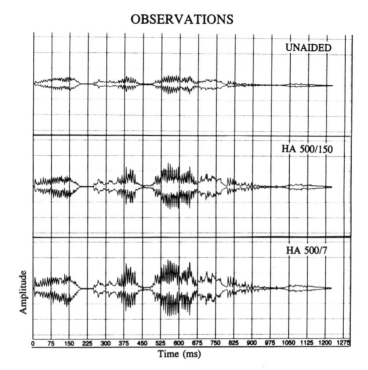

Figure 15–1.   Time waveform mesured at the output of a two-channel AGC hearing aid for the word *observations*. (**A**) Unamplified signal, (**B**) amplified waveform when the high pass channel utilizes a 150 msec release time from compression; and (**C**) amplified waveform when the high pass channel utilizes a 7 msec release time from compression. (From Tyler et al.[14])

Figure 15–2 is the effect of the compression circuit on the formant trajectories. The lower panels indicate that the inter-formant energy has been amplified, while the peaks appear to be compressed. In view of the dynamic changes in the response that are dependent on input stimulus in many current circuits, future electroacoustic measures of hearing aid performance may consider using "real" speech dynamics in their measurement procedures. Pure tones, narrow bands of noise, and speech-shaped complexes provide a picture of the static response of the hearing aid. Speech is not static, and its interaction with nonlinear circuitry may significantly impact the fidelity and, consequently, the quality and quantity of the message to the user.

Improved Speech Recognition Ability

Audibility of the Speech Signal

In addition to verifying high fidelity reproduction, strategies aimed at verification of the audibility of the speech signal are gaining attention. Numerous prescriptive hearing aid fitting strategies have been proposed over the past

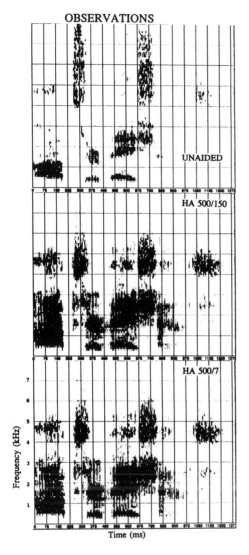

Figure 15–2. Spectrogram from the word *observations* unaided and processed through a two-channel AGC hearing aid with release times of 500 msec low pass channel and 150 msec high pass channel and 500 msec low pass channel and 7 msec high pass channel. (From Tyler et al.[14])

several years, based on threshold or suprathreshold measures. These prescriptions include the prescription of gain and output (POGO),[16] National Acoustic Laboratories (NAL),[17] Version 3.1 of the Memphis State University Hearing Instrument Prescription Formula (MSUv3),[18] and the Central Institute for the Deaf Phase IV Method (CID).[19–21] More recently, several strategies, including Version 3.1 of the Desired Sensation Level (DSL),[22] have been proposed with the goal of amplifying the average speech spectrum to a predetermined sensation level. While it is not possible to ensure audibility of the entire speech spectrum under all listening conditions, consideration of the audibility of the average speech spectrum affords more promise of attaining the goal of improved speech recognition. ("Although it is true that mere detection of a

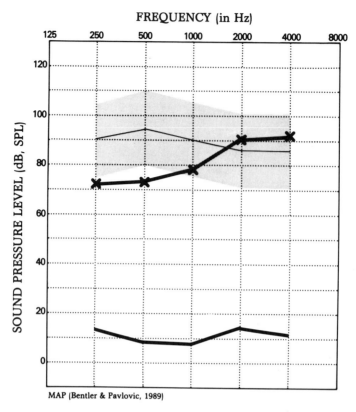

FREQUENCY (in Hz)

MAP (Bentler & Pavlovic, 1989)

Figure 15–3. An example of a hearing aid fitting. Unaided thresholds (x–x) and amplified speech spectrum (– – –) indicated that little of the spectrum is audible above 1500 Hz, although the prescriptive target was matched.

sound does not ensure its recognition, it is even more true that without detection the probabilities of correct identification are greatly diminished."[23])

Figure 15–3 illustrates an example in which the frequency-gain response of a hearing aid was adjusted to provide real-ear gain approximating one-half the hearing loss or a match to a half-gain prescriptive formula. All measures are shown with the eardrum as the referent. Thresholds in hearing level (HL) (ANSI[24]) were converted to sound pressure level (SPL) at the eardrum using the MAP derivation as described by Bentler and Pavlovic.[25] When that amount of gain is applied to a typical speech spectrum, a strategy proposed by Seewald et al.,[26,27] it becomes more apparent that significant portions of the amplified speech spectrum may not actually be audible. For example, assuming a speech spectrum similar to the one presented by Cox and Moore[28,29] and shown as one-third octave values in Table 15–1, many of the high frequency components of the amplified speech signal shown in Figure 15–3 are not within the range of audibility for that individual. The half-gain prescriptive target was achieved, but a portion of the average conversational speech spectrum is not audible. A similar result occurs when the output is unduly limited and the hearing aid

Table 15-1. Comparison of One-Third Octave Levels of Speech (in dB SPL)

Frequency (Hz)	Formula*			
	NAL	*MSU*	*DSL*	*CID*
100	0.0	0.0	39.1	
125	0.0	0.0	39.9	
160	0.0	0.0	46.3	
200	63.0	0.0	59.6	
250	62.0	60.0	62.8	62.0
315	60.0	57.0	60.1	
400	62.0	61.0	61.6	
500	61.0	62.0	64.3	66.0
630	58.0	59.0	63.1	
800	55.0	56.5	60.1	
1000	50.0	55.0	56.4	56.0
1250	51.0	54.5	53.7	
1600	51.0	52.0	52.1	
2000	49.0	49.0	51.0	50.0
2500	48.0	48.0	48.8	
3150	47.0	46.5	45.0	
4000	48.0	46.0	42.3	49.0
5000	45.0	44.0	41.5	
6300	46.0	45.5	42.1	
8000	0.0	0.0	40.9	
10 000	0.0	0.0	38.0	
Overall	70.0	70.0	70.9	70

* NAL, National Acoustics Laboratories; MSU, Memphis State University Version 3.0; DSL, Desired Sensation Level, Version 3.0; CID, Central Institute of the Deaf, Phase IV.

(From Bentler.[28])

reaches saturation for soft input levels, thus limiting the range of amplification for all levels of the input signal. The potential for such error is even more pronounced for individuals with severe to profound hearing impairment (refer to Ch. 13).

In assessing the audibility of speech, it is also possible that the speech spectrum chosen for graphic manipulation as is done in Figure 15-3 may not be representative of any one patient's listening experience. As shown in Table 15-1, several investigators have proposed different speech spectra as being "average." Olsen et al.[30] reviewed the various published average speech spectra and acknowledged that the particular spectral characteristics of any speech signal are dependent on a number of factors, including the age and gender of the talker, the speech material used, the length of time over which the sample is obtained, and the location of the measuring microphone, to mention a few. For application in pediatric fittings, Seewald et al.[26] have proposed utilizing an average speech spectrum that is more representative of that which is measured at the ear-level of the child to whom the hearing aid is being fit.

Cornelisse et al.[31] obtained ear-level measures of the long-term average speech spectrum (LTASS) for three groups of subjects (adult males, adult females, and children). They reported that more low frequency energy (below 1000 Hz) and less high frequency energy (above 2500 Hz) was present than was previously reported by investigators whose measurements were obtained directly in front of the speaker(s). Incorporated into their LTASS estimate is the spectrum of the child's own voice obtained at ear level.

Other investigators continue to define an average speech spectrum that may be more appropriate to the fitting needs of the individual. Stelmachowicz[32] has attempted to measure speech spectra for a variety of parent–child positions. Future verification strategies that attempt to validate audibility of the "average" speech spectrum must consider and define the particular spectral characteristics of the speech signal being amplified.

Of perhaps greater importance than the choice of speech spectrum may be the choice of vocal effort used in the verification of the audibility of speech. As shown in Figure 15–4, the spectral characteristics of speech are known to vary depending on the vocal effect of the talker(s). One futuristic verification strategy proposed by Humes[13] accounts for both spectral content of the speech sounds and vocal effort of production. A plot called a *phon-gram* (shown in Figure 15–5) is generated during the hearing aid evaluation. The phon-gram is a plot of the SPL generated at the eardrum for seven speech sounds that "encompass a spectral range from approximately 300 to 10 000 Hz and almost the full range of amplitudes in conversational speech"[13] (p. 102). (Only the first and second formants of the vowels were considered in order to maintain

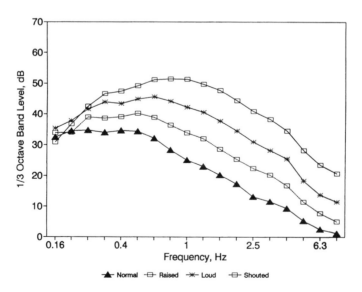

Figure 15–4. Speech spectra for four vocal efforts: normal (62.35 dB SPL), raised (68.34 dB SPL), loud (74.85 dB SPL), and shouted (82.30 dB SPL). (Derived from the Proposed American National Standard Methods for the Calculation of the Speech Intelligibility Index.[62])

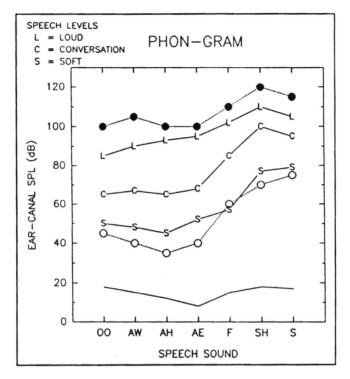

Figure 15–5. Illustration of an aided phon-gram for a hypothetical hearing impaired listener. Letters connected by solid lines represent ear canal sound pressure levels of each speech sound (from Table 15–2) presented at sound field levels corresponding to soft (S), conversational (C), and loud (L) speech. (From Humes.[33])

Table 15–2. Acoustic Parameters of Speech Sounds
Used in Phon-Gram for Figure 15–5

Speech Sound	Region (Hz) of Spectral Concentration	Relative Amplitude (dB)
/u/	300, 870	58.3
/ɔ/	570, 840	60.0
/e/	730, 1090	59.6
/æ/	600, 1720	58.6
/f/	1000–10 000	38.7
/ʃ/	2000–5000	50.7
/s/	4000–8000	43.7

(From Humes.[33])

frequency specificity.) The acoustic characteristics of those speech sounds were derived from Hodgson[34] and are shown in Table 15–2. Threshold and discomfort levels are initially obtained using the speech sounds as stimuli. The ear canal SPL for each stimuli at threshold and discomfort can be plotted using any commercially available probe microphone system. Subsequently, the chosen hearing aid is inserted, and probe microphone measures of SPL at the eardrum are obtained for varying levels of vocal effort (soft, conversational, and loud) for each of the seven speech sounds. As is apparent in Figure 15–5, the results suggest audibility (and yet no discomfort) for all but high frequency speech sound. Manipulation of the high frequency gain may alter the audibility of that particular sound. Implementation of this verification procedure can be accomplished with current computer capability.[35]

Measures of Speech Recognition

Without actually measuring audibility across the speech spectrum, objective measures of speech recognition are currently being obtained in many clinics. Presumably, those measures are obtained for one of two reasons: (1) to determine some aided performance level that is *predictive* of actual performance in everyday situations or (2) to determine the aided *improvement* in speech recognition performance.

Of related interest is the issue of maturation of hearing aid benefit[3] or acclimatization to the speech signal.[36] If speech recognition performance changes in the weeks following the fitting of the hearing, then verification measures should also be obtained at some time after the initial fitting. At least one investigation has shown aided speech recognition performance to remain relatively stable over a 1 year period. Bentler et al.[1,2] measured speech recognition ability in quiet and noise over a 1 year postfitting period. The tests employed were the Speech Perception in Noise test[37,38] and the CUNY Nonsense Syllable Test.[39] Performance level was found to be relatively constant for 65 subjects with varying degrees and configurations of hearing loss. These investigators chose the revised National Acoustic Laboratories' (NAL-R) gain-based prescriptive formula[17] for adjusting the frequency-gain response of the hearing aids. Baseline speech recognition scores were measured with the volume control adjusted to provide an NAL-R fitting. Subsequent measures of speech recognition were obtained over the year, with the subjects setting the volume control at preferred use gain. While preferred use gain settings at 6 months and 1 year postfitting did not vary significantly from prescribed settings, it is possible that, had the subjects been allowed to adjust the volume control for the initial tests, the speech recognition scores may have reflected lower gain settings. In addition, all hearing aids used in that investigation were single channel hearing aids with relatively linear function; newer signal processing schemes may require a practice or training period to optimize the benefit. Cox and Alexander[3] also reported no change in speech recognition ability over a 10 week time period in noisy and reverberant environments with visual cues present. In environments with low background noise levels, or where visual cues were not available, improvement in performance increased through the same 10 week post-fitting time period.

It is doubtful that future verification strategies will employ repeated and time-consuming speech recognition tests of the sort that are currently being used. Rather, tests that represent more realistic listening situations will continue to be developed and normative data generated. The obvious difficulty lies in reproducing the exact acoustic environments experienced by the hearing impaired listener. Alternatively, incorporation of some of the sources of speech degradation may result in a more realistic approximation of the actual performance with the hearing aid by the listener. For many years, speech recognition testing has been attempted in a background of various noises, ranging from a speech-weighted wide-band random or complex noise to multi-talker babble of 4, 12, or more speakers. Whether the purpose of presenting speech-in-noise tasks is to predict everyday performance or verify optimal fit, the selection of the type of noise must be carefully considered in that outcome measures are closely tied to the type of noise used to obtain those measures.[40–43]

Another possible means of validating the test design is to incorporate reverberation effects into the test. *Reverberation* refers to the persistence of sound within a room as a result of the sound waves reflecting off of walls and other hard surfaces. *Reverberation time* (T) is the length of time in seconds it takes for a sound to decrease 60 dB in level once it has ended. The measure, originally proposed by Sabine,[44,45] has been shown to vary with frequency. For simplicity, T is typically represented by a single number, the mean of Ts for 500, 1000 and 2000 Hz. The effect of reverberation time on speech perception has been studied extensively, and the negative impact of noise and reverberation are well documented.[45–47]

Incorporation of the reverberation coefficient into clinical measures of speech recognition ability has also been reported. Gordon-Salant and Fitzgibbons[48] utilized temporally "distorted" speech recognition tasks in a series of studies with elderly listeners. In one condition, the Speech Perception in Noise[37,38] low-predictability sentences were mathematically convolved with an impulse response simulating four conditions of reverberation. Four groups of ten listeners (normal hearing elderly, hearing impaired elderly, normal hearing young, and hearing impaired young) exhibited similar performance for the quiet condition. For the four reverberation conditions (T = 0.2, 0.3, 0.4, and 0.6 seconds), significant main effects for age and hearing loss were found. Since a typical complaint of many hearing impaired listeners is that standardized tests do not approximate "real-life" listening in terms of interference from background noise, future tests of speech recognition could allow for simulating different reverberant environments. Conversely, provided a typical reverberation time for a typical office or classroom, the clinician may opt to compare a number of the current signal processing circuits in one particular reverberant "environment" to determine if, in fact, one circuit provides greater benefit than another or other circuits.

Prediction of Speech Recognition Performance

Rather than actually test the speech recognition ability, a prediction of performance based on Articulation Index (AI) theory may be used. As Studebaker[49] notes, "It seems probable that such theories will receive substantially increased attention in the immediate future". According to this theoretical model, "audible speech energy in a frequency band determines the intelligibility of the band"[50] and is based on work done at the Bell Telephone Laboratories after World War I. The AI relates audible energy of the speech signal to intelligibility and is calculated with the following equation:

$$AI = P\int_0 I(f)W(f)df^{[50]}$$

where P refers to the proficiency factor, or experience of the talker and listener. "By definition, P equals 1.00 when communication involves average, normal hearing talkers and listeners who speak the same dialect" (Fletcher and Galt[51] in Studebaker and Sherbecoe,[50]). I(f) refers to the frequency importance function and is derived from results reporting speech recognition performance for a wide range of speech materials, including nonsense syllables,[51–53] monosyllabic words,[50,54,55,56] high and low context sentences,[57] and continuous discourse.[58,59] W(f) refers to the weighting or audibility function and "expresses how much of the available information given by I(f) is actually delivered to the listener under conditions that are less than optimal".[60]

As outlined in ANSI S3.5-1969 (A newly proposed ANSI standard[61] has changes the name of the AI to *Speech Intelligibility Index*. Various changes in the proposed standard reflect more recent understanding and manipulation of the input variables, methods of measurement, and computer implementation.)[62] and Dillon,[63] an individual's speech test score can be predicted utilizing the following protocol:

1. The maximum short-term root mean square (RMS) level of speech that is audible is determined for each one-third octave band (referred to as the sensation level of the speech).
2. The sensation levels are subsequently multiplied by the "importance function," which specifies the relative importance of each one-third octave band to the predicted score.
3. The resulting scores are summed.
4. Using a "transfer function" for a particular type of speech material, a prediction of speech recognition performance is made.

The transfer functions can be very dissimilar, depending on the speech material used. Dillon[63] notes that the "shape of the transfer function depends upon a large number of factors including the type of material used (sentence versus words versus nonsense syllables), the number of response alternatives available, the clarity of the individual talker, the experience of the listener with the test and the degree of hearing loss of the listener."

Computer implementation of the AI has made its application in the clinic more feasible. It remains that calibration and accuracy of measuring real-ear gain can cause considerable error in prediction of the AI. In an effort to simplify the calculations for clinical implementation, Humes,[64] Mueller and Killion,[65] and Pavlovic[66] have proposed count-the-dot approaches toward measuring the amount of speech cue information that is available to the listener. All of these authors concur that the term *Audibility Index* rather than *Articulation Index* should be used to refer to the AI obtained in this manner.[67]

Unlike the Mueller and Killion procedure, which uses an importance weighting function for nonsense syllables, Pavlovic[66] contends that average "everyday" speech importance function weighting results in an aided AI that is "proportional to the efficiency of the auditory channel (plus hearing instrument) in dealing with the information content of everyday or 'average' speech" (p. 20). Called the A_d, calculations can be made for unaided and aided conditions in the following manner:

1. The audiogram obtained using standard clinical procedures and calibration (ANSI, 1989) is plotted on the audiogram shown in Figure 15–6.

2. Insertion gain measures are obtained, and the resultant shifted audiogram (which should be differentiated from the "aided audiogram") is plotted in a similar manner.

3. For both the shifted and unaided audiogram, the number of dots that exceed threshold (or fall below the threshold markings on the audiogram) are counted and divided by 100. If the unaided or shifted threshold line falls on top of any dot, the dot is still counted if half or more falls below the marked threshold.

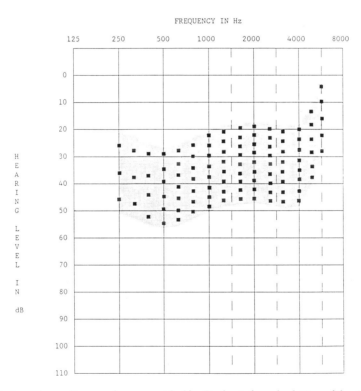

Figure 15–6. The audiogram form provided by Pavlovic for calculation of the Articulation Index by the A_d method. (From Pavlovic.[66])

As Pavlovic notes, however, such a visual representation and calculation may be misleading to the patient and the audiologist in two ways: (1) The impact of the thresholds of discomfort to the dynamic range of speech is not apparent using this audiogram format, and (2) by making the thresholds "better" by the amount of measured real-ear gain, it appears that the threshold has changed rather than that the speech spectrum has been shifted to a more audible range. Care should be taken in this procedure so as not to confuse the "shifted" and "aided" thresholds. The *shifted threshold*, which is used for these calculations, refers to thresholds shifted by the amount of real-ear gain, while for an aided audiogram thresholds are obtained in a sound field using warble tone or narrowband stimuli in unaided and aided conditions. In case of nonlinear aids, these two may not be the same.[68] Since functional gain, or aided thresholds, has traditionally been placed onto the audiogram form, misinterpretation (and potential error) of the A_d graphical representation is possible.

Despite its apparent resurgence into the clinical domain, the limitations of the AI must be acknowledged. As pointed out by Pavlovic,[66] an AI of 1.0 "does not mean that the auditory system with the hearing instrument is functioning normally, . . . [but] for most hearing impaired individuals, indicates that the hearing instrument is optimally matched to the hearing impaired system for maximizing speech intelligibility" (p. 23). Although a number of investigators have shown that actual speech recognition scores are lower than predicted by the AI,[69–72] the relationship has been shown to be a monotonic one.

The application of AI theory to the nonlinear circuits and speech enhancement strategies that are discussed in Chapter 14 remains unclear. Since the measured real-ear gain for nonlinear hearing aids may be dependent on the intensity level, the spectral composition, and/or duration of the input signal (as in the case of adaptive compression), the logistics of calculating an AI for a nonlinear hearing aid circuit coupled to the listener's ear can be rather cumbersome. Nonetheless, clinical applications of the AI theory continue to emerge.

Recently, Dillon[63] suggested the use of hearing aid "speech gain" as a verification of the fitting method employed. *Speech gain* is defined as "the difference in level between the aided and unaided performance–intensity functions measured at any specific value of percentage of items correct." In his investigation, the AI was used to predict speech gain for 11 subjects based on unaided sound field thresholds, ambient noise, internal noise generated by the hearing aid, measured real-ear insertion gain, and unaided performance–intensity (PI) functions. Insertion gain measures were obtained and averaged at one-third octave center frequencies from 1250 to 8000 Hz. Subsequently, the subjects were tested with monosyllabic iso-phonemic AB word lists[73] and a series of short stories (continuous discourse) read by a male speaker. Aided and unaided PI functions were obtained and hearing levels at the 25%, 50%, and 75% correct points were computed. Predicted speech gain was calculated "as the level difference between the curve fitted to the unaided data and the curve predicted for the aided PI function" based on insertion gain manipulations of the speech spectrum. These calculations agreed with measured speech gain with an RMS error of 3 dB for each of the 25%, 50%, and 75% correct points.

Dillon[63] points out that the prediction of speech gain has a number of advantages over the more traditional method of obtaining speech recognition measures: (1) Real-ear insertion gain measures can be more quickly obtained than speech measures (different levels of presentation, lists, and reliability) and (2) choice of importance function is not critical to the outcome. The author did point out that those subjects with more hearing aid experience tended to obtain speech gains "higher than predicted," while those with less than 2 months experience tended to have speech gain lower than predicted. Although this difference was not statistically significant, it does lend support to the concept of maturation of hearing aid benefit over the initial months of use.

Another, though indirect, attempt has been made to ascertain benefit from amplification in communicative situations using measures of reaction or response time. Reaction time was investigated 50 years ago relative to the loudness of a stimulus.[74] Cox, Alexander and Gilmore[80] have reported on the use of response time measures to differentiate between three frequency responses in three typical environments, including living room, lecture hall, and "cocktail party." She found a significant relationship between speech intelligibility and reaction time ($r = 0.67$, $p < 0.01$). Intelligibility measures showed a difference in benefit across environments, whereas reaction time measures showed a difference across the different frequency responses, at least in the "cocktail party" environment. Intelligibility benefit data further confirmed that differing frequency response characteristics (such as those provided by different prescriptive formulas) do *not* "produce differing benefits in daily life," which the authors have attributed to the use of the volume control wheel.[3] Other investigators[75,76] found reaction time to increase with increasing complexity of the speech recognition task. Levitt[77] cautions that since individual differences in reaction time have been shown to be very large across subjects, comparisons within observers rather than between observers should be made. In view of error in measurement due to the subject guessing with very difficult test material, Levitt[77] further suggests a task whereby the listener is required to verify whether a test sentence is true or false. Besides providing reaction time data, inherent in those results would be a measure of the speech understanding ability of the listener.

Enhanced Self-Perception of Communication Ability

Self-Report Inventories

Although not explicitly stated in the 1990 Consensus Statement for "Recommended Components of a Hearing Aid Selection Procedure for Adults,"[78] verification should be made that the use of a hearing aid has enhanced the individual's communication ability. Self-report inventories, satisfaction ratings, and/or open-ended questionnaires have been used to verify the appropriateness of the hearing aid fitting for many years (refer to Alpiner[79] for a review of tests). It has been shown that objective measures of benefit (e.g., speech recognition measures) are not accurate predictors of self-perception of benefit from amplification.[1,2] For this reason, future verification strategies must incorporate the individual's perception of benefit obtained from the amplification as well. Success in the eyes of the dispenser does not always equate to success in the eyes of the hearing aid user. As Cox et al.[80] note, "In the long run, the verdict of the hearing aid consumer determines whether or not the amplification strategy has been successful" (p. 206). Unfortunately, the myriad of subjective self-perception scales yield different, and often contradicting, views of the actual outcome of a particular hearing aid fitting. More standardized methods of obtaining the information will surface in the future. Specific areas of self-perception that will receive additional focus over the next decade include expectations and quality-of-life measures.

Expectation Measures

An alternative approach toward predicting rather than measuring the effectiveness of amplification was considered by Seyfried.[81] She attempted to discern whether an individual's expectations related to hearing aid use would predict (or influence) their success with amplification. Prior to the fitting of a hearing aid, subjects were given a 12 item Expectation Checklist and asked to indicate the response category that most applied:

- Practically Always
- Frequently
- About Half the Time
- Occasionally
- Almost Never.

Examples of items from the checklist include:

1.   I will have difficulty operating the controls on my hearing aid(s).
2.   My hearing aid(s) will fit comfortably.
3.   My hearing aid(s) will make speech sounds more distinct.
4.   My family believes my hearing aid(s) will help me communicate better.
5.   I will have difficulty inserting and removing my hearing aids.
6.   I will adjust slowly to my hearing aid(s).

However, in her study and a subsequent study utilizing the same Expectation Checklist,[2] little relationship could be found between the expectations of the subjective and objective measures of performance or self-reports of hearing aid benefit. Even though the usefulness of that particular checklist is not apparent, clinicians concur that expectations, biases, and a variety of preconceived notions held by potential hearing aid users have considerable impact on the success of the fitting. How to measure those "notions" remains a research need.

Quality-of-Life Measures

Of equal importance may be the use of broader quality-of-life ratings. Many current self-rating scales are designed to measure the impact of hearing loss and hearing aids on social, emotional, occupational, and other communication demands. Future outcome measures might include scales not specifically designed to measure communication effects, but the effect of amplification on the individual's perceived quality of life.[82]

While hearing performance is known to change with the introduction of amplification, does amplification result in an improved self image, less depression, or increased assertiveness, in addition to enhanced communication ability? Little attention has been focused on such outcome measures to date. In a single large-scale study reported by Mulrow et al.,[83] improved psychosocial function was maintained for the 12-month interval after amplification was introduced. Changes in the areas of social and emotional handicap were measured with the Hearing Handicap Inventory for the Elderly.[84–86] Changes in perceived communication were assessed with the Quantified Denver Scale of Communication.[87,88] The authors point out that the subjects were elderly veterans, and thus the findings may not be generalizable to other populations. Further studies aimed at assessing the outcome of amplification efforts are necessary. Consideration for counseling sessions during the follow-up period may further enhance the measurable benefits.

Conclusion

In view of all the choices presented to the clinician in terms of circuitry and measurement tools, verification of the appropriateness of each decision involved in the fitting of a hearing aid is not possible. Yet the impact of those decisions on user performance and satisfaction has not changed with the introduction of current technology. Outcome measures need to be developed and used to verify both short- and long-term benefit from amplification. Objective tools to assess performance of the hearing and its user must remain operative. In addition, subjective measures of perceived performance will continue to offer insight into the individual rehabilitative needs.

References

1. Bentler RA, Niebuhr DP, Getta JP, et al.: Longitudinal study of hearing aid effectiveness. I: Objective measures. *J Speech Hear Res* 1993; 36:808–819.
2. Bentler RA, Niebuhr DP, Getta JP, et al.: Longitudinal study of hearing aid effectiveness. II: Subjective measures. *J Speech Hear Res* 1993; 36:820–831.
3. Cox RM, Alexander GC: Maturation of hearing aid benefit: Objective and subjective measurements. *Ear Hear* 1992; 13:131–141.
4. Haggard MP, Foster JR, Iredale FE: Use and benefit of postaural aids in sensory hearing loss. *Scand Audiol* 1981; 10:45–52.
5. Stround DJ, Hamill TA: A multidimensional evaluation of three hearing aid prescription formulae. *ASHA* 1989; 31:60.
6. Surr RK, Schuchman GI, Montgomery AA: Factors influencing use of hearing aids. *Arch Otolaryngol* 1978; 104:732–736.
7. Killion MC: Transducers and acoustic couplings: The hearing aid problem that is mostly solved, in Studebaker GA, Hochberg I (eds): *Acoustical Factors Affecting Hearing Aid Performance*, ed 2. Boston, MA: Allyn and Bacon, 1993, pp 31–50.
8. Reddy SN, Kirlin RL: Evaluation of hearing aid and auditory response using pseudorandom noise, in Larson V, Egolf D, Kirlin R, Stile S (eds): *Auditory and Hearing Prosthetics Research*. New York: Grune & Stratton, 1979, pp 377–410.
9. ANSI S3.22: *Specification of Hearing Aid Characteristics*. New York: American National Standards Institute, Inc., 1987.

10. Hawkins DB, Naidoo S: A comparison of sound quality and clarity with asymmetrical peak clipping and output limiting compression. J Am Acad Audio 1993; 4:221–228.
11. Preves DA: Expressing hearing aid noise and distortion with coherence measurements. *ASHA* 1990; 56–59.
12. Dyrlund O: Characterization of non-linear distortion in hearing aids using coherence analysis. *Scand Audiol* 1989; 18:143–148.
13. Kates J: New development in hearing aid measurements, in Studebaker G, Bess F, Beck L (eds): *The Vanderbilt Hearing-Aid Report II*. Parkton, MD: York Press, 1992, pp 149–164.
14. Tyler RS, Schum DJ, Opie JM, et al.: Acoustical measurements of hearing aid processed speech. Paper presented at the annual American Speech-Language-Hearing Association, 1992, San Antonio, TX.
15. Revoile SG, Holden-Pitt LD: Some acoustic enhancements of speech and their effects on consonant identification by the hearing impaired, in Studebaker GA, Hochberg I (eds): *Acoustical Factors Affecting Hearing Aid Performance*, ed 2. Boston, MA: Allyn and Bacon, 1993, pp 373–385.
16. McCandless G, Lyregaard PE: Prescription of gain/output (POGO) for hearing aids. *Hear Instrum* 1983; 34(1):16–21.
17. Byrne D, Dillon H: The National Acoustic Laboratories (NAL) new procedure for selecting the gain and frequency response of a hearing aid. *Ear Hear* 1986; 7:257–265.
18. Cox RM: The MSU hearing instrument prescriptive procedure. *Hear Instrum* 1988; 39(1):6–10.
19. Popelka GR: *Program for Hearing Aid Selection and Evaluation: PHASE IV*. St. Louis: Central Institute for the Deaf Publication, 1983.
20. Popelka GR: The CID method: Phase IV. *Hear Instrum* 1988; 39(7):15–16, 18.
21. Popelka GR, Engebretson AM: A computer-based system for hearing aid assessment. *Hear Instrum* 1983; 34(7):6–9, 44.
22. Seewald RC, Ross M, Spiro MK: Selecting amplification characteristics for young hearing-impaired children. *Ear Hear* 1985; 6:48–53.
23. Pascoe DP: Clinical implications of nonverbal method of hearing aid selection and fitting. *Semin Speech Language Hear* 1980; 1:217–229.
24. ANSI S3.6: *Specification for Audiometers*. New York: American National Standards Institute, Inc., 1989.
25. Bentler RA, Pavlovic CV: Transfer functions and correction factors used in hearing aid evaluation and research. *Ear Hear* 1989; 10:58–63.
26. Seewald RC, Zelisko DLC, Ramji K, et al.: Computer assisted implementation of the DSL approach: Version 3.0. Poster presentation at the International Hearing Aids Conference, 1991a, Iowa City, IA.
27. Seewald RC, Zelisko DLC, Ramji K, et al.: *DSL (Version 3.0) Users Manual 1991b*. London, Ontario: The University of Western Ontario.
28. Bentler RA: Amplification for the hearing impaired child, in Alpiner JG, McCarthy PA (eds): *Rehabilitative Audiology: Children and Adults*. Baltimore, MD: Williams & Wilkins, 1993, p 72–105.
29. Cox RM, Moore JN: Composite speech spectrum for hearing aid gain prescriptions. *J Speech Hear Res* 1988; 31:102–107.
30. Olsen WO, Hawkins DB, Van Tasell DJ: Representations of the long-term spectra of speech. *Ear Hear* 1987; 8(Suppl 5):100S–107S.
31. Cornelisse LE, Gagne JP, Seewald RC: Ear level recordings of the long-term average spectrum of speech. *Ear Hear* 1991; 12:47–54.
32. Stelmachowicz PG: Current issues in pediatric amplification. Paper presented at the Conference on Pediatric Amplification, 1991, Omaha, NE.
33. Humes LE: Hearing aid selection and evaluation in the year 2000. *J Speech–Language Pathol Audiol* 1993; 1(Suppl):98–106.
34. Hodgson WR: Speech acoustics and intelligibility, in Hodgson WR (ed): *Hearing Aid Assessment and Use in Audiologic Habilitation*. Baltimore, MD: Williams & Wilkins, 1986, pp 109–127.
35. Humes LE, Houghton R: Beyond insertion gain. *Hear Instrum* 1992; 43(3):32–35.
36. Gatehouse S: Acclimatization to amplified speech. Paper presented at the International Hearing Aid Conference, 1991, Iowa City, IA.
37. Kalikow DN, Stevens KN, Elliot LL: Development of a test of speech intelligibility in noise using sentence materials with controlled word predictability. *J Acoust Soc Am* 1977; 61:1337–1351.
38. Bilger RC, Neutzel JM, Rabinowitz WM, et al.: Standardization of a test of speech perception in noise. *J Speech Hear Res* 1984; 27:32–48.
39. Levitt H, Resnick S: Speech reception by the hearing impaired: Methods of testing and development of new tests. *Scand Audiol* 1978; 6:107–129.
40. Carhart R, Tillman T, Gretis E: Perceptual masking in multiple sound backgrounds. *J Acoust Soc Am* 1969; 45:694–703.

41. Danhauer JL, Doyle PC, Lucks L: Effects of noise on NST and NU-6 stimuli. *Ear Hear* 1985; 6:266–269.
42. Dirks DD, Wilson R, Bower D: Effect of pulsed masking on selected speech materials. *J Acoust Soc Am* 1969; 46:898–906.
43. Horii Y, House A, Hughes G: A masking noise with speech-envelope characteristics for studying intelligibility. *J Acoust Soc Am* 1971; 49:1849–1856.
44. Sabine KC: *Collected Papers on Acoustics*. Cambridge, MA: Harvard University Press, 1927, pp 43–45. [Note: This book is out of print. It has been reprinted by Dover Press in New York, 1964.]
45. Nabelek AK: Communication in noisy and reverberant environments, in Studebaker GA, Hochberg I (eds): *Acoustical Factors Affecting Hearing Aid Performance*, ed 2. Boston, MA: Allyn and Bacon, 1993, pp 15–28.
46. Nabelek AK, Pickett JM: Reception of consonants in a classroom as affected by monaural and binaural listening, noise, reverberation, and hearing aids. *J Acoust Soc Am* 1974; 56:628–639.
47. Nabelek AK: Identification of vowels in quiet, noise, and reverberation: Relationships with age and hearing loss. *J Acoust Soc Am* 1988; 84:476–484.
48. Gordon-Salant S, Fitzgibbons P: Perception of temporally degraded speech by elderly listeners. Poster presented at the annual meeting of the American Speech-Language-Hearing Association, 1992, San Antonio, TX.
49. Studebaker GA: Preface statements, in Studebaker GA, Hochberg I: *Acoustical Factors Affecting Hearing Aid Performance*, ed 2. Boston MA: Allyn and Bacon, 1993.
50. Studebaker GA, Sherbecoe RL: Frequency-importance functions for speech recognition, in Studebaker GA, Hochberg I (eds): *Acoustical Factors Affecting Hearing Aid Performance*, ed 2. Boston, MA: Allyn and Bacon, 1993, pp 185–204.
51. Fletcher H, Galt RH: The perception of speech and its relation to telephony. *J Acoust Soc Am* 1950; 22:89–151.
52. Beranek LL: The design of speech communication systems. *Proc IRE* 1947; 35:880–890.
53. French NR, Steinberg JC: Factors governing the intelligibility of speech sounds. *J Acoust Soc Am* 1947; 19:90–119.
54. Black JW: Equally contributing frequency bands in intelligibility testing. *J Speech Hear Res* 1959; 2:81–83.
55. Duggirala Y: *Derivation of Frequency Importance Functions for a Feature Recognition Test Material.* Doctoral dissertation, 1986, Memphis State University.
56. Studebaker GA, Sherbecoe RL: Frequency-importance and transfer functions for recorded CID W-22 word lists. *J Speech Hear Res* 1991; 34:427–438.
57. Dirks DD, Bell TS, Trine T, et al.: Articulation index importance functions for contextual speech materials. Paper presented at the annual meeting of the American Speech-Language-Hearing Association, 1989, St. Louis, MO.
58. Studebaker GA, Pavlovic CV, Sherbecoe RL: A frequency importance function for continuous discourse. *J Acoust Soc Am* 1987; 81:1130–1138.
59. Dirks DD, Dubno JR, Ahlstrom JB, et al.: Articulation index importance and transfer functions for several speech materials. Poster presented at the annual meeting of the American Speech-Language-Hearing Association, 1990, Seattle, WA.
60. Pavlovic CV, Studebaker GA: An evaluation of some assumptions underlying the articulation index. *J Acoust Soc Am* 1984; 75:1606–1612.
61. ANSI S3.5: *Methods for Calculation of the Articulation Index.* New York: American National Standards Institute, Inc., 1969.
62. ANSI S3.5: *Methods for Calculation of the Speech Intelligibility Index* (Proposed V3). New York: American National Standards Institute, Inc., 1993.
63. Dillon H: Hearing aid evaluation: Predicting speech gain from insertion gain. *J Speech Hear Res* 1993; 36:621–633.
64. Humes LE: Understanding the speech-understanding problems of the hearing impaired. *J Am Acad Audiol* 1991; 2:59–69.
65. Mueller GH, Killion MC: An easy method for calculating the articulation index. *Hear J* 1990; 43(9):14–17.
66. Pavlovic CV: Speech recognition and five articulation indexes. *Hear Instrum* 1991; 42(9):20–23.
67. Killion MC, Mueller HG, Pavlovic CV, Humes LE: A is for audibility. *Hear J* 1993; 43:14–17.
68. Seewald RC, Hudson SP, Gagne J-P, Zelisko DLC: Comparison of two methods for estimating the sensation level of amplified speech. *Ear Hear* 1992; 13:142–149.
69. Dubno JR, Dirks DD, Schaefer AB: Stop-consonant recognition for normal-hearing listeners and listeners with high frequency hearing loss. II: Articulation index predictions. *J Acoust Soc Am* 1989; 85:355–364.

70. Kamm CA, Dirks DD, Bell TS: Speech recognition and the Articulation Index for normal and hearing-impaired listeners. *J Acoust Soc Am* 1985; 77:281–288.
71. Pavlovic CV: Use of the articulation index for assessing residual auditory function in listeners with sensorineural hearing impairment. *J Acoust Soc Am* 1984; 75:1253–1258.
72. Pavlovic CV: Articulation index predictions of speech intelligibility in hearing aid selection. *ASHA* 1988; 30:63–65.
73. Boothroyd A: Developments in speech audiometry. *Sound* 1968; 2:3–10.
74. Chochelle R: Variation des temps de reaction auditifs en fonction de l'intensite a diverses frequences. *Anee Psychol* 1940; 41:65–124.
75. Gatehouse S, Gordon J: Response times to speech stimuli as measures of benefit from amplification. *Br J Audiol* 1990; 24:63–68.
76. Pratt RL: On the use of reaction time as a measure of intelligibility. *Br J Audiol* 1981; 15:253–255.
77. Levitt H: Future directions in hearing aid research. *J Speech–Language Pathol Audiol* 1993; 1(Suppl):107–124.
78. Vanderbilt/VA Hearing Aid Conference 1990 Consensus Statement: Recommended components of a hearing aid selection, procedure for adults, in Studebaker GA, Bess FH, Beck LB (eds): *The Vanderbilt Hearing-Aid Report II*. Parkton, MD: York Press, 1991, pp 321–323.
79. Alpiner JG: Evaluation of adult communication function, in Alpiner JG, McCarthy PA (eds): *Rehabilitative Audiology Children and Adults*. Baltimore, MD: Williams & Wilkins, 1987, pp 44–114.
80. Cox RM, Alexander GC, Gilmore CG: Objective and self-report measures of hearing aid benefit, in Studebaker GA, Bess F, Beck L (eds): *The Vanderbilt Hearing Aid Report II*. Parkton, MD: York Press, 1991, pp 201–214.
81. Seyfried DA: Use of a communication self report inventory to measure hearing aid counseling effects. Ph.D. Dissertation, 1990, University of Iowa.
82. Bess F: Hearing impairment in the Elderly: Common grounds and conflicts. Paper presented at Scott Haug Foundation Audiology Retreat, 1992, San Antonio, TX.
83. Mulrow CD, Tuley MR, Aguilar C: Sustained benefits of hearing aids. *J Speech Hear Res* 1992; 35:1402–1405.
84. Newman CW, Weinstein BE: The Hearing Handicap Inventory for the Elderly as a measure of hearing aid benefit. *Ear Hear* 1988; 9:81–85.
85. Ventry IM, Weinstein BE: The Hearing Handicap Inventory for the Elderly: A new tool. *Ear Hear* 1982; 3:128–134.
86. Weinstein BE, Spitzer JB, Ventry IM: Test–retest reliability of the Hearing Handicap Inventory for the Elderly. *Ear Hear* 1986; 7:295–299.
87. Alpiner JG: Evaluation of communication function, in Alpiner JG (ed): *Handbook of Adult Rehabilitative Audiology*. Baltimore, MD: Williams & Wilkins, 1982, pp 44–114.
88. Tuley MR, Mulrow CD, Aguilar C, Velez R: Sustained benefits of hearing aids. *J Speech Hear Res* 1992; 35:1402–1405.

16

Future Trends in Hearing Aid Technology

DAVID A. PREVES

Introduction

Although advances in hearing aid technology are rapidly improving the effectiveness of hearing aid fittings, several major problems still exist: Many currently produced hearing aids have poor sound quality, limited capability for shaping the frequency response to a target prescription, produce squealing as a result of acoustic feedback oscillation, and amplify undesirable noises. These problems frequently can be so severe that they lead to rejection of hearing aids. With hearing aids generally having the reputation for not performing very well, many people who might benefit from amplification choose not to avail themselves of it. This chapter will explore the technical limitations underlying these current problems in hearing aids and how further improvements in hearing aid technology can be used to solve them.

Hearing Aid Sound Quality

One of the most important technological challenges for future hearing aids is improving the sound quality of their processed signals. The sound quality of many hearing aids is frequently judged to be inferior to that of high fidelity audio systems or, for that matter, even to the sound quality of the unaided signal. This problem is partially caused by inadequate headroom resulting from the low battery voltage (1.3 V) used in hearing aids. (*Headroom* is the difference between the sound pressure level [SPL] at which peak clipping due to saturation begins in the hearing aid and the sum of input SPL and hearing aid gain.) Recent statistics (e.g., the data from Kranmer that appear each year in *Hearing Instruments*) show that approximately 80% of the hearing aids fitted in the United States are in-the-ear (ITE) or in-the-canal (ITC) types, and approximately 82% of the hearing aids fitted use linear amplifiers.[1] To keep amplified signals from peak clipping, the saturation sound pressure level (SSPL90) created by the hearing aid amplifier, receiver, and battery must be greater than the sum of the peak input signal SPL and the gain provided by the amplifier. For example, at a specific frequency, if the hearing aid wearer's own voice produces a long-term root mean square (RMS) input level to the hearing aid of 75 dB SPL with a peak level of 87 dB SPL, and the gain is 30 dB, the SSPL90 must be greater than 117 dB SPL to prevent saturation from occurring during the peaks. Since SSPL90 is not always this high, many linear hearing aids operating with 1.3 V batteries may produce poor sound quality because of the nonlinear distortion created by peak clipping during saturation.[2]

Certain types of nonlinear distortion can reduce sound quality.[3] In particular, the presence of nonlinear harmonic and intermodulation distortion in adverse listening conditions results in reports of poor sound quality and reduced clarity.[4] These distortions typically occur when hearing aids are driven into saturation while processing speech in high levels of environmental noise. Because speech and many environmental sounds have significant crest factors, hearing aids can easily be driven into saturation at even moderate input levels.[5] (*Crest factor* is the difference in decibels between the peak signal level and the RMS signal level.) As mentioned above, a common input signal (75–80 dB SPL) of moderate intensity that can easily drive linear hearing aids into saturation is the hearing aid wearer's own voice. Saturation produces nonlinear distortion that in turn decreases the signal-to-noise ratio of hearing aid–processed signals. These distortions can sometimes make the sound quality of processed speech so poor and the listening experience so annoying and fatiguing that, in noisy environments, hearing aids are turned off or are even taken out. One study investigating if adaptive frequency response shaping would reduce upward spread of masking in comparison to linear amplification discovered that it was not possible to perform the experiment with actual hearing aids because extra masking was created by saturation-induced distortion in the linear condition.[6]

Increasing Headroom to Improve Sound Quality

The type of distortion discussed above arises from inadequate headroom, a condition resulting from relatively low SSPL90 combined with high gain, causing peak clipping at moderate and high input levels. One way to preserve head-room is to lower the gain with the volume control. However, this may be undesirable since the wearer may not receive sufficient gain at lower input levels. Reducing the gain at higher input levels can be automated using compression or adaptive frequency response (AFR) circuits, both of which can increase headroom by automatically reducing gain at higher input levels.[7] Headroom can also be preserved by increasing the SSPL90. Higher SSPL90 for extending headroom may be achieved with the use of push–pull (Class B) and Class D output stages with lower battery drain than Class A output stages having a higher SSPL90.[8] To maximize headroom and improve sound quality, hearing aids of the future will incorporate more Class B and Class D output stages and fewer Class A output stages.

Coherence as an Indicator of Sound Quality

In the future, the coherence function may present a way to quantify sound quality in hearing aids. The coherence function measurement is currently available in many dual channel spectrum analyzers incorporating fast-Fourier transform analysis. The coherence function for hearing aids may be obtained using the broadband noise input signal specified in ANSI S3.42-1992. This signal is a more viable input signal than pure tones for measuring harmonic and intermodulation distortion, because many combinations of input frequencies are formed simultaneously within the hearing aid. Coherence is a direct measure of the linearity of a hearing aid and represents, in a number from 0 to 1, what part of the output signal is due only to the input signal.[9] A coherence of 1.0 would signify perfect reproduction of the input signal, while a coherence of 0 would represent total degradation of the input signal. A coherence of 0.5 would indicate that there is an equal amount of distortion and noise in the hearing aid output as there is input signal. At low input levels (e.g., 50 dB SPL), low coherence indicates high levels of hearing aid amplifier noise.[10] At high input levels (e.g., 90 dB SPL), low coherence is due mainly to harmonic and intermodulation distortion resulting from inadequate headroom. Signal-to-distortion ratio, and hence percent distortion, can be calculated from coherence measures. Signal-to-distortion ratio is calculated as follows:

$$\text{Signal/Distortion} = \sqrt{\frac{\text{coherence}}{1 - \text{coherence}}}$$

Thus, a coherence of 0.99 corresponds to 10% distortion. A coherence of 0.90 corresponds to approximately 30% distortion. Lower coherence values (e.g. 0.5), at high input levels appear to be a good indicator of a hearing aid with poor sound quality, particularly in listening situations with competing noise.[11,12]

As an example of the use of coherence in comparing hearing aids, Figure 16–1a shows a family of frequency–response curves for a linear ITE (hearing aid A) having a widely used amplifier with a Class A output stage. The components and performance for this instrument are representative of hearing aid designs of 10–15 years ago. Frequency–response curves were obtained on an HA-1 2 cc coupler as the input level of a continuous, broadband, speech-shaped random noise signal was varied from 50 to 80 dB SPL in 10 dB steps. When the input signal increased to 80 dB SPL, the gain was significantly reduced across the frequency range as a result of clipping. In Figure 16–1b the same measurements were made at slightly higher gain for a newer generation linear ITE (hearing aid B) having an amplifier with a Class D output stage. For this hearing aid, even at the 80 dB SPL input level, gain is not reduced and jaggedness in the frequency responses is not seen. These results are consistent with the coherence function plots shown in Figures 16–1c and 16–1d (with 70 and 80 dB SPL input levels, respectively) in which mid and high frequency coherence is much higher for hearing aid B than for hearing aid A. Listening tests by the author in competing noise with hearing aids A and B revealed that hearing aid B had much better speech clarity and overall sound quality in high levels of background noise than hearing aid A. The probable reason for this

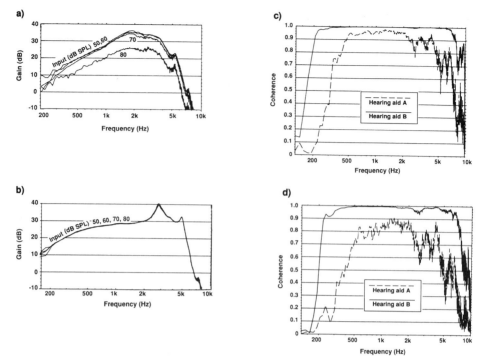

Figure 16–1.   Family of frequency response curves obtained on an HA-182 cm³ coupler using speech-shaped random noise input levels ranging from 50 to 80 dB SPL in 10 dB steps for an ITE hearing aid (A) with (**a**) a widely used linear circuit having a Class A output stage and (**b**) ITE hearing aid (B) with a linear circuit with Class D output stage (Argosy Linear Plus). Coherence functions for hearing aids A and B are shown with speech-shaped random noise inputs at (**c**) 70 dB SPL and (**d**) 80 dB SPL. (From Preves and Woodruff.[7])

improvement was that hearing aid B had significantly greater headroom: The high frequency average (HFA) SSPL90 for hearing aid A (110 dB SPL) was 8 dB lower than that for hearing aid B (118 dB SPL).

Headroom for Linear Amplification, Coherence, and Aided Loudness Discomfort Level (LDL)

Currently, a common practice is to set the SSPL90 below a patient's loudness discomfort level (LDL) as measured with an audiometer under headphones with speech or tonal stimuli. However, successful linear hearing aid fittings of the future may not always require that SSPL90 be below the LDL. Recently, there have been some indications that LDL is not an appropriate measure with which to set the SSPL90 of a hearing aid.[13] For conversational speech at 75 dB SPL, it has been found that *aided* LDL may be lower than the LDL obtained with an audiometer and headphones, particularly for linear hearing aids with limited headroom (i.e., those that easily saturate as a result of high gain and low HFA SSPL90 values).[14] While audiometers and headphones are capable of producing virtually distortion-free signals at very high levels, this is rarely the case with linear hearing aids that saturate at relatively low levels. Additionally, linear hearing aids with a class D output stage having high SSPL90s appear to produce higher real-ear SPLs at the levels that LDL occur than those with a Class A output stage having a lower SSPL90. Thus, it appears that saturation-induced distortion can affect the sensation of loudness in hearing aid fittings. While the same results may not be found for different types of stimuli (e.g., impulsive sounds), the use of output limiting via peak clipping in a linear circuit in order to conform with an LDL determined with an audiometer using headphones may result in decreased wearer satisfaction. The occurrence of excessively loud sounds and excessively distorted sounds can be prevented by using compression or AFR-type circuits or, in the case of linear hearing aids, by maintaining SSPL90 at relatively high levels.

Certainly the possibility exists that linear hearing aids with HFA SSPL90 exceeding LDL will be rejected by some wearers as being excessively loud. An analysis of Class A and Class D linear hearing aids (of the same types as that shown in Fig. 16–1 and in the LDL study described above) that were returned to the factory for adjustment was conducted in order to determine whether relationships exist between LDLs for speech reported by the dispenser on the order form, HFA SSPL90s of the hearing aids, and the reasons for dispensers returning these hearing aids for adjustment.[15] Tables 16–1 and 16–2, respectively, show data for some of the ITE hearing aids produced in 1990 (number in each LDL category indicated by N) made with Class D output stage amplifiers (Argosy Linear Plus) and for some made with Class A output stage amplifiers. By design, the Class D Linear Plus has an HFA SSPL90 that does not vary, except when rotating the volume control. As a result, most hearing aid wearers were either "overfit" or "underfit" in HFA SSPL90 by varying amounts if one were to consider the speech LDL obtained with an audiometer under headphones to be the appropriate indicator. For example, the second column of Table 16–1 shows that the mean HFA SSPL90 of the Class D hearing aids considered in the analysis ranged from 116 to 118 dB SPL for each LDL category. Therefore, hearing aid wearers with low LDLs were "overfit" in HFA SSPL90 by as much as 11 dB, while those with very high LDLs were "underfit" in HFA SSPL90 by as much as 12 dB. The last three columns in Tables 16–1 and 16–2 show three common reasons among the many possible for hearing aids being returned to the factory. Individual weighted means were calculated for each of these three common reasons for return from the number of hearing aids in each row combined with the percent returned in that row. The overall weighted means were calculated from the three individual weighted means. For the Class D hearing aids, these data show that few had been returned for distortion, and a low percentage had been returned for being too strong despite the fact that many individuals had a HFA SSPL90 that exceeded LDL. For example, in Table 16–1 none of the hearing aids from the 105 dB SPL LDL group were returned for being too strong despite the fact that these individuals were "overfit" in HFA SSPL90 by an average of 11 dB. However, 5% of the Class D aids in this LDL category were returned for being too weak. In general,

Table 16–1. Class D Linear Plus returns as a Function of LDL

LDL (dB SPL)	Mean HFA SSPL90 (dB SPL)	No. of Hearing Aids	HFA SSPL90 Minus LDL (dB)	Mean HFA FOG (dB)	Est. Max. Undistorted Input Level (dB SPL)	Returned for (%)		
						Distorted	Strong	Weak
105	116	65	11	33	83	0	0	5
110	117	117	7	36	81	0	1	3
115	118	281	3	37	81	1	0	3
120	118	450	-2	38	80	0	0	2
125	118	240	-7	40	78	0	0	3
130	118	184	-12	39	79	0	1	7
Individual weighted means						0.2	0.3	3.0

Overall weighted mean: 1.2%.

(From Fortone et al.[15])

Table 16–2. Class A returns as a Function of LDL

LDL (dB SPL)	Mean HFA SSPL90 (dB SPL)	No. of Hearing Aids (N)	HFA SSPL90 Minus LDL (dB)	Mean HFA FOG (dB)	Est. Max. Undistorted Input Level (dB SPL)	Returned for (%)		
						Distorted	Strong	Weak
105	107	792	2	32	75	1	2	2
110	108	1,203	-2	33	75	0	2	2
115	111	1,450	-4	34	77	0	2	4
120	110	2,073	-10	35	75	0	1	3
125	110	1,073	-15	35	75	1	1	3
130	111	529	-19	36	75	0	1	2
Individual weighted means						0.3	1.0	3.0

Overall weighted mean: 1.4%.

(From Fortone et al.[15])

for any LDL value, Class D hearing aids were returned far more often than Class A hearing aids for being too weak than for being too strong, whether the HFA SSPL90 values of these aids exceeded the LDL or not.

The SSPL90 for the Class A hearing aids may be preset at the factory or adjusted by the dispenser with a peak-clipping output limit potentiometer. Accordingly, as shown in Table 16–2, for low reported speech LDLs, HFA SSPL90 was preset near the LDL values provided by dispensers. However, the first two rows and first two columns in Table 16–2 show that individuals with LDLs greater than 105 dB were underfit in HFA SSPL90 relative to LDL by up to 19 dB because a Class A output stage with reasonable battery life cannot produce as high an SSPL90 as a Class D output stage. Despite this fact, the last two columns in Table 16–2 show that a higher percentage of Class A hearing aids than Class D hearing aids were returned for being too strong. This result is consistent with the assumption that many hearing aids with Class A output stages easily saturate, producing distortion that may contribute to the sensation of loudness discomfort. However, the return rate specifically for distortion was about the same for both Class A and Class D hearing aids.

These results are consistent with the hypothesis that hearing-impaired persons with low audiometer/headphone LDLs may be successfully fit with linear hearing aids having an HFA SSPL90 considerably exceeding these LDL values. The assumption is that aided LDLs with this higher SSPL90 will exceed those measured had a hearing aid with lower SSPL90 been used, because the latter would produce greater distortion. This apparent violation of basic hearing aid fitting principles may be due to the fact that in order to process signals cleanly so that the aided LDL is as high as the audiometer/headphone LDL, the HFA SSPL90 of a hearing aid must allow the peak values of amplified signals to pass unclipped. For example, with a speech signal having a crest factor of 17 dB, if the audiometer/headphone LDL is 100 dB SPL, the HFA SSPL90 of the hearing aid must be at least 117 dB SPL to have the aided LDL near 100 dB SPL. This scenario could have applied to the Class D Linear Plus results given above. If this is true, if clipping occurs in the hearing aid on the peaks for amplified signals whose RMS values are near the audiometer/headphone LDL, then the aided LDL for these signals will be considerably less than the audiometer/headphone LDL. This was the case for the Class A hearing aid results given above. Taking all of this together, it seems that the audiometer/headphone LDL may be indicative of the RMS value of the speech signal rather than the peaks of the speech signal.

Hearing aid fittings of the future will use more amplifiers with Class D output stages, which will result in improved headroom and better sound quality. Such hearing aids may not necessarily maintain SSPL90 below LDL as determined on an audiometer with headphones.

Frequency Response Shaping

For many hearing aid fittings, real-ear probe microphone measurements are used to verify performance specified by prescription formulae. However, precise matching of the prescribed targets with the actual gain by frequency produced by hearing aids has often been difficult with older analog hearing aid technology.[16] Finer control of gain by frequency for selectively producing peaks or troughs in REIG is required in the future to match more exactly an electroacoustic prescription.

Solving Past Technologic Limitations

Two major limitations in hearing aid technology were the main causes for a limited capability to match ITE hearing aid frequency responses to target prescription frequency responses: (1) Older hearing aid receivers that produced a primary frequency response peak between 1600 and 2200 Hz and had inadequate high frequency sensitivity: This limitation usually resulted in a large reduction in the real ear insertion response (REIR), usually at about 2800 Hz, and inadequate high frequency REIR above 3000 Hz. (2) The limited range of variability provided by adjustable tone controls: Until recently, probably because of physical space limitations, most ITE hearing aids had low frequency tone controls consisting of a single pole high pass filter. With these low frequency tone controls having a slope of only 6 dB per octave with which to vary the frequency response, it was possible to reduce gain at 500 Hz, for example, by only about 10 dB. These limitations often combined to produce hearing aids providing greater than prescribed low and mid frequency REIR when they were able to achieve the prescribed high frequency target insertion gain.[17] Often the high frequency insertion gain target could not be achieved anyway even with the highest possible overall gain provided, especially for persons with steeply sloping, high frequency hearing loss.

Most older generation ITE hearing aids had a Class A power output stage in the amplifier, which was often associated with a narrowband receiver response and limited tone control variability and, hence, poor flexibility in the insertion gain frequency response. Many current ITE hearing aids employ either a Class D or Class B output stage in the amplifier and a receiver with a wider band frequency response. These hearing aids typically have a primary frequency response peak at about 3000 Hz and adequate high frequency gain above that frequency. Thus, although not necessarily directly related, many ITE hearing aids with good insertion frequency responses are associated with amplifiers that have Class D and Class B output stages. In addition, more and more current ITE hearing aids employ active tone controls consisting of two- or even four-pole filters, having slopes of 12 and 24 dB/octave, respectively. These higher order filters provide greater flexibility in varying the frequency response. It is not uncommon to have low frequency tone controls providing up to 40 dB variation in gain at 500 Hz.

Frequency Response Shaping with Multi-band Hearing Aids

In the past, most hearing aid amplifiers have been single band, broadband devices. One of the most recent technological advances in hearing aids has been the incorporation of a graphic or parametric equalizer within the hearing aid amplifier. Multi-band amplifiers give much finer resolution in frequency response shaping than single band amplifiers, because gain is controllable in

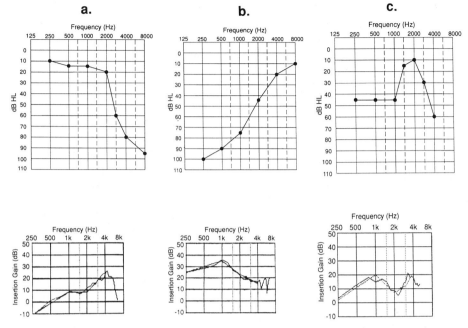

Figure 16–2. Examples of frequency–response matching achieved with a three-band ITE hearing aid (Argosy 3-Channel-Clock) on a real ear. For each case, the audiogram is the upper part of the figure, and the NAL-R REIR prescription is the smoother line in the lower part of the figure.

each frequency band. With a parametric equalizer, gain is controllable in each frequency band, and the cross-over frequencies of the bands can be shifted. Three examples of precise frequency response matching to prescription targets with a three-band parametric equalizer hearing aid amplifier in an ITE hearing aid (Argosy 3-Channel-Clock) are shown in Figure 16–2a–c.

Analog Versus Digital Processing

In the past, most hearing aid amplifiers have been implemented with bipolar analog semiconductor technology. Bipolar analog circuitry, which is still widely used in hearing aids, meets the important requirements of low noise and the capability to produce high output drive. Bipolar analog circuitry inherently uses relatively large value capacitors (one per filter pole). These capacitors limit the amount of multi-band filtering and signal processing possible because of size constraints of small hearing aids. Recent advances in complementary metal oxide semiconductor (CMOS) integrated circuit semiconductor technology have considerably extended the capability of analog circuitry for hearing aids. CMOS integrated circuitry is very high density, permitting more transistors, resistors, and capacitors per unit chip area than most bipolar integrated circuitry. Switched capacitor filters are made with CMOS integrated circuitry implemented on smaller chip sizes and with fewer components external to the chip than with bipolar semiconductor technology. Sophisticated analog signal processors employ switched capacitor filters for greater filter slope. Unfortunately, CMOS semiconductor circuitry tends to be noisier than bipolar semiconductor circuitry. Consequently, hearing aid circuits are beginning to be made with a combination of bipolar and CMOS circuitry on one chip—called BICMOS circuitry. Inherent with BICMOS semiconductor technology are the advantages of low noise bipolar circuitry for hearing aid preamplifiers together with higher order switched capacitor filters with on-chip capacitors to provide the maximum possible signal processing capability for small hearing aid sizes. More and more future hearing aid designs will utilize multi-band analog amplifiers implemented with CMOS switched capacitor filters.

While work with true digital hearing aids has been reported by various organizations and laboratories,[18–20] few have been marketed. Certainly, digital signal processing (DSP) will offer significant improvement in the performance of hearing aids in the future.[21,22] Various ratios of the amount of digital electronics relative to the amount of analog electronics are encountered in what some persons now call *digital* hearing aids. These range from hybrid analog–digital hearing aids, in which an analog form of the signal is controlled digitally, to true digital hearing aids, in which digital processing is performed on a digital representation of the signal. To have "true" digital processing, the incoming signal must first be converted from analog to digital format so that a digital computer can perform the signal processing algorithms.[23]

As mentioned previously, the U.S. hearing aid marketplace has been dominated by ITE-and ITC-type hearing aids. The challenge of incorporating true digital technology into these devices is much more difficult than it is to package it into behind-the-ear (BTE) hearing aids. Several commercial efforts for true digital processing hearing aids have not been successful. One digital hearing aid consisted of a body-worn processor connected with a cord to a BTE housing containing the microphone and receiver. Four batteries were required, three in the body-worn processor and one in the BTE housing. Although published information is lacking as to how effective this true digital hearing aid was, one study concluded that it provided more benefit and was preferred by some hearing aid wearers over their own hearing aids.[24] However, this hearing aid was eventually withdrawn from the market. It appears that the failure of this digital hearing aid may have been due to a combination of factors, including large size, high operating cost, and perhaps high selling price without sufficient offsetting performance benefit compared with conventional hearing aids.

Another effort in digital processing involved an integrated circuit that attempted to separate speech from background noise.[25] In this CMOS combination analog–digital chip, the incoming signal was converted to digital form and a digital signal processing algorithm made a decision as to whether speech or noise was present. This information was then used to control the frequency ranges and bandpass gains of analog-switched capacitor filters. Although the algorithm performed by the chip seemed to make a great deal of sense from a theoretical standpoint, many hearing aids utilizing this chip were not generally considered successful fittings. One primary reason for this failure was the introduction by the chip of undesirable audible artifacts in processing fluctuating environmental sounds. These annoying pumping sounds were produced by the chip when it made large adaptive reductions and increases in gain in response to small changes in environmental noises. This device has subsequently also been removed from the marketplace. These examples show that the real problem underlying the use of true digital processing for noise reduction in hearing aids may be the absence of viable digital signal processing algorithms that are significantly more effective than the less costly and more miniature existing analog-based algorithms.

Consequently, current efforts have centered on providing partially digital, "programmable" hearing aids. In the last few years, there has been a proliferation of such digitally programmed analog hearing aids in the maketplace. Some of these hybrid analog–digital hearing aids offer significant performance features as compared with those of purely analog hearing aids without a significant increase in size or operating cost. Although these devices are rich in new fitting features,[22] since they do not process the signal in a digital form, the real promise of digital technology in hearing aids has yet to be fulfilled.

One important advantage of true DSP in hearing aids derives from its software base. With software, several sophisticated algorithms can be performed simultaneously once the digital computer hardware is in place and more performance features can be offered within a given hardware package than with analog processing. Conceivably, with the proper DSP software in conjunction with a powerful digital computer, precise frequency response shaping as well as acoustic feedback reduction and noise reduction can all be accomplished simultaneously. However, analog technology will likely never become obsolete, even in hearing aids performing true DSP, because analog input and output circuitry must still be present to provide the electroacoustic interface into and out of the hearing aid.

While the prospects of improved performance offered by digital technology in hearing aids are exciting, true digital processing should not be regarded as the solution for all the problems associated with current hearing aids. The analog preamplifier and power amplifier may produce distortion that can degrade the sound quality of true digital hearing aids. The use of digital processing in hearing aids can also introduce three types of distortions: (1) *aliasing*—signals in a band centered at the sampling frequency overlapping the original baseband signal at a lower frequency, caused by too low a sampling rate versus the spectral bandwidth of the incoming signal; (2) *quantization error*—too gross an approximation of the analog signal by the analog–digital converter, caused by too large a digital step size, resulting from too few bits; and (3) *imaging*—a jagged rather than a smooth analog output waveform, caused by inadequate smoothing of the output signal from the digital to analog converter after digital processing.[26]

Packaging Considerations for Digital Electronics

One requirement for a DSP hearing aid is performing all its functions in real time, as opposed to off-line as is sometimes used in computer simulations of hearing aids. At this time, it has only been possible to package a true DSP hearing aid in a large BTE housing. However, by using specially designed, custom DSP integrated circuit chips, it may be possible in the future to have true DSP ITE hearing aids. Because of their generalized application capabilities, standard, off-the-shelf DSP chips that are sufficiently high speed to perform all of the required signal processing functions in real time are too large and require too much current drain. However, if budgetary considerations permit it, in the future, custom DSP chips can be designed that would meet hearing aid performance, packaging size, and battery requirements while performing algorithms specifically intended for hearing aids.[26,27]

Applications of True Digital Processing for Hearing Aids

Brief overviews of applications of digital technology for hearing aids have been published by Murray and Hanson[28] and Levitt.[29] The following discussion considers several of these applications for solving some of the major problems of many existing hearing aid fittings that were outlined at the beginning of this chapter.

Frequency Response Shaping With Digital Technology

The ability to control with fine resolution the peaks and troughs in the REIR is required in order to match a prescriptive target. Such a requirement can easily be provided with a digital filter and to a much higher degree of accuracy than with analog switched capacitor filtering. Highly effective algorithms have been developed for controlling with great precision the frequency response and phase of hearing aids via a digital filter.[30-32] This is among the most straight-forward applications of DSP. For example, Figure 16–3 shows the precision possible with digital filtering in matching a prescribed frequency response and phase for a steeply sloping high frequency hearing loss. Controlling the phase is important for suppressing spurious peaks in the frequency response and for preventing acoustic feedback oscillation. To achieve such a high degree of accuracy with current analog circuitry would require many transistors, capacitors, and resistors with a resulting large-sized hearing aid.

Digital Algorithms for Reducing Acoustic Feedback Oscillation

Overviews of methods for preventing acoustical feedback oscillation in hearing aids have been published by Egolf,[33] Preves,[34] and Harjani and Wang.[35] Techniques for feedback reduction in hearing aids have been patterned after methods that have been used for preventing squealing in public address systems. Included are reducing amplification in the frequency range of the acoustic feedback oscillation with low pass filtering or notch filtering,[36] frequency shifting,[37,38] phase shifting,[34,35] and phase warbling.[39] While many of these techniques have used analog technology, digital technology also lends itself to solving this bothersome problem. For example, cancelling the feedback path has been suggested via an adaptive filter in the forward path of the hearing aid that is tuned to the inverse frequency response and phase of the acoustic feedback path.[40] An earlier version of this approach used a second microphone with an

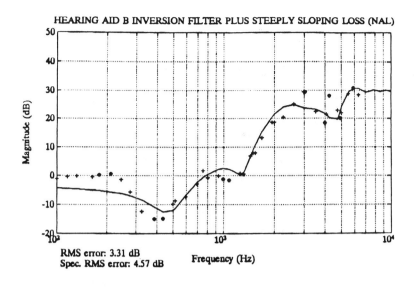

HEARING AID B INVERSION FILTER PLUS STEEPLY SLOPING LOSS (NAL)

RMS error: 3.31 dB
Spec. RMS error: 4.57 dB

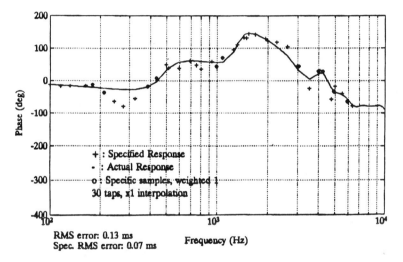

RMS error: 0.13 ms
Spec. RMS error: 0.07 ms

Figure 16–3. Ability of digital filtering to match precisely the NAL-R target frequency–response (upper) and desired phase (lower) for subjects with steeply sloping hearing loss. (From Nielsen et al.[32])

adaptive filter to synthesize an inverse of the acoustic feedback path.[41] An adaptive filter is used rather than a fixed-parameter filter to compensate for variations in the acoustic feedback path caused by distance changing between objects and the hearing aid.[42]

The first step is to determine the open loop transfer function of the acoustic feedback path[43] by disconnecting the forward path and injecting a noise probe signal, as shown in Figure 16–4. The probe signal must be of very short

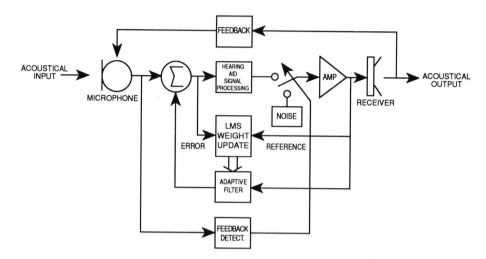

Figure 16–4. Block diagram of a hearing aid feedback cancellation system showing adaptive Wiener filter and noise probe injected into broken loop to determine acoustic feedback path transfer function. (From Kates.[44])

duration and not repeated too often so that it is not audible to the wearer. The acoustic feedback path can be attenuated by up to 50 dB as a result of this approach.[44] In another study,[39] the inverse of the feedback path was implemented as a fixed delay of about 0.85 msec, followed by an adaptive filter. With this approach, maximum stable gain obtained on KEMAR increased by as much as 10 dB with little sacrifice in sound quality. With a pocket processor coupled to a BTE earpiece with a cord, hearing aid wearers reported that oscillation due to feedback was suppressed in most situations in which oscillation would have been present while using conventional hearing aids.

Dyrlund and Bisgaard[45] evaluated a digital implementation of the feedback path subtraction approach for a high gain BTE hearing aid connected to a body-worn processing device with a cord. The system was "trained" periodically by re-estimating the acoustic feedback path transfer function with an injected noise signal. Ten to 15 dB improvement in feedback margin was achieved,

Table 16–3.   Maximum Attainable Insertion Gain Before
Feedback (Average 500, 1000, 2000 Hz) With a Danavox
DFS True Digital Antifeedback Hearing Aid

DFS (dB)	Own Aid (dB)	Diff (dB)
63	48	+15
63	53	+10
65	52	+13
59	51	+8
50	37	+13
65	55	+10

which the authors believed would be achieved regardless of the amount of earmold venting. In a significant technical achievement of a true digital anti-feedback algorithm, this approach has subsequently been introduced as a commercial BTE hearing aid operating from a single 1.3 V battery (Danavox DFS). Table 16–3 shows that the maximum insertion gain (averaged at 500, 1000, and 2000 Hz) achievable before feedback with this instrument on six subjects was 8–15 dB higher than that obtained with their own hearing aids.

Enhancing Speech With Analog and Digital Processing

Two areas may be considered when attempting to design hearing aids for improved speech intelligibility: improvement in signal-to-noise (S/N) ratio and enhancement of the speech signal itself. Hearing aid wearers miss or confuse unvoiced stop consonants and fricatives more than any other speech phoneme, especially in noise. Thus, to a certain point, as much consonant emphasis as possible, relative to vowel amplification, may be desirable in a hearing aid fitting. Many efforts in speech enhancement have therefore concentrated on improving the intelligibility of unvoiced fricatives and plosive sounds.

Reviews of speech enhancement techniques are abundant in the literature.[46–49] From the literature, a simple categorization of speech enhancement techniques may include (1) consonant–vowel ratio enhancement, (2) spectral contrast enhancement, (3) duration enhancement, and (4) temporal envelope expansion. Investigators have digitally manipulated the speech waveform to alter such features as the duration and amplitude of vowels and consonants, size of formant transitions, voice onset time and burst amplitude of stop consonants, and the amount of frication noise for voiceless fricatives. Since many of these techniques have been implemented with large digital computers and have not been employed in commercially available hearing aids, they represent possible future approaches and will be briefly reviewed here.

CONSONANT–VOWEL RATIO (CVR) ENHANCEMENT

CVR enhancement involves increasing the acoustic energy of consonants relative to vowels. Some researchers have attempted in improve intelligibility by enhancing the CVR beyond the values in unaided speech. In the past, most efforts to increase CVR have been research studies, implemented using large digital computers rather than subminiature components suitable for packaging in headworn hearing aids. Because of the cosmetic pressures currently driving the hearing aid marketplace, only consonant enhancement algorithms implemented with subminiature circuitry will receive widespread use. Another important goal is to accomplish an increase in CVR without introducing audible artifacts so that the hearing aid–processed signals do not sound distorted or artificial. It is possible that the benefit of CVR enhancement may be that it simply results in audibility of consonants. Thus, enhancing consonant audibility may be more important for good speech perception than actually enhancing the CVR per se.[50,51]

Some fairly simple signal processing algorithms, utilized for many years in analog headworn hearing aids, provide CVR enhancement. Enhancing the

CVR is one result of compression[52,53] and adaptive high pass filtering.[54] For example, significant improvement in speech recognition in high levels of competing noise were found when high pass filtering followed by automatic amplitude recognition of (syllabic compression) was employed in comparison to the intelligibility for unprocessed speech.[55] CVR was increased due to the rapid attack and release times in the compressor resulting in attenuating higher level vowel energy. A multi-band compressor having independent compression circuits for each frequency band eliminates the problem of most single band compressors that reduce gain across the entire frequency range in response to low frequency noise.[56] However, some researchers contend that high compression ratios with multi-band compression may degrade the relative intensity cues required to identify speech.[57,58] In spite of this possible disadvantage, the future of multi-band compression in hearing aids is virtually assured, if only for providing superior capability to achieve prescribed frequency responses.

Expansion, in contrast to compression, produces a greater change in output SPL for a given change in input SPL. Use of expansion for increasing the perception of low level consonants has been suggested.[59] For example, after determining the presence of a consonant by sensing the level of high frequency energy in a number of bandpass channels, the system reported by Kates[59] applies a 3:1 dynamic range expansion in these high frequency bands in which the speech level has exceeded a pre-selected threshold. Walker et al.[60] reported equivalent or reduced speech intelligibility for a six-band expander/compressor relative to a six-band linear processor for a small group of hearing impaired subjects. Their expander operated only on low level signals in the high frequency bands, while the compressor was used for high level signals.

A combination of adaptive high pass filtering followed by expansion as shown in the block diagram in Figure 16–5a has been investigated for potentially increasing CVR with analog circuitry small enough to be packaged in ITE hearing aids.[61,62] The intent of this algorithm was initially to attenuate the higher energy vowels via adaptive high pass filtering, leaving mainly low energy consonants to be amplified. After the low frequency energy was attenuated, the residual high frequency-dominant signal was expanded as shown in Figure 16–5B to increase the CVR further. Higher CVRs were found with this combination algorithm than with adaptive high pass filtering alone for some, but not all consonants. Fortune and Preves[63] and Tezeli et al.[51] obtained higher Nonsense Syllable Test scores for some, but not all consonants with adaptive high pass filtering followed by expansion than with adaptive high pass filtering alone for persons with sharply sloping hearing losses.

With digital laboratory instrumentation for hearing impaired listeners with mild to moderate gradually sloping and sharply sloping audiometric configurations, Gordon-Salant[64] reported that a 10 dB increase in the CVR resulted in a mean improvement of 14% in the recognition of 19 consonants paired with three vowels in a competing babble presented at +6 dB S/N ratio. Using a similar protocol, consonants from the California Consonant Test were amplified by 10–21 dB to yield a CVR of 0 dB. This protocol produced a mean improvement of 10% in intelligibility.[65] In another study,[66] improved recognition was reported with normal-hearing listeners for voiced stops in competing white noise as a result of amplifying consonants by 10 dB. These authors

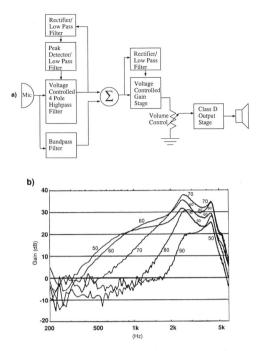

Figure 16–5. (a) Block diagram of a hearing aid with adaptive high pass filter followed by expansion. (b) Family of frequency–response curves with speech-shaped noise input levels ranging from 50 to 90 dB SPL in 10 dB steps. (From Preves et al.[61])

theorized that the improvement may have been the result of amplification of the burst release that resulted in emphasized modulation envelope cues. However, for other types of consonants, recognition was reduced, presumably because of modulation envelope distortion. Kennedy and Levitt,[67] recognizing that the optimal CVR may vary on an individual basis, obtained a mean improvement of 15% in Nonsense Syllable Test scores for nine hearing impaired listeners with 3, 6, 9, and 12 dB increase in the level of the consonant energy. However, too much amplification of certain consonants for some subjects resulted in a decrease in intelligibility from that obtained for the "ideal" amount of enhancement.

SPECTRAL CONTRAST ENHANCEMENT

Spectral sharpening or spectral contrast enhancement has been evaluated to help compensate for reduced frequency selectivity of impaired auditory systems.[68] Several researchers have investigated spectral contrast enhancement by using formant bandwidth reduction and principal components compression. For example, Summerfield et al.[69] evaluated the effect on stop consonant recognition of narrowing and broadening the formant bandwidths of synthetic speech by 0.25–8 times normal as shown in Figure 16–6. Broadening the formant bandwidths (lower three examples) produced lower percent correct stop consonant identification for both hearing impaired and normal-hearing subjects. Although no mean increase in correct identification resulted from the

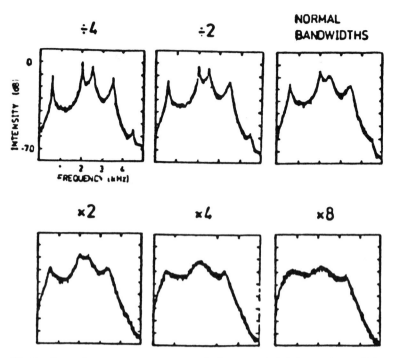

Figure 16–6. Long-term power spectra of the vowel /e/ from the syllables "get," "debt," and "bet" showing the effects of varying formant bandwidths from 0.25 to 8.0 times normal values. (From Summerfield et al.[69])

narrower formant bandwidths provided by spectral sharpening, some persons in both groups benefitted from one-half the normal formant bandwidths (top center example).

Bustamante and Braida[70] investigated a principal components compression technique for reducing gross speech amplitude changes while maintaining spectral contrast. They compressed only the first two principal components, corresponding to overall level (PC1) and spectral tilt (PC2) to preserve rapid fluctuations of speech while reducing overall band level variation. In another study, Bustamante and Braida[71] evaluated wideband compression with sharpening of short-term spectral shape by expanding the component weights responsible for peak–valley ratio. This algorithm produced either no change or reduced intelligibility for a CVC nonsense syllable recognition task relative to wideband compression alone and only a modest benefit over linear amplification. In a third study,[72] these authors found that compressing PC1 produced improved intelligibility for four hearing-impaired listeners, as did wideband compression, relative to linear processing. However, compressing both PC1 and PC2 reduced intelligibility relative to linear processing. The effect of selectively manipulating spectral tilt has also been evaluated.[73] Haggard et al.[73] found a decrement in performance when spectral tilt was slowly switched between flat and rising responses relative to a fixed spectral tilt. The idea

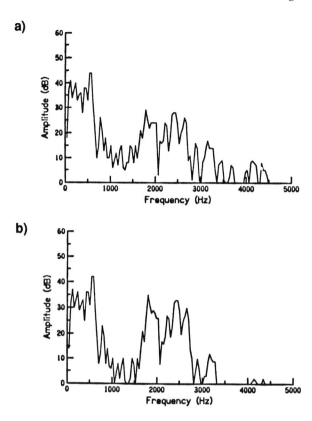

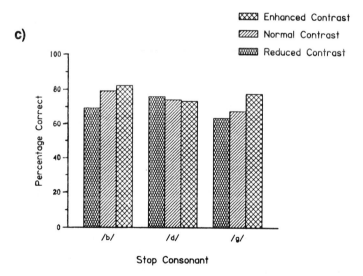

Figure 16–7. Examples of unprocessed (**a**) and contrast-enhanced (**b**) spectra. The enhancement was applied only to midfrequency peaks. (**c**) Percent correct identification of three stop consonants with three spectral contrast conditions. (From Bunnell.[74])

behind this type of compression was to narrow the distribution of spectral tilt relative to that of the unprocessed signal. A rising response was provided for speech segments having a falling long-term spectrum (voiced sounds) while a flat response was given to those with a flat spectrum (voiceless sounds). It was thought that the decrement in performance was caused by the importance of maintaining the spectral envelope contour within individual frequency bands. Bunnell[74] investigated reducing and enhancing spectral contrasts via principal components compression for F2 and F3 formants, but not for F1. Figure 16–7a shows an unprocessed example and Figure 16–7b the result of enhancing F2 and F3 for the same speech segment. With reduced spectral contrast, correct identifications of stop consonants by ten hearing-impaired persons were reduced. As shown in Figure 16–7c, enhancing spectral contrast raised the number of correct identifications for /b/and/g/, but not for /d/. In summary, in comparison to wideband compression, it appears that the benefits provided with spectral contrast enhancement and manipulation of spectral tilt are somewhat doubtful, since reduced or, at best, only slightly improved intelligibility resulted in most of the investigations.

DURATION ENHANCEMENT

To compensate for reduced temporal resolution of impaired auditory systems, several researchers have investigated varying the duration of speech components. In one study, the duration of the preceding vowel was lengthened for syllables with a final /z/ or /v/ and shortened for syllables with a final /s/ or /f/. This strategy provided substantial increases in consonant recognition for 25 moderately to profoundly hearing impaired listeners.[75] However, Gordon-Salant[64] found that 100% increases in consonant duration did not generally produce an increase in consonant recognition scores for elderly listeners with mild to moderate hearing impairments at two presentation levels. Similarly, for consonant duration increases of up to 30 msec, Montgomery and Edge[65] reported no increase in California Consonant Test scores at a 65 dB SPL presentation level and only a mean 5% increase at 95 dB SPL for subjects having near-normal low frequency hearing sensitivity accompanied by a moderate to severe high frequency loss. From this work, it appears that such manipulations of duration are helpful for more severely hearing impaired persons but not for more mildly hearing impaired persons.

TEMPORAL ENVELOPE EXPANSION

The purpose of temporal envelope expansion is to increase the contrast or modulation index in the temporal speech waveform. It is thought that selective exaggeration or compression of the modulation envelope may improve speech recognition for hearing impaired persons.[58,76] Testing this idea, as compared to the unprocessed condition, Langhans and Strube[77] reported a 30% improvement in recognition by applying either 20:1 compression, 5 dB expansion or linear amplification if the modulation frequency in the temporal envelope was less than 2 Hz, between 2 and 5 Hz, or greater than 18 Hz, respectively. As shown in the block diagram in Figure 16–8, after determining the short time

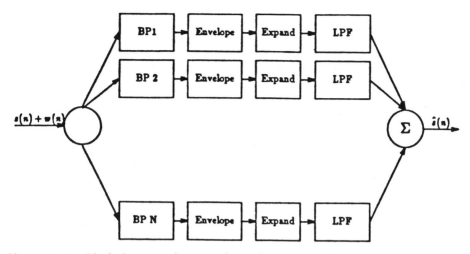

Figure 16–8. Block diagram of system that enhances speech using temporal envelope expansion. BPF, band pass filtering; LPF, low-pass filtering. x(n) is the input consisting of signal s(n) and noise w(n), and $\hat{S}(n)$ is the enhanced output. (From Clarkson and Bahgat.[78])

spectrum in 20 band pass filters Clarkson and Bahgat,[78] using a similar expansion algorithm to that of Langhans and Strube[77] with normal hearing listeners, reported a 6% mean improvement in Modified Rhyme Test scores with competing white noise at a 0 dB S/N ratio. Based on the results of these few studies, the use of temporal envelope expansion in hearing aids of the future appears promising.

Digital Noise Reduction Algorithms

Separating speech from noise is a difficult task even for large laboratory computers that are processing off-line rather than in real time as is required for hearing aids. Because of the continually varying nature of common background noises, many of the techniques found in the literature for reduction of steady-state noise need to be modified to be applicable for hearing aids. The following brief review of digital noise reduction algorithms is intended as a sampling of the type of techniques that might be used in hearing aids of the future. A simple way of classifying noise reduction algorithms is to divide them into single microphone approaches and multiple microphone approaches.

SINGLE MICROPHONE APPROACHES

In most single microphone noise reduction approaches, the contribution of a specific frequency band within the overall frequency spectrum is attenuated if the measured speech level in that band is more than a specified amount below an estimate of the background noise level in that band. Examples of single microphone noise reduction approaches are *spectral power subtraction, adaptive Wiener filtering,* and *active noise reduction.*

Spectral Power Subtraction. In this approach, the short-time spectral magnitude of speech is estimated from a sample of speech mixed with noise and then combined with the phase of the speech and noise to produce enhanced speech.[79,80] To determine the average noise power, there is a need to know if speech is present. To aid in this decision, the temporal differences between the transients in speech and the comparatively steady-state nature of noise can be exploited: The characteristics of the noise are estimated during the silent intervals in the speech. A major problem occurs if the spectrum of the noise is similar to that of speech, as in the case of competing speech babble, because simply subtracting the noise spectrum from the incoming signal will also subtract a signifiant amount of the speech itself.[81] In one evaluation of this technique, using nonsense sentences mixed with wideband random noise, recognition scores were not improved, but the processed speech sounded less noisy and provided improved sound quality compared with the unprocessed speech.[82] For high S/N ratios, it is "most likely" (a decision made by the algorithm) that speech is present and that the speech envelope is more easily extracted from the noise. McAulay and Malpass[83] used an algorithm that suppressed noise effectively for low speech S/N ratios, a condition "most likely" corresponding to noise alone. However, when attempting to suppress noise for low SNR's, other investigators have noted considerable distortion when using spectral subtraction, resulting in a music-like residual noise.[84]

Adaptive Wiener Filtering. The output of an ideal adaptive Wiener filter yields an estimate of speech without the presence of any noise. Qualitatively, an adaptive, multi-band Wiener filter reduces the gain from moment to moment in a band if noise is predominately present in that band. The parameters of the digital filter are adaptively changed to estimate the noise during silent periods in the speech signal. Adaptive Wiener filtering works well when the noise does not vary much (quasi-steady-state noise), but performance of the filter degrades if the noise changes in character or if the long-time spectrum of the noise is similar to that of speech (e.g., speech of several competing talkers mixed together). Also, some knowledge is required about the speech and noise signals and their transmission paths from the source to the hearing aid microphone. One laboratory study,[85] using a multi-band adaptive Wiener filter reported a remarkable improvement in the quality of processed speech by increasing the number of bands to 24. For S/N ratios greater than 6 dB, the device "nearly eliminated" (a 32 dB noise reduction) disturbing noise while introducing negligible distortion in the speech. As is frequently the case with other single microphone processors, this noise reduction system was not as effective in lower SNR conditions.

The Zeta Noise Blocker (ZNB), which is the noise reduction chip referred to previously, is an implementation of an adaptive Wiener filter that was small enough to be marketed in ITE hearing aids. It consisted of a custom-designed special-purpose digital computer implemented with a combination analog–digital CMOS integrated circuit.[25] The ZNB used analog-switched capacitor filters and attempted to separate speech from noise in several frequency bands using temporal differences between speech and quasi-steady-state noise. The

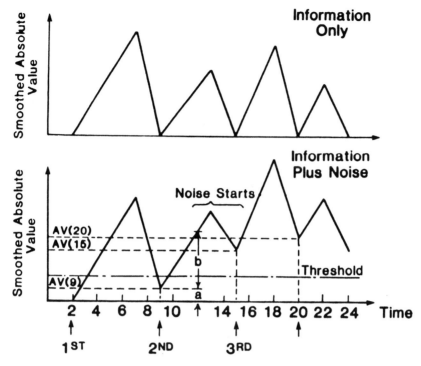

Figure 16–9. Temporal processing of the Zeta Noise Blocker. Time representation of energy of smoothed speech pulses without additive noise (upper) and with additive noise (lower). Sampling to identify noise occurs during the pauses in the speech pulses as indicated by the arrows.

noise was sensed during the silent intervals between vocal cord pulses of speech, as shown in the lower graph of Figure 16–9. As indicated in the figure, when noise starts, these silent periods would "fill up," and, as a result, the ZNB would reduce the gain in the corresponding frequency band. The frequency response of a ZNB hearing aid did not change very much for pulsing signals like speech in quiet[86] (e.g., upper graph in Fig. 16–9), but for a pulsing signal mixed with steady-state noise, gain was attenuated in the frequency range of the noise. In spite of this sophisticated algorithm and its availability from a number of hearing aid manufacturers in ITE hearing aid models, the ZNB did not achieve widespread success as a noise suppression circuit. As mentioned before, it may be that it produced too-noticeable, drastic changes in the frequency response from only small changes in the listening environment.

Active Noise Reduction.   A possible future technique for reducing noise in hearing aid fittings might utilize active noise reduction (ANR), sometimes called *active noise control*. As shown in Figure 16–10, ANR involves sensing the noise in a restricted cavity and cancelling the noise by injecting an equal magnitude signal having the opposite phase of the noise into the cavity. This technique has been used successfully to cancel noises that do not have the

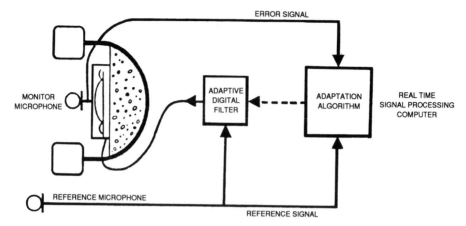

Figure 16–10.   Block diagram of adaptive digital noise reduction system for an airforce flight helmet. Filter adapts until the error signal (residual noise) is minimized. (From Carter.[87])

same spectral characteristics as speech (e.g., in headphones and helmets for aviation and military applications[87]). It has also been used in consumer application for attenuating road and exhaust noise in vehicles[88] and for reducing air conditioner duct and fan noises.[89] The methodology of ANR for application to hearing aids would entail controlling an adaptive digital filter with an error signal indicative of the noise remaining in the ear canal after cancellation. A key question that must be addressed is whether this technique could be effective enough for separating speech-like noises (e.g., babble) from the desired speech signal.

MULTIPLE MICROPHONE APPROACHES

The effectiveness of many conventional DSP algorithms for S/N ratio enhancement using one microphone is limited primarily because they attempt to subtract the noise from the speech, with the result often being a significant reduction of the speech energy as well as the noise energy. With two or more microphones, more sophisticated algorithms providing superior noise cancellation can be utilized because each microphone receives a different representation of the desired (target) signal and the interfering noise.

ADAPTIVE NOISE CANCELLING

One popular two microphone noise reduction technique uses the correlation of the noise signal in two microphones and has been called *adaptive noise cancelling*.[90] An adaptive noise canceller (ANC) in hearing aids of the future might consist of two microphones in the same housing or a microphone in each side of a binaural hearing aid fitting. Referring to Figure 16–11, the signal (S) in the primary microphone is the desired input, with the noise signal (N2) from the second microphone used as a reference for the adaptive filter. The reference

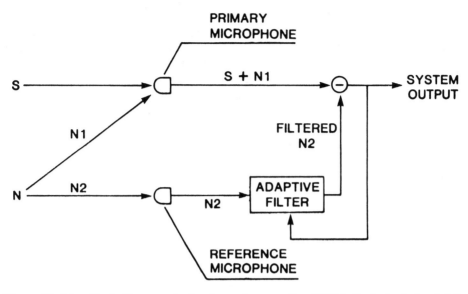

Figure 16–11.   Block diagram of adaptive noise canceller (ANC). S, desired signal; N1, noise in the primary microphone; N2 noise in the reference microphone. (From Weiss.[94])

microphone is placed some distance away from the primary microphone and, ideally, as close as possible to interfering noise sources. The object of this noise reduction scheme is to obtain a good estimate of the desired speech signal in the primary microphone. The adaptive filter parameters are updated periodically to eliminate the difference between the noise signals in the primary and reference microphones. This filtering algorithm has also been termed *least mean squares* (LMS), referring to minimizing the error between the two inputs by adjusting the adaptive filter coefficients. Unlike single microphone noise reduction systems that perform Wiener filtering, this technique has the advantage that no prior knowledge is required of the speech and noise signals to set up the adaptive filter. The ideal situation for two microphone adaptive noise cancellation to work perfectly is to have the same noise signal in both microphones, but to have only speech in the primary microphone. Ideally, therefore, the input to the primary microphone is speech and noise while the only input to the reference microphone is noise correlated to the noise in the primary microphone. Then, much of the noise will be cancelled in the summing junction, and as much as 20 dB improvement in the S/N ratio is possible. Realizing these ideal requirements in practice, however, necessitates a large spacing between the two microphones and requires having the reference microphone close to the interfering noise source(s)—both unrealistic in hearing aid applications. In real-world implementations, the reference microphone output contains some speech as well as noise, causing partial cancellation of the desired speech. Additionally, reverberation can invalidate another important ideal criterion— that the signal and the noise are uncorrelated.[91]

Many of the references cited herein that have investigated adaptive noise cancellation have employed computer simulations and/or large, laboratory-grade components instead of hearing aid-size components housed in actual hearing aids and worn by hearing impaired listeners in real-world listening environments. For example, in one study,[92] a microphone was used to pick up speech and noise for the primary channel, but the reference channel input was taken from the electrical output of a speech noise generator passed through a low pass filter rather than from a second microphone. This artifactual experimental design formed the perfect input for the reference channel—the speech signal was totally absent, and only a correlated noise signal was present. Another investigation[20] of the two microphone ANC technique reported an 18–22 dB reduction in speech babble or speech-weighted noise and a resulting 27–40% improvement in CID W-22 word recognition for hearing impaired listeners. However, for this study, two loudspeakers separated by 2 m were used. One loudspeaker output had only the desired speech signal with the primary microphone placed close by; the second loudspeaker output had only the undesired noise with the reference microphone positioned close by. This is obviously not a practical simulation of the spacing of wearable hearing aid microphones, but was evidently done to ensure that the speech signal would be much stronger in the primary channel than in the reference channel. The excellent results of this study therefore reflect the best improvements obtainable under idealized conditions. Although promising, perhaps test results from such experimental protocols should be regarded as having only academic interest until such algorithms and the required instrumentation can be made available and evaluated in actual hearing aid applications in situ.

Investigators have utilized directional microphones as another way of dealing with the effects of the physical environment on the input signal, to ensure that only noise is present in the second microphone.[93–95] In these approaches, a directional microphone facing backwards was employed to help ensure that only noise was sensed for the reference channel. In the Weiss[94] study, non-hearing aid–sized components were employed for the high grade microphones and the adaptive noise canceller, and the microphone output signals were tape recorded for off-line presentation to the adaptive filter. Weiss[94] concluded that in real-world reverberant environments the advantage provided by this relatively complicated system would be minimal compared with that provided by a single directional microphone facing forward in a conventional hearing aid.

BEAMFORMING

A beamformer is a noise canceller that utilizes the spacial orientation of microphones relative to the locations of the desired signal and the undesired noises. A beamformer consists of two or more microphones, which, in combination with a fixed or an adaptive filter, emphasizes desired signals while producing sharp nulls in the polar directivity pattern to cancel noise. Beamformers have been advocated to compensate for the loss of the directionally-selective noise reduction capacity reported in hearing impaired auditory systems. With N microphones, $N - 1$ nulls can be generated to attenuate noises originating

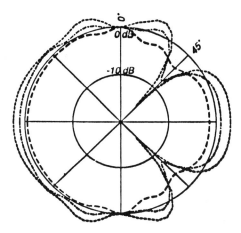

Figure 16–12. Polar directivity patterns of a two-microphone beamformer averaged across a 4.3 kHz passband. Simulated environments are indicated by short dash, anechoic; dot–dash, living room; long dash, a reverberant conference room; Desired signal is at 0° azimuth, and undesired noise is at 45°. (From Peterson.[91])

from several directions. For example, in theory, two microphones can cancel one noise source adaptively by moving the null direction provided by the canceller automatically to the direction of the undesired noise. Beamformers are usually designed to provide maximum gain at 0° azimuth (called the *look* direction).

One question that arises about the possible use of beamformers in hearing aids of the future is whether they can provide better directivity than a simple directional microphone. For example, Figure 16–12 shows the polar directivity patterns achieved with a two-microphone beamformer[91] with desired signal at 0° and undesired noise at 45° azimuth for three environments having different amounts of reverberation. For comparative purposes, the range of polar directivity patterns possible with first-order gradient directional microphones are reproduced by Marshall and Harry[96] and shown in Figure 16–13. These polar directivity patterns are similar to those produced by first-order gradient directional microphones used in hearing aids beginning in the early 1970s. The amount of directivity achieved with only a single directional microphone (e.g., lower left polar pattern) is greater than that in Figure 16–12 obtained with the much more complicated two-microphone beamformer. Also, unlike a directional microphone in a hearing aid, a beamformer having two omni-directional microphones (with one worn on each ear) has the disadvantage of not being able to determine which direction is front and which is back. However, unlike the fixed directionality provided by a directional microphone, an adaptive beamformer has the advantage that the direction of the null(s) in its polar directivity pattern can adapt to changes in the direction of the undesirable noise sources. However, if the "look" direction always follows the line of sight of the hearing aid wearer, the directivity pattern of a directional microphone, as worn, will adapt to a certain degree from movements of the hearing aid wearer's head.

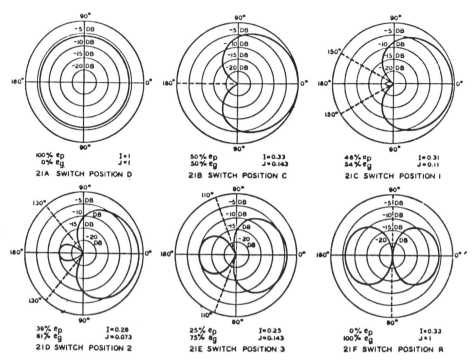

Figure 16–13. Directivity patterns obtainable in free space with a first-order gradient directional microphone of the type used in hearing aids. (From Marshall and Harry.[96])

A even higher degree of directivity with directional microphones would be possible[97] with second-order gradient directional microphones, as shown in Figure 16–14. Note the extreme reduction of energy in these polar patterns in the rear hemisphere (from 90° to 270°). Hearing aids have not utilized second-order gradient directional microphones because they are usually implemented with long parallel tubes bundled together. Lengths in excess of one foot are necessary to provide good directionality at low frequencies. Obviously, such a packaging approach would not be cosmetically acceptable for headworn hearing aids. To create two arbitrarily spaced nulls in the polar directivity pattern, something a directional microphone cannot do, a beamformer must be designed with a third microphone, as shown in Figure 16–15a, which could be added at the center of the front of a hearing aid wearer's head.[98] This three-microphone beamformer produced a double-null directivity pattern as shown in Figure 16–15b for noise sources at +40° and −60°. Locating three microphones in this configuration is obviously not practical in the conventional sense of hearing aid packaging except perhaps in an eyeglass hearing aid.

With still more microphones, it is also possible to achieve polar directivity patterns having a greater degree of directionality[99,100] with fixed-direction (non-adaptive) beamformers having four omnidirectional and five directional microphones, respectively. For example, Hoffman and Buckley[101] evaluated five omni-directional microphones located symmetrically around the head at 45°

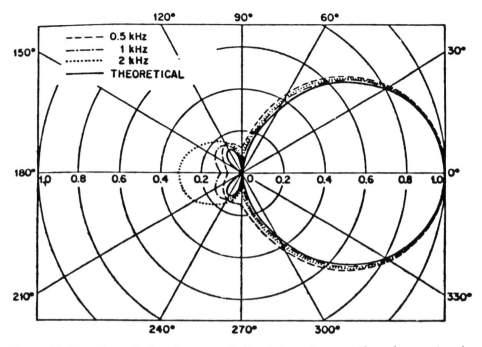

Figure 16–14. Theoretical and measured directivity patterns at three frequencies obtainable with a second-order gradient directional microphone in free space. (From Sessler and West.[97])

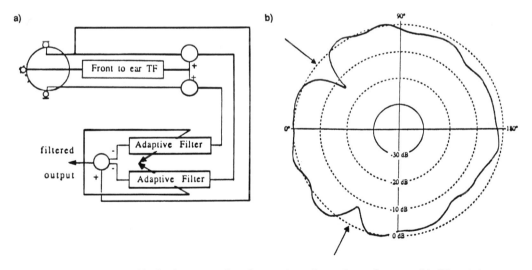

Figure 16–15. (a) Block diagram of a three-microphone beamformer. (b) Directivity pattern produces two nulls with this configuration in response to uncorrelated noises at 40° and at −60°. (From Farassopoulos.[98])

intervals from $-90°$ to $+90°$ with a beamformer response fixed in the look direction. They reported a 30 dB attenuation of speech-shaped noise in the presence of two 0 dB S/N ratio interfering sources located at $-60°$ and $+30°$. In another study,[102] improved speech reception threshold estimates were reported for two- and four-microphone adaptive beamformers operating on one or two interfering noises in simulated anechoic and living room environments for negative S/N ratios. The performance of their system[102] degraded for S/N ratios greater than 0 dB and when the target signals in the microphones were not equal due to reverberation, two conditions that would be commonly encountered by hearing aid wearers. At high S/N ratio, due to imperfect cancellation of the target signal in the two microphones, the target may be stronger in the reference signal than the noise, resulting in more target cancellation than noise cancellation. This study did not include the effects of diffraction from a hearing aid wearer, which would add to the array misalignment problem. At the same laboratory, real-time measurements, as opposed to beamformer simulation, have been made with the same stimuli for a two-microphone array on KEMAR using an Ariel DSP board communicating with a personal computer for the adaptive filter.[103] In this study, the microphones were located on the KEMAR head for one test in an eyeglass frame (broadside configuration) and for another test in one eyeglass temple (endfire configuration). Tests were run with one and two SPIN babble interfering noises from several directions. It was found that in a reverberant environment, a broadside microphone location (e.g., across the front of an eyeglass frame) with a fixed beamformer generally provided superior performance in comparison to an endfire microphone array on an eyeglass temple with an adaptive beamformer.

A word must be said about packaging considerations. Since beamformers consist of two or more microphones connecting to an adaptive filter, the outputs of the microphones need to be forwarded to the central computer processing location. This can be done by direct wiring or, to be more cosmetically acceptable, without any wires. Thus, a practical implementation of a beamformer implies wireless transmission from the microphones to the digital filter. Packaging the circuitry for this wireless communication link presents a significant problem as it would add to the already difficult task of cosmetically packaging standard hearing aid components.

Conclusion

Digital signal processing offers the promise of superior performance with hearing aids compared with processing with the current analog technology. However, proven digital algorithms that are much more effective than those used in analog hearing aids are not yet available in miniaturized form to enhance speech and reduce environmental noise without introducing undesirable audible artifacts.

Dramatic improvements in current hearing aid sound quality continue to be made using important technological advances such as amplifiers with Class D output stages. Effective digitally based algorithms do currently exist for reducing acoustic feedback oscillation but need to be miniaturized sufficiently before they can receive widespread use in hearing aids. In the meantime, the capabilities of CMOS integrated circuitry are just beginning to be used in analog and in hybrid analog–digital type hearing aids for solving these problems and for providing superior frequency shaping capability.

References

1. Hawkins D, Naidov S: A comparison of sound quality and clarity with peak clipping and compression output limiting. Paper presented at the convention of the American Academy of Audiology, 1992, Nashville, TN.
2. Preves DA, Newton JR: The headroom problem and hearing aid performance. *Hear J* 1989; 42(10):21.
3. Corliss E, Burnett E, Kobal M, Bassin M: The relative importance of frequency distortion and changes in time constants in the intelligibility of speech. *IEEE Trans Audio Electroacoustics* 1968; 16:36–39.
4. Agnew J: Hearing instrument distortion: What does it mean for the listener? *Hear Instrum* 1988; 39(10):10–20.
5. Frye G: Crest factor and composite signals for hearing aid testing. *Hear J* 1987; 40(10):15–18.
6. Van Tasell D, Crain T: Noise reduction hearing aids: release from masking and release from distortion. *Ear Hear* 1992; 13:114–121.
7. Preves D, Woodruff B: Some methods of improving and assessing hearing aid headroom. *Audecibel* 1990; 39(3):8–13.
8. Carlson EV: An output amplifier whose time has come. *Hear Instrum* 1988; 39(10):30–32.
9. Reddy SN, Kirlin RL: Evaluation of hearing aid and auditory response using pseudorandom noise, in Larson V, Egolf D, Kirlin R, Stile S (eds): *Auditory and Hearing Prosthetics Research*. New York: Grune and Stratton, 1979, pp 377–410.
10. Preves D: Expressing hearing aid noise and distortion with the coherence measurement. *ASHA* 1990; 32(6):56–59.
11. Schweitzer H, Grim M, Preves D, Kubichek R: Qualitative assessment of hearing aid performance by an expert pattern recognition system. Poster presented at the convention of the American Academy of Audiology Denver, CO 1991.
12. Hawkins D: A comparison of sound quality and clarity with peak clipping and compression output limiting. Poster presented at the convention of the American Academy of Audiology, 1992, Nashville, TN.
13. Filion P, Margolis R: Comparison of clinical and real-life judgments of loudness discomfort. *J Am Acad Audiol* 1992; 3:193–199.
14. Fortune T, Preves D: Hearing aid saturation and aided loudness discomfort. *J Speech Hear Res* 1992; 35:175–185.
15. Fortune T, Preves D, Woodruff B: Saturation-induced distortion and its effects on aided LDL. *Hear Instrum* 1991; 42(10):37–42.
16. Sammeth C, Bess F, Bratt G, et al.: The Vanderbilt/VA hearing aid selection study: interim report. Poster presented at the convention of the American Speech–Language–Hearing Association, 1989, St. Louis, MO.
17. Sammeth C, Preves D, Bratt G, et al.: Achieving prescribed gain/frequency responses with advances in hearing aid technology. *J Rehab Res Dev* 1993 (in press).
18. Nunley J, Staab W, Steadman J, et al.: A wearable digital hearing aid. *Hear J* 1983; 36(10): 29–35.
19. Morely R, Engel G, Sullivan T, Natarajan S: VLSI based design of a battery-operated digital hearing aid. *Proceedings of IEEE Conference on Acoustics, Speech and Signal Processing*, 1988.
20. Harris R, Brey R, Robinette M, et al.: Use of adaptive digital signal processing to improve speech communication for normally hearing and hearing-impaired subjects. *J Speech Hear Res* 1988; 31:265–271.
21. Miller E: Digital signal processing in hearing aids: implications and applications. *Hear J* 1988; 41(4):22–26.
22. Widin G: The meaning of digital technology. *Hear Instrum* 1987; 38(11):28–33.
23. Staab W: Digital hearing aids. *Hear Instrum* 1985; 36(11):14.
24. Roeser R, Taylor K: Audiometric and field testing with a digital hearing instrument. *Hear Instrum* 1988; 39(4):14.
25. Graupe D, Causey D: Method of and means for adaptively filtering near-stationary noise from speech. U.S. Patent 4,025,721, 1977.
26. Levitt H: Digital hearing aids: A tutorial review. *J Rehab Res Dev* 1987; 24:7–20.

27. Preves D: Digital hearing aids. *ASHA* 1987; 29:45–47.
28. Murray D, Hanson J: Application of digital signal processing to hearing aids: A critical survey. *J Am Acad Audiol* 1992; 3:145–152.
29. Levitt H: Advanced signal processing techniques for hearing aids, in Studebaker G, Bess F, Beck L (eds): *The Vanderbilt Hearing-Aid Report II*. Parkton, MD: York Press, 1991, pp 93–99.
30. French-St George M: Central Institute for the Deaf digital hearing aid project. Paper presented at Amplification in the 90's/International Hearing Aid Conference, 1992, St. Louis, MO.
31. Lunner T, Hellgren J: A digital filterbank hearing aid-design, implementation and evaluation. *Proceedings of IEEE Conference on Acoustics, Speech and Signal Processing, 1991, pp 3661–3664.*
32. Nielsen L, Wu E, Hoffman M, et al.: Design and evaluation of FIR filters for digital hearing aids with arbitrary amplitude and phase response. *J Acoust Soc Am* 1990; 87(Suppl 1) S24.
33. Egolf D: Review of the acoustic feedback literature from a control systems point of view, in Studebaker G, Bess F (eds): *The Vanderbilt Hearing-Aid Report: State of the Art—Research Needs.* Upper Darby, PA: Monographs in Contemporary Audiology, 1992, pp 94–103.
34. Preves D: Principles of Signal Processing, in Sandlin R (ed): *Handbook of Hearing Aid Amplification*, vol 1. 1988, pp 81–120. College-Hill Press, Little, Brown and Company; Boston, MA.
35. Harjani R, Wang R: *The Elimination of Acoustic Oscillations in Hearing Aids Using Phase Equalization.* Minneapolis. MN: University of Minnesota, Department of Electrical Engineering 1992.
36. Beex A: Moving-average notch filter. U.S. Patent 4,232,192, 1980.
37. Schroeder M: Improvement of acoustic feedback stability by freqeuncy shifting. *J Acoust Soc Am* 1961; 33:1718–1724.
38. Bennett M, Srikandan S, Browne L: A controlled feedback hearing aid. *Hear Aid J* 1980; 12:42–43.
39. Bustamante D, Worrall T, Williamson M: Measurement and adaptive suppression of acoustic feedback in hearing aids, in *Proceedings of the IEEE Conference on Acoustics, Speech and Signal Processing,* 1989, pp 2017–2020.
40. Levitt H, Dugot R, Kopper K: Programmable digital hearing aid system. U.S. Patent 4,731,850, 1988.
41. Egolf D, Larson V, Ahlstrom C, Rainbolt H, McConnell: The development and evaluation of a prototype acoustic feedback suppressor. Poster presented at the convention of the American Speech–Language–Hearing Association, New Orleans, LA, 1987.
42. Best L: *Digital Suppression of Acoustic Feedback in Hearing Aids.* Master's thesis. Laramie, WY: University of Wyoming, Department of Electrical Engineering, 1985.
43. Egolf D, Howell H, Weaver K, Barker SD: The hearing aid feedback path: Mathematical simulations and experimental verification. *J Acoust Soc Am* 1985; 78:1578–1587.
44. Kates J: Feedback cancellation in hearing aids: Results from a computer simulation. *IEEE Trans Acoustics Speech Signal Processing* 1991; 39:553–562.
45. Dyrlund O, Bisgaard N: Acoustic feedback margin improvements in hearing instruments using a prototype DFS (digital feedback suppresion) system. *Scand Audiol* 1991; 20:49–53.
46. Lim J: *Speech Enhancement.* Englewood Cliffs, NJ: Prentice-Hall, 1983.
47. Montgomery A: A review of speech signal enhancement for the hearing impaired, in *Proceedings of Symposium on Hearing Aid Technology.* Gallaudet University, 1984.
48. Revoile S, Holden-Pitt L: Some acoustic enhancements of speech and their effect on consonant identification by the hearing impaired. Paper presented at Arrowhead Conference, 1990. Lake Arrowhead, CA.
49. Williamson M, Punch J: Speech enhancement in digital hearing aids. *Semin Hear* 1990; 11:68–77.
50. Freyman R, Nerbonne G: The importance of consonant–vowel intensity ratio in the intelligibility of voiceless consonants. *J Speech Hear Res* 1989; 32:524–535.
51. Tetzeli M, Sammeth C, Ochs M: Effects of nonlinear amplification on speech intelligibility and sound quality. Paper presented at the convention of the American Speech–Language–Hearing Association, Atlanta, GA, 1991.
52. Villchur E: Signal processing to improve speech intelligibility in perceptive deafness. *J Acoust Soc Am* 1973; 53:1646–1657.
53. Dillon H: Hearing aid amplification method and apparatus. U.S. Patent 4,803,732, 1989.
54. Preves D: Output limiting and speech enhancement, in Studebaker G, Bess F, Beck L (eds): *The Vanderbilt Hearing-Aid Report II.* Parkton, MD: York Press, 1991, pp 36–39.
55. Niederjohn R, Grotelueschen J: The enhancement of speech intelligibility in high noise levels by high-pass filtering followed by rapid amplitude compression. *IEEE Trans Acoustics Speech Signal Processing,* 1976; 24:277–282.
56. Kates J: Signal processing for hearing aids. *Hear Instrum* 1986; 37(2):19–22.

57. DeGennaro S, Braida L, Durlach N: Multiband syllabic compression for severely impaired listeners. *J Rehab Res Dev* 1986; 23:17–24.
58. Plomp R: The negative effect of amplitude compression in multichannel hearing aids in the light of the modulation-transfer function. *J Acoust Soc Am* 1988; 83:2322–2327.
59. Kates J: Speech intelligibility enhancement. U.S. Patent 4,454,609, 1984.
60. Walker G, Byrne D, Dillon H: The effects of multichannel compression/expansion amplificationon the intelligibility of nonsense syllables in noise. *J Acoust Soc Am* 1984; 73:746–757.
61. Preves D, Fortune T, Woodruff B, Newton J: Strategies for enhancing the consonant to vowel ratio with in the ear hearing aids. *Ear Hear* 1991; 6(Suppl 12): 139s–153s.
62. Ochs M, Sammeth C, Tetzeli M: Acoustic analysis of syllables processed by linear and nonlinear hearing aid circuits. Poster presented at the convention of the American Acadedmy Audiology of Nashville, TN, April 1991.
63. Fortune T, Preves D: Consonant perception and the modifiation of real ear consonant-to-vowel ratios produced by analog in-the-ear hearing aids. Paper presented at the convention of the American Speech–Language–Hearing Association, Atlanta, GA, 1991.
64. Gordon-Salant S: Effects of acoustic modification on consonant recognition by elderly hearing-impaired subjects. *J Acoust Soc AM* 1987; 81:1199–1202.
65. Montgomery A, Edge R: Evaluation of two speech enhancement techniques to improve intelligibility for hearing-impaired adults. *J Speech Hear Res* 1988; 31:386–393.
66. Freyman R, Nerbonne G, Cole H: Effect of consonant-vowel-ratio modification on amplitude envelope cues for consonant recognition. *J Speech Hear Res* 1991; 34:415–426.
67. Kennedy E, Levitt H: Optimal C/V intensity ratio at MCL. Presented at the convention of the American Speech–Language–Hearing *Association*, Seattle WA, 1990.
68. Boers P: *Formant Enhancement of Speech of Listeners With Sensorineural Hearing Loss.* I.P.O. Annual Progress Report. The Netherlands: Institut voor Perceptie Onderzoek, 1980, 15:21–28.
69. Summerfield Q, Foster J, Tyler R: Influences of formant bandwidth and auditory frequency selectivity on identification of place of articulation in stop consonants. *Speech Comm* 1985; 4:213–229.
70. Bustamante D, Braida L: Principal component amplitude compression. Paper presented at the meeting of the Acoustics Society of America, 1983.
71. Bustamante D, Braida L: Wideband compression and spectral sharpening for hearing-impaired listeners. *J Acoust Soc Am* 1986; 80(Suppl 1):S12–S13.
72. Bustamante D, Braida L: Principal-component amplitude compression for the hearing impaired. *J Acoust Soc Am* 1987; 82:1227–1242.
73. Haggard M, Trinder J, Foster J, Lindblad A: Two-state compression of spectral tilt: Individual differences and psychoacoustical limitations to the benefit from compression. *J Rehab Res Dev* 1987; 24:193–206.
74. Bunnell T: On enhancement of spectral contrast in speech for hearing-impaired listeners. *J Acoust Soc Am* 1990; 88:2546–2556.
75. Revoile S, Holden-Pitt L, Edward D, Pickett J: Some rehabilitative considerations for future speech-processing hearing aids. *J Rehab Res Dev* 1986; 23:89–94.
76. Schroeder M: Acoustics in human communications. Plenary lecture, meeting of the Acoustics Society of America, Cambridge, MA, 1979.
77. Langhans T, Strube H: Speech enhancement by nonlinear multiband envelope expansion, in *Proceedings of IEEE Conference on Acoustics, Speech and Signal Processing,* 1982, pp 156–159.
78. Clarkson P, Bahgat S: Envelope expansion methods for speech enhancement. *J Acoust Soc Am* 1991; 89:1378–1382.
79. Berouti M, Schwartz R, Makhoul J: Enhancement of speech corrupted by acoustic noise, in *Proceedings of IEEE Conference on Acoustics, Speech and Signal Processing,* Washington, DC, 1979.
80. Boll S: Suppression of acoustic noise in speech using spectral subtraction. *IEEE Trans Acoustics Speech Signal Processing,* 1979; 29:113–120.
81. Lim J: Signal processing for speech enhancement, in Studebaker G, Bess F (eds): *The Vanderbilt Hearing-Aid Report.* Upper Darby, PA: Monographs in Coantemporary Audiology, 1982, pp 124–130.
82. Lim J: Evaluation of a correlation subtraction method for enhancing speech degraded by additive white noise. *IEEE Trans Acoustics Speech Signal Processing* 1979; 26:471–472.
83. McAulay R, Malpass M: Speech enhancement using a soft-decision noise suppresion filter. *IEEE Trans Acoustics Speech Signal Processing* 1980; 29:137–145.
84. Ephraim Y, Malah D: Speech enhancement using a minimum mean-square error short-time spectral amplitude estimator. *IEEE Trans Acoustics Speech Signal Processing* 1984; 32:1109–1120.

85. Doblinger G: "Optimum" filter for speech enhancement using integrated digital signal processors, *Proceedings of the IEEE Conference on Acoustics, Speech and Signal Processing*, Paris, France, 1982.
86. Bareham J: Part 3. Hearing aid measurements using dual channel signal analysis. *Hear Instrum* 1990; 41(3):34–36.
87. Carter J: *Active Noise Reduction.* Report MRL-TR-84-003. Daytor, OH: Wright-Patterson Air Force Base, 1984.
88. Landgarten H: The cancellation of repetitive noise and vibration by active methods. *Sound Vibration* 1987; 6–10.
89. Eriksson L, Allie M, Bremigan C, Gilbert J: Active noise control on systems with time-varying sources and parameters. *Sound Vibration* 1989; 16–21.
90. Widrow B, Glover J, McCool J, et al.: Adaptive noise cancelling: principles and applications, in *Proceedings of the IEEE Conference on Acoustics, Speech and Signal Processing*, 1975, pp 1692–1716.
91. Peterson P, Durlach N, Rabinowitz W, Zurek P: Multimicrophone adaptive beamforming for interference reduction in hearing aids. *J Rehab Res Dev* 1987; 24:103–110.
92. Brey R, Robinette M, Chabries D, Christiansen R: Improvement in speech intelligibility in noise employing an adaptive filter with normal and hearing-impaired subjects. *J Rehab Res Develop* 1987; 24:75–86.
93. Miller H: Electronic noise-reducing system. U.S. Patent 4,589,137, 1986.
94. Weiss M: Use of an adaptive noise canceler as an input preprocessor for a hearing aid. *J Rehab Res Dev* 1987; 24:93–102.
95. Staab W: Digital/programmable hearing aids—an eye towards the future. *Br J Audiol* 1990; 24:243–256.
96. Marshall R, Harry W: A new microphone providing uniform directivity over an extended frequency range. *J Acoust Soc Am* 1941; 12:481–498.
97. Sessler G, West J: Second order gradient unidirectional microphones utilizing an electret transducer. *J Acoust Soc Am* 1975; 58:278.
98. Farassopoulos A: Speech enhancement for hearing aids using adaptive beamformers, in *Proceedings of the IEEE Conference on Acoustics, Speech and Signal Processing*, 1989, pp 1322–1325.
99. Beex A, DeBrunner V: Restricted geometry acoustic arrays for highly directional patterns. *Appl Acoust* 1991; 33:63–77.
100. Soede W: *Improvement of Speech Intelligibility in Noise. Development and Evaluation of a New Directional Hearing Instrument Based on Array Technology.* Doctoral thesis, Delft, The Netherlands: Delft Univeristy of Technology 1990.
101. Hoffman M, Buckley K: Constrained optimum filtering for multi-microphone digital hearing aids, in *Proceedings of the IEEE Conference on Acoustics, Speech and Signal Processing*, March 1990.
102. Peterson P, Wei S, Rabinowitz W, Zurek P: Robustness of an adaptive beamforming method for hearing aids. *Acta Otolaryngol* 1990; 469(Suppl):85–90.
103. Greenberg J: *A Real-Time Adaptive-Beamforming Hearing Aid.* Masters thesis, Massachusetts Institute of Technology, Department of Electrical Engineering, 1989.

Glossary

Acquired hearing loss: hearing loss occurring sometime after birth.

Adaptation: a decrease in the perception of a prolonged auditory signal. Test used during promontory stimulation of cochlear implant candidates to determine if there is a decrease in the auditory perception of the electrical signal during a one minute interval.

Adaptive frequency response (AFR): the type of hearing aid whose frequency response changes as input level changes.

Adaptive high-frequency filter: a non-linear process in which the gain at high frequencies decreases as the input level increases; also called "BILL," for "bass increases at low levels."

Adaptive low-frequency filter: a non-linear process in which the gain at low frequencies decreases as the input level increases; also called "TILL," for "treble increases at low levels."

Adaptive noise canceller: a system of two or more microphones with an adaptive filter that attempts to cancel noise by moving one or more polar pattern sensitivity nulls to the direction(s) of the noise(s).

Adaptive procedure: an estimation procedure (e.g., of thresholds, optimal setting on hearing aids etc) in which the manner of stimulus change is determined by the listener's response.

Adenoidectomy: removal of the adenoid, a collection of lymphatic tissue in the nasopharynx; part of the treatment of patients presenting otitis media with effusion.

AGC: automatic gain control; a non-linear process in which the gain changes as a function of changing signal levels (see also "compression amplification").

AGC-I: input-controlled AGC (see "input compression").

AGC-O: output-controlled AGC (see "output compression").

Air-bone gap: the difference in air-conduction and bone-conduction thresholds; used as a measure of the magnitude of a conductive hearing loss.

Air conduction hearing aid: a hearing aid which transmits the amplified signal to the inner ear through the ear canal and middle ear.

Alerting devices: assistive devices that alert a person to the presence of a particular sound. For example, a vibrating alarm clock or light flashing to a doorbell or telephone ring.

Algorithm: a set of instructions describing a specific way to perform a certain task.

Anacusic: without any measurable hearing.

Analog: the natural, continuous amplitude versus continuous time form of a signal.

Anterior footplate: the site of prediliction for otosclerosis.

Anti-aliasing filter: low-pass filter (usually with a sharp cut-off) designed to prevent corruption of an analog signal. It is used prior to conversion of the signal to a digital format.

Articulation Index: AI theory is used in an attempt to quantify how much of the speech signal is available to a listener. In general, the AI is computed on the basis of speech importance weightings in various frequency bands and yields a number from 0.00 (no speech sounds are audible) to 1.00 (all speech sounds are audible).

Aspiration: aperiodic speech sound created by relatively unconstricted flow of air through the vocal tract (e.g., "h" sound).

Atresia: absence of the external auditory canal; may be congenital or acquired.

Attack and release times: the time required for a dynamic non-linear process to reach its steady-state value.

Audiant: the implantable electromagnetic bone conductor manufactured by XOMED-Treace.

Azimuth: the direction of a sound source, measured in degrees. 0° is directly in front of the listener, +90° is to the right, 180° is directly behind.

Beamformer: a spacially-oriented system of two or more microphones with either a fixed or an adaptive filter. For hearing aid applications, a fixed beamformer would maximize the desired signal in the look-ahead direction while providing a fixed pattern of sensitivity nulls in the direction of undesired noises. An adaptive beamformer attempts to cancel noise by moving one or more polar pattern sensitivity nulls to the direction(s) of the noise(s).

BILL: bass increase at low levels.

Bipolar: the type of low noise integrated circuitry used in older hearing aid designs that uses large off-chip capacitors. The resulting size limitations cause bipolar amplifiers for subminiature hearing aids to have only limited range tone controls.

Binaural: listening with two ears, typically taken to imply that the two ears are receiving different signals, although this is not a necessary condition.

Binaural summation: an advantage (in dB) of binaural over monaural listening. Binaural threshold is approximately 3 dB better than the monaural threshold (assuming the ears are symmetrical). The binaural advantage increases to 6 dB at suprathreshold levels and to almost 10 dB when the signal(s) is presented at 90 dB sensation level (SL).

Binaural squelch: the improvement, relative to monaural, in speech intelligibility in a noisy sound field listening condition resulting from interaural phase and intensity differences but not including the head shadow effect.

Biphasic pulse: a square wave stimulus having equal negative and positive charge. The stimulus delivered to the electrodes for the Nucleus 22 Channel Cochlear Implant System.

Bone-conduction hearing aid: hearing aid in which the amplified signal directly stimulates the inner ear via a bone vibrator placed on the mastoid process; the bone vibrator can be coupled to a body aid via a cord or can be placed within the frame of an eyeglass hearing aid.

CHIP/IC: an integrated circuit. A miniature electronic unit of components and conductors which is manufactured as a single module.

Cholesteatoma: a mass of keratinizing squamous epithelium that grows into the middle ear from chronic negative middle ear pressure. The mass expands silently over time and will erode bone from pressure and enzymatic activity.

Chronic suppurative otitis media (CSOM): presence of a non-healing perforation of the tympanic membrane due to infection; may be active or inactive.

Circuit noise: the unwanted signal present at the output of a system which is not part of or due to the input signal. This signal is solely due to the activation of the system.

Closed captioning (CC): text of some television shows or videotapes printed at the bottom of the screen and visible with a closed caption decoder (adapter) purchased separately from the television set or with a special circuit installed in the television set.

CMOS: complementary metal oxide semiconductor. The type of integrated circuitry used in newer hearing aid designs which uses small on-chip capacitors. As a result, CMOS multi-band amplifiers with sharp filter slopes are possible in subminiature hearing aids.

Cochlear nucleus: location on each side of the lower brainstem where the cell bodies of second order auditory neurons are found. First order neurons from the auditory nerve synapse on the second order neurons in this nucleus.

Cochlear nucleus implant: an experimental device specifically designed for those profoundly hearing impaired individuals whose auditory nerve is not functioning (i.e., the auditory nerve has been cut during removal of an acoustic neuroma). The device is implanted on the cochlear nucleus located in the brainstem and directly stimulates neurons in the cochlear nucleus.

Coherence: coherence is measured on a simple linear magnitude scale of 0.0 (no coherence) to 1.0 (perfect coherence). There are no vertical units. The horizontal scale indicates frequency. A 1.0 value means that all of the output of the device under test at a particular frequency was caused by the input to the device. In contrast, a value of 0.0 means that all of the output at the measurement frequency as caused by something other than the input to the device (e.g., due to distortion or oscillation within the device). Coherence is measured in the frequency domain.

Communicative assertiveness: behavior exhibited by a person with a hearing impairment that incorporates the use of communication strategies to improve understanding in all situations.

Composite: see *harmonic tone complex*.

Compression amplification: a type of automatic gain control (AGC) whereby a given change in the input level is associated with a reduced change in the output level.

Compression limiting: see *output-limiting compression*.

Compression ratio: ratio of the change in output level resulting from a given change in input level in a compression amplifier.

Congenital hearing loss: hearing loss present at birth.

Consonant-vowel-ratio: the difference in decibels between the level of a consonant and the level of a neighboring vowel in a syllable.

CORFIG: coupler response for flat insertion gain; the transformation added to a prescribed real-ear insertion response to obtain a prescribed 2-cc coupler response; arithmetic inverse of "GIFROC."

CPU: central processing unit. The part of a computer that interprets and executes instructions.

Crest factor: the difference in decibels between the peak sound pressure level and the root mean square sound pressure level.

CROS (contralateral routing of signals) amplification: a hearing aid for patients with unilateral hearing loss. A microphone is placed at or near the poor ear and the signal is routed to the better ear via an open earmold.

CROS-plus: traditional CROS amplification to the good ear combined with a second hearing aid (in-the-ear, behind-the-ear or eyeglass) providing direct amplification to the poor ear.

Crossover frequency: the frequency or frequencies which represent the cut-off frequencies of the filters used to separate the frequency range into separate bands. Analog signal manipulation of this type is limited by the steepness of the filter skirts. Consequently, there is some overlap of the bands on either side of the crossover frequency.

CRT: cathode ray tube. The display component of a computer monitor (i.e., the glass tube).

Current amplitude: the intensity of electrical current delivered to an electrode(s) intended to cause a hearing percept.

Daisy-chain: to interconnect a number of devices via a serial cable arrangement. Each device sends and receive information over the same cable. The functions of all devices on the daisy-chain are available to the controlling device via a single I/O port.

dB gain: decibels gain; comparison of an observed output sound pressure with an observed input sound pressure; dB gain $= 20 \log_{10}$ (output sound pressure $\div$ input sound pressure); also, dB gain $=$ (output dB SPL) $-$ (input dB SPL).

dB SPL: decibels sound pressure level; a comparison of an observed rms sound pressure with a standard reference sound pressure; dB SPL $= 20 \log_{10}$ (observed rms sound pressure $\div$ $20\,\mu$Pa).

Dichotic: binaural listening with different signals at the two ears.

Digital: a discrete amplitude versus discrete time representation of a signal using numbers.

Digital filter: a filter which is implimented in computer software.

Digital signal processing (DSP): a hearing aid that processes the signal in numerical rather than analog form.

Diotic: binaural listening with exactly the same signal at the two ears.

Direct audio-input (DAI): circuit available in some hearing aids that allows direct connection to certain assistive listening devices as well as stereos, television, and radio.

Double-elimination tournament: a paired comparison technique to determine which one of several hearing aids (or settings) is the most preferable. A hearing aid (or setting) loses the tournament if it loses two comparisons.

Download: transfer data from a computer file, or database, to a connected device.

Dropouts: momentary disruptions in audibility associated with transient input signals and a compression amplifier having an inappropriately long release time.

DSP: digital signal processor.

EEPROM: electrically erasable programmable read only memory.

EPROM: (ultra-violet) erasable programmable read only memory.

Expansion: expansion in the intensity domain refers to increasing (by a fixed ratio) the range of variation in the output SPL in relation to the input SPL. Like compression, expansion is invoked in a system when the incoming signal exceeds some pre-determined threshold.

Far ear or Monaural indirect: desired signal presented on the side of the head opposite the aided ear.

FFT: fast fourier transform. A mathematical method of determining frequency components of a signal.

Fibrosis: scar tissue formation due to disease or injury.

Final estimate: the combination of settings on a hearing aid that is chosen by the listener as the best under specific listening condition and judgment criteria.

Firmware: computer programming instructions and data stored in programmed read only memory.

FM system: an assistive listening device consisting of a microphone, transmitter and receiver. It can be used for one-to-one communication, but is especially helpful in a large group, such as a classroom, because of the excellent signal-to-noise ratio that it can provide. The microphone and transmitter are worn by the speaker and the receiver is worn by the listener. The signal is transmitted by FM radio waves.

FOG: full on gain.

Formant: a resonance formed by the vocal tract, often contributing to the distinguishing features of a voiced speech sound.

Formant frequencies (F1, F2): each voiced speech sound has concentrations of acoustic energy in several frequency regions, the peak frequencies (Hz) of which are the formant frequencies.

Frequency discrimination: test used during promontory stimulation of cochlear implant candidates to assess their ability to distinguish between a high and a low pitched signal.

Frication: aperiodic, high-frequency speech sound created, in part, by the friction of air passing through a constriction in the vocal tract (e.g., "f" sound).

Full dynamic range compression: feature of a hearing aid or amplification system for which the amplified output levels are compressed into a narrower range than the range of input levels, and the compression occurs over an input range from approximately 45 to 90 dB SPL.

Fundamental frequency: the lowest frequency in a harmonic tone complex (also called *first harmonic*); determines the minimum number of Hz separating the components of a harmonic tone complex; determines the perceived pitch of a harmonic tone complex.

Fuzzy logic: circuitry which responds to comparative models rather than binary ones. Parameters can assume a wide range of values. Fuzzy logic is used to approximate some of the characteristics of human reasoning based on comparisons of available data. An example is the classic "If-Then-Else" statement in which one decision is made if the logical expression is true and another decision is made if the expression is false. With fuzzy logic, however, the logical expression can be comparative: "If conditions A and B are greater than condition C, then do X rather than Y". (This type of reasoning can be extended, for example, by changing the first part of the statement to, "If conditions A and B are approximately equal AND greater than. . . ."). The inherent ability of fuzzy logic to deal effectively with nebulous information facilitates operation in cases of noisy and/or changing data.

Gap detection: test used during promontory stimulation of cochlear implant candidates to assess their temporal processing skills by measuring their ability to detect the smallest gap between two signals.

GIFROC: the arithmetic inverse of CORFIG; GIFROC is the transformation added to a 2 cc coupler response to predict the real-ear insertion response.

HA-1 coupler: standard, direct-access, 2 cc coupler for testing in-the-ear and in-the-canal hearing aids; can also be used to test behind-the-ear hearing aids with a custom earmold attached.

HA-2 coupler: standard 2 cc coupler for testing hearing aids having non-integrated earpieces (e.g., behind-the-ear, eyeglass, and body aids); includes a standard earmold simulator.

Harmonic: a component of a harmonic tone complex; the frequency of a given harmonic is an integer multiple of the fundamental frequency; e.g., 2nd harmonic = (fundamental frequency) × 2.

Harmonic Distortion: the addition of spurious harmonic components to a signal that either lacked harmonics originally or did not have them in such strength. It is expressed as a percentage of the total signal at the point of measurement.

Harmonic tone complex (composite): a signal consisting of at least two frequency components, where all components are separated in frequency by integer multiples of the fundamental frequency.

Headroom: the difference in SPL between the intensity of the sum of the average incoming signal (speech) to a hearing aid and its gain at user settings and that intensity which causes saturation of the aid.

Head shadow effect: when a stimulus is presented to one side of the head (i.e., near ear), the intensity is decreased (attenuated) by an average of 6.4 dB to the ear on the opposite side of the head (i.e., far ear). That is, the far ear is in the "shadow of the head."

Hearing aid effect: the negative attitude the hearing aid wearer perceives to be elicited in others by the presence of the hearing aid.

HFA: high-frequency average; in ANSI S3.22[1], the average of the decibel response values at 1000, 1600, and 2500 Hz.

Hybrid: a mixture of analog and digital electronics in a hearing aid.

Idiopathic hearing loss: no known cause for the existing hearing loss.

Impulse blanking: suppression of transient noises by shutting off the audio circuit for the duration of a brief noise (such as the noise made when a dinner fork is dropped from a height to a china dinner plate).

Incidence: the degree or range of occurrence.

Infrared system: an assistive listening device for television viewing or wide area use, such as a movie or a concert, that utilizes an infrared light signal to carry the sound from a transmitter to a headset receiver worn by a hearing impaired person. This permits the hearing impaired person to set the volume to a level that is comfortable without bothering others while maintaining an excellent signal-to-noise ratio.

Initial estimate: the first combination of settings on a hearing aid that will be used to compare with other settings in order to estimate optimal setting.

Input compression: compression amplification whose degree of gain reduction depends on the input level and the kneepoint. A form of *AGC-I*.

Interaural attenuation: the loss of energy (in decibels) when a sound is presented to one ear by headset or a bone conduction vibrator, but is heard in cochlea of the opposite ear.

Interface: the point(s) of interconnection between two devices. A hardware or software mechanism which facilitates the interconnection of two devices or systems.

Interformant energy: that energy which is present between the energy peaks (formants) of the speech signal. In general this value is revealed by calculating a ratio of formant power (harmonics) with respect to the noise floor.

Intermodulation (IM) distortion: distortion of a complex waveform associated with sums and differences among frequency components.

Iterative: repetitive.

Kneepoint (compression threshold): the point on an input/output curve at which the slope digresses from unity, indicating the signal level at which a non-linear process begins to take effect.

LCD: liquid crystal display. A thin, planar information display (such as that seen on a digital watch or lap-top computer). It is not a vacuum tube structure like the CRT.

Linear amplification: a hearing aid or amplification system for which there is the same gain for all input levels until the maximum output of the device is reached.

Localization: finding the azimuth of a sound source by comparing time and intensity differences between the ears, or by noting spectral differences in the case of monaural localization.

Long-term spectrum of speech (LTSS): the overall level and configuration of speech energy chosen to represent everyday speech. Pascoe's (1978) speech spectrum represents the sensation level at which normal hearing listeners hear speech babble at an overall level of 65 dB SPL.

Loop system: an assistive listening device that uses magnetic induction to carry a signal from a microphone/amplifier to a loop. The signal is picked up from the loop by a hearing aid set to the telecoil position or by a receiver with built-in telecoil, volume control, and earpiece. Loops are either worn around an individual's neck or can encircle a room, such as a classroom, permitting an excellent signal-to-noise ratio.

Loudness recruitment: the abnormally rapid growth of loudness above threshold as the physical intensity of sound increases or a normal loudness sensation at moderate to high intensity levels despite loss of hearing sensation for softer sounds.

Loudness summation: occurs when the bandwidth of a complex sound is increased so that it exceeds a critical bandwidth and the loudness increases even though the sound pressure level of the complex sound is kept constant.

LTASS: longterm average speech spectrum.

Masking level difference (MLD): the improvement in binaural masked thresholds when differences in the signal and/or masker are present between ears (i.e., dichotic listening) in comparison to when these differences are not present (i.e., diotic listening). The differences between ears can be in intensity, time, phase and/or spectrum.

Miniaturize: make small. Use advanced electronic production techniques to reduce the size of an electronic circuit or component.

Modified simplex: a modification of the original simplex procedure in that relative subjective judgments (of speech intelligibility, clarity etc.) are used instead of absolute speech recognition scores for estimating optimal hearing aid settings.

Monaural: listening with one ear.

Mondini deformity: incomplete development and malformation of the cochlea.

mSTI: modified speech transmission index; an acoustic index that combines some features of the articulation index and the speech transmission index— STI. The mSTI was proposed by Humes et al. 1986.

Multi-electrode intracochlear implant: system consisting of a surgically implanted internal device (multi-electrode array) and an externally worn device (microphone, transmitter, and processor) designed specifically for severely to profoundly hearing impaired individuals who no longer receive benefit from hearing aids. The system provides this population of hearing impaired individuals with sound as well as varying degrees of speech understanding.

Near ear or Monaural direct: desired signal presented on the side of the head of the aided ear.

Necrosis: tissue death. The most common site in CSOM is the long process of the incus.

Neoplasm: a benign or malignant new growth that continues to enlarge and cause tissue damage by pressure or infiltration.

Neural networks: an adaptive system which solves problems by imitating the architecture of the biological neural systems. Multiple groupings of artificial neurons are interconnected with different weightings representing the relative strengths of interconnections between the neurons. It is possible to construct operational neural networks in both hardware and software.

Non-linear hearing aid: a hearing aid whose overall gain and/or frequency-response change as a function of changing input signals.

Open captioning: printed text of certain television shows or videotapes that is visible on the screen without the use of a decoder, adapter, or special circuit.

Oral/aural communication: a mode of communication that utilizes hearing, the spoken word and speechreading.

Oscillation: in audiology, refers to the undesired tonal output of an amplifier behaving unstably as a result of feedback; whistling.

Otitis media with effusion: the most common cause of hearing loss in children. Results from bacterial infection in the middle ear with secondary formation of infected fluid in the middle ear space.

Otosclerosis: formation of spongy bone around the stapes. It is an hereditary condition that causes hearing loss in the early adult years. In late stages it may invade the cochlear to cause sensorineural loss as well. Also called otospongiosis.

Output compression: compression amplification whose degree of gain reduction depends on the output level and the kneepoint. A form of *AGC-O*.

Output-limiting compression (compression limiting): a form of output compression that limits the maximum output of a hearing aid by reducing the gain automatically as a function of the output level and a pre-set kneepoint (threshold).

Paired comparison: data collection technique whereby a listener compares two hearing aids (or settings) to decide on the one that meets the criteria set by the clinician and/or listener.

Peak-clipping: distortion of a waveform resulting from amplifier saturation.

Periodic waveform: a waveform that repeats; in audiology, a waveform that repeats at audible frequencies.

Personality module: a plug-in module which contains stored digital information to configure an instrument or device for operation in a particular manner. An example is a hearing aid programming device which receives different personality modules to configure the device to program hearing aids from different manufacturers.

Phase: relative position in time of a point within a periodic waveform.

Polar directivity pattern: a plot that shows the relative amplitude output as a function of angle of sound incidence from a directionally sensitive device.

Pole: referring to the slope of a tone control filter. Each pole in a filter provides about 6 dB per octave slope.

Prevalence: the widespread occurrence.

Primary auditory neurons: the first order neurons with cell bodies in the modiolus or VIIIth cranial nerve, dendrites in the cochlea, and axons that synapse with second order auditory neurons in the cochlear nucleus.

PROM: Programmed Read Only Memory. Storage that can be easily read, but not easily written to; usually nonvolatile. Some types of ROM can be erased by special electrical signals or by exposure to ultra-violet light.

Pulse width: the width of a biphasic pulse stimulus delivered to the implant. Varying the width of the pulse is one way to change the perceived loudness.

For example, if the pulse width is increased, the electrical charge is increased as well as the loudness percept.

Pumping and breathing: audible fluctuations in background noise associated with pulsating input signals and a compression amplifier having an inappropriately short release time.

Pure tone: a signal containing one, and only one, frequency; a sinusoidal acoustic signal.

RAM: Random Access Memory. Volatile storage (stored information is lost when power is removed). Storage in which any address can be accessed as easily and quickly as any other. It can be written to, or read, with equal ease and speed.

Random waveform: a waveform, whose amplitudes, frequencies, and phases vary randomly over time.

REAR: real-ear aided response; the difference, in decibels, between the sound pressure level at a reference point outside the ear and that in the earcanal, with a hearing aid in place and turned on.

RECD: real-ear-to-coupler level difference; difference between the SPL developed in an earcanal versus a coupler owing to differing acoustic load impedances.

Reference, sound-field: the calibration point of a sound-field measurement.

REIR: real-ear insertion response; the net increase in sound pressure level (SPL) provided to the earcanal by a hearing aid, as compared to the SPL in the natural open ear, for a given sound source outside the ear. REIR = REAR − REUR.

Repair strategies: compensatory strategies used by hearing impaired individuals directed at fixing or clarifying missed or misunderstood utterances.

RETSPL: reference equivalent thresholds in decibels sound pressure level.

REUR: real-ear unaided response; the difference, in decibels, between the sound pressure level at a reference point outside the ear and that in the open earcanal.

Reversal: a change in the direction of preference during adaptive testing.

RMS: root-mean-square; the long-term, overall, effective level of a signal; the square-root of the mean of the squared instantaneous values of a signal integrated over a time period long enough so that the result is not sensitive to small changes in the integration period. For periodic signals, the integration period can be any integer multiple of the period of the signal.

Round-robin tournament: a paired comparison technique whereby each hearing aid (or setting on a hearing aid) is compared to all other hearing aids (or settings) in order to obtain ranking information.

Run: a series of comparisons in which settings are changed in the same direction.

Saturation: the condition caused by peak clipping in a hearing aid that prevents an increase in input sound pressure level from causing the same change in output sound pressure level.

SCF: switched capacitor filter; an IC that can be used as a lowpass, highpass, band-pass, or notch filter with as many as five or more poles on a single chip. Characteristics of SCFs, such as filter type, Q, and bandwidth, are determined by external resistors. The filter center frequency is determined by an external clock signal. The frequency and bandwidth can be controlled digitally. Presently available SCF devices have dynamic ranges of about 80 dB, Qs up to 50, and usable center frequencies up to 250 kHz.

Seeding rules: guidelines that are used to determine the order in which available hearing aids (or settings) are compared in either a single- or double-elimination tournament.

Signal-to-distortion ratio (SDR): the difference in decibels between the signal level and the distortion level.

Simple up-down procedure: an adaptive procedure that allows one to estimate the best setting on a hearing aid in one electroacoustic dimension.

Simplex procedure: an adaptive procedure designed to estimate the electroacoustic settings on more than one dimension of a hearing aid in order to maximize speech recognition score.

Single-elimination tournament: a paired comparison technique to determine which one of several comparison hearing aids (or settings) is most preferred. A hearing aid (or setting) will be eliminated from further comparisons if it loses once.

Small fenestra stapedectomy, stapedotomy: a surgical procedure to bypass the conductive hearing loss of otosclerosis. A small opening is made in the footplate into which a piston is inserted and crimped around the long process of the incus.

Socially adequate hearing: an average pure-tone threshold (0.5, 1.0, 2.0 kHz) of 25 dB HL or better with normal word recognition.

Speech weighted composite signal: a broadband, complex sound that has the same crest factor as speech (12 dB).

Spectral contrast: the difference in decibels between the peaks and the valleys of the formants in the spectrum of a short term sample of speech.

Spectrum: analysis of the amplitudes of the frequencies comprising a signal.

Squamous epithelium: this lines the ear canal and outer surface of the tympanic membrane.

Square wave: a waveform consisting of a voltage that is constant in amplitude but reverses its polarity at regular intervals.

Stapediovestibular joint: the connection between oval window and the stapes. Fixation of the joint produces conductive hearing loss.

Steady state: in a circuit whose response changes over time, the response level reached after which no appreciable changes occur over additional time.

Stenosis: narrowing of a passageway producing obstruction.

Step size: represents the magnitude of change in electroacoustic settings between two comparisons.

Superior olivary complex: part of the central auditory system in the brain. After leaving the cochlear nucleus, the afferent fibers of the auditory nerve travel to both the ipsilateral and contralateral superior olive. The superior olivary complex is the point at which the auditory system processes information from both ears (binaurally).

Symmetrical hearing loss: The audiometric configuration (flat, sloping, etc.) is the same in the two ears. Usually, the implication is that the degree of hearing loss is the same in the two ears, but it may be different.

Telecommunication device for the deaf (TDD): A telephone system for those with severe hearing impairment with which a typewritten message is transmitted over telephone lines and is received as a printed message.

Temporal envelope: the modulation formed by the amplitude versus time relationship of a signal.

Temporal envelope expansion: enlarging the differences between levels of the peaks and the valleys in the modulation formed by the amplitude versus time relationship of a signal.

Temporal pattern: a pattern of changes that occur over time.

TILL: treble increase at low levels.

Transcranial CROS: coupling a high gain/high output in-the-ear or behind-the-ear hearing aid to the poor ear so the amplified sound can be transferred transcranially across the skull to the cochlea of the good ear.

Transducer: a device which is used to transport energy from one system (electrical, mechanical, or acoustical) to another. Example: A microphone or a telephone audio magnetic pick-up coil.

True digital: a hearing aid in which the signal is converted to digital form for digital signal processing and then reconverted back to analog form.

Two-channel AGC hearing aid: a hearing aid in which the signal is separated into two frequency bands, each band having a separate AGC circuit.

Tympanostomy tube: a plastic or metal tube surgically inserted into the tympanic membrane to promote prolonged aeration, ventilation, and pressure equalization of the middle ear in cases of chronic otitis media with effusion.

Unilateral hearing loss: one ear is unaidable and the hearing in the opposite ear is ±15 dB (HL) at 250–8000 Hz.

Vertex: the setting (as represented on a simplex matrix) to which other comparison settings that deviate from this setting in one (and only one) parametric value is compared.

Virtual environment: a computer generated acoustic/visual stimulus set presented to the subject via a sophisticated head-worn assembly. It yields a perception of three dimensional visual and acoustical space through which the headgear wearer "moves" by actuating various electronic controls. The perspective of the auditory and visual presentations changes as the position in the computer generated space changes.

Warble tone: a frequency-modulated pure tone, also called "FM tone."

Index

and self-perception of communication
  ability, 357–359
and speech recognition ability, 346–
  357
trends in, 343–359
see also Asymmetrical hearing loss;
  Conductive hearing loss; Noise-
  induced hearing loss; Symmetrical
  hearing loss; Unilateral hearing loss
Vertex, 412
Virtual environment, 325, 412
Voiced sound, 71
Volume control wheel (VCW), 56, 57

Warble tone, 73, 412
Waveform
  periodic, 408
  random, 409
  square wave, 411
Weighting *see* Speech shaping
White noise *see* Random noise
Wiener filter, 384
Word recognition *see* Speech recognition

Zeta Noise Blocker (ZNB), 384–385
ZNB *see* Zeta Noise Blocker